Peri-Implant Therapy for the Dental Hygienist

Peri-Implant Therapy for the Dental Hygienist

Second Edition

Susan S. Wingrove, BS, RDH

International Speaker, Writer, Researcher
Wingrove Dynamics LLC
Missoula, MT, USA

WILEY Blackwell

Registered Office
John Wiley & Sons, Inc., 111 River Street, Hoboken, NJ 07030, USA

Editorial Office
111 River Street, Hoboken, NJ 07030, USA

For details of our global editorial offices, customer services, and more information about Wiley products visit us at www.wiley.com.

Wiley also publishes its books in a variety of electronic formats and by print-on-demand. Some content that appears in standard print versions of this book may not be available in other formats.

Library of Congress Cataloging-in-Publication Data

Names: Wingrove, Susan S., author.
Title: Peri-implant therapy for the dental hygienist / Susan S. Wingrove.
Description: Second edition. | Hoboken, NJ : Wiley-Blackwell, 2022. |
    Includes bibliographical references and index.
Identifiers: LCCN 2021058899 (print) | LCCN 2021058900 (ebook) |
    ISBN 9781119766186 (paperback) | ISBN 9781119766209 (Adobe PDF) |
    ISBN 9781119766223 (epub)
Subjects: MESH: Dental Implants | Dental Implantation–adverse effects |
    Dental Implants–adverse effects | Dental Hygienists
Classification: LCC RK667.I45 (print) | LCC RK667.I45 (ebook) | NLM WU
    640 | DDC 617.6/93–dc23/eng/20211227
LC record available at https://lccn.loc.gov/2021058899
LC ebook record available at https://lccn.loc.gov/2021058900

Cover Design: Wiley
Cover Images: Marc Swanson Photography/Design, Dr. Tom Lambert and Wingrove Dynamics LLC

Set in 10/12.5pt Palatino by Straive, Pondicherry, India

Printed in Singapore
M003501_150322

I would like to dedicate this book to my dental colleagues and friends
in Italy who inspire me with their passion in life and learning.
This book is my passion on paper!

Time is like a river. You cannot touch the same water twice, because
the flow that has passed will never pass again.
Enjoy every moment in life!

Contents

Foreword

Dental implants are a viable option for natural tooth replacement with predictable long-term survival rates. Implant survival alone is an inadequate predictor of success according to modern standards. Careful implant position, prosthetic design, and soft-tissue management can result in superior aesthetic and functional outcomes. Preservation of peri-implant soft tissues, optimal function and aesthetics, and implant survival has become the parameters that define success. As such, the partnership of the implant surgeon, restorative dentist, and dental hygienist is essential to preserve these outcomes.

The success of an implant-supported restoration is promoted by a prosthetically driven treatment plan. The days of placing implants *where the bone is*, without consideration for tooth position or the planned prosthesis, are long gone. Implant position is ideally determined by the position of the teeth and by the type of prosthesis to be planned. Moreover, the amount of vertical space required for the planned prosthesis must be assessed prior to implant placement. Modern technology facilitates this planning; CBCT machines allow accurate 3-D visualization of patients' anatomy, proposed implant positions, and the prosthesis. Surgical guides can be fabricated quickly and economically using 3-D printing or with CAD/CAM technology. Although this technology is used routinely in planning dental implants, it is critical that the implant surgeon utilizes this technology correctly for accurate implant placement, especially if an immediate prosthesis is planned. Moreover, meticulous surgical technique is vital for healing and implant survival.

Paying particular attention to prosthetic design will promote a favorable outcome. The number of implants, antero-posterior spread, implant-to-prosthesis ratios, lip support, the condition of the opposing arch, and functional requirements are considerations when planning an implant prosthesis. An important and sometimes overlooked consideration is the cleanability of the final prosthesis. Creating a prosthesis that harmonizes function, aesthetics, respect for biology, and cleanability should be the primary objective when planning and carrying out fixed and removable implant therapies. If tooth position, function, implant positions, and/or lip support results in a fixed prosthesis that is not conducive to proper and complete oral hygiene practices, a different prosthetic design must be considered.

The necessity for complete and responsible implant maintenance transcends the traditional goal of calculus removal. Oral biofilm is not only responsible for localized and generalized dental, periodontal, and implant disease but is also implicated in the exacerbation of many systemic conditions, including, but not limited to cardiovascular disease, metabolic imbalances, rheumatoid arthritis, and Alzheimer's disease. Complete biofilm disruption has been shown to promote a favorable oral environment and to reduce the risk of the oral contribution to systemic disease. Technology is available to facilitate efficient and effective biofilm disruption in a way that is safe for dental implants. Conversely, there are instruments and medicaments that can be damaging to dental implant surfaces and prosthetic materials and can compromise longevity. The titanium surface on dental implants has been proven to be biocompatible and corrosion-resistant, but common preventive practices have been implicated in its degradation, including topical medicaments to prevent dental caries, a general or local acidic pH and instruments used to remove biofilm, plaque, and calculus. This dissolution, degradation or permanent deformation of the implant surface may contribute to peri-implant inflammation, bone loss or eventual loss of osseointegration.

Collaboration between the dentist and dental hygienist is fundamental to promote successful long-term implant outcomes. A restoration that is not only maintainable for the patient but also the dental hygienist will encourage health in the oral environment and peri-implant tissues. Dental hygienists that have a general understanding about implant restorations, dental materials, and appropriate preventive measures are invaluable. First, the dental hygienist can educate patients about available prostheses and assess the patient's motivation to pursue implant therapy. This can begin a fruitful discussion for the dentist and the patient. In addition, when dental hygienists understand dental materials and basic prosthetic design, they can select the appropriate armamentarium for maintenance appointments and properly educate patients to practice optimal at-home maintenance.

To provide safe and appropriate care for implant patients, attention to all of the points previously introduced is crucial. Collaboration between the dentist and dental hygienist will produce superior patient care and a satisfying clinical environment. The dental hygienist has a profound responsibility to be equipped with the knowledge, instruments, technology, and materials to successfully contribute to this collaboration. This text is a culmination of decades of research and will educate and ultimately empower the dental hygienist to provide exceptional care for patients considering, undergoing, or have completed implant therapy.

Dr. Pam Maragliano-Muniz
BSDH, DMD, FACP
Board-certified Prosthodontist
Chief Editor, Dental Economics
Salem, MA, USA

Acknowledgments

Over this past year, many colleagues, friends, and companies have contributed to this update of *Peri-Implant Therapy for the Dental Hygienist*. It has been an exciting journey for me that I know will continue to lead me into more learning adventures in the future.

A very heartfelt thank you goes to the following:

To my contributors, Drs. Maria L. Geisinger, Robert Horowitz, Pam Maragliano-Muniz, Gerrarda O'Beirne, Luciana Safioti, and Robert Schneider who supported me in this update of the textbook with their expertise and writing. They are all role models in our profession that support and promote our hygiene profession in this very important challenge of peri-implant therapy.

To my fellow dental colleagues and friends nationally and internationally, who have supported me, adding their research, critiqued chapters, and encouraged me on this year-long journey: Boris Atlas, Wendy Birtles, Richelle Braun, Kathi and Jeff Carlson, Anne Christophersen, Stancey Coughlan, Sarah Crow, Lisa Darrow, Diane Daubert, John DeAngelo, Catherine Fairfield, Carla Frey, Stephanie Gans, Annamaria Genovesi, Liz Graham, Debbie and Paul Harrison, Tracy Hull, Implant Consortium, Alessia Iommiello, Carol Jahn, Beth Jordan, Claire Jeong, Heather Kelley, Amy Kinnamon, Sherri Lukes, Deborah Lyle, Tabetha Magnuszewski, Linda Miller, Michelle Miller, Carie Miskell, Paolo Modena, Gianna Nardi, Trisha O'Hehir, Michaela O'Neill, Noel and Rich Paschke, Michele Petre, Tom Raish, Birgit Renggli, Heather Rogers, Consuelo Sanavia, Silva Savatini, Kandra Sellers, Alison Stahl, Lynette Thompson, Lori Totten, Linda Turner, Melissa Vandyke, Leslie Winston, and Debbie Zafiropoulos.

Special thank you to Alison Stahl for her expertise and knowledge to collaborate on the "Mastering the Arch" protocols. To Dr. Kevin Frawley, Dr. Peter Fritz, Dr. Amita Gorur, Dr. Georgios Kotsakis, Dr. Tom Lambert, Dr. Marco Montevecchi, Dr. Marco Padilla, Dr. John Remien, Dr. Sam St. John, Marc Swanson, Dr. Caspar Wohlfahrt for their support and outstanding photographs.

To the companies that have generously provided photos, illustrations, and information: Acteon, BioHorizons, Crest + Oral-B (P & G), Directa, EMS, GC America, Glidewell Dental, Guidor, Ivoclar Vivadent, Keystone Dental, Labrida, Mectron, Nobel Biocare, Neoss, Orsing, Parkell, Paradise Dental Technologies (PDT), Preventech, Rowpar (CloSYS), Salvin Dental Specialties, SDS, StellaLife, Straumann, Sunstar, Surgical Esthetics, TePe, Waterpik, W & H, Zeramex, and Zest Dental Solutions.

To Tanya McMullin, Erica Judisch, Susan Engelken, Angela Cohen, and Selvakumar Gunakundru at Wiley Blackwell, for their expertise and encouragement.

Susan S. Wingrove.

About the Author

Susan Wingrove BS, RDH. International speaker, researcher, writer, consultant, and RDH Award of Distinction Recipient. Instrument co-designer of the Wingrove Titanium Implant Series, ACE probes, and Queen of Hearts instruments. Susan specializes in sorting through the science to develop protocols for healthy teeth, implants, and disease treatment. She does medical research on regenerative wound healing and dental research on biofilm-focused care for long-term disease prevention. Published author ACP Clinical Practice Guidelines Scientific Panel, Doctor Clinical Implant Maintenance White Papers, American and International journals on peri-implant therapy, regeneration, and advanced instrumentation. Resides in Missoula, Montana, USA and enjoys fly fishing, hiking, and snowshoeing.

List of Contributors

Dr. Maria L. Geisinger, DDS, MS
Diplomate, American Board of
Periodontology
Professor / Director, Advanced Education
Program in Periodontology
Department of Periodontology
University of Alabama at Birmingham
Birmingham, AL, USA

Dr. Robert Horowitz, DDS
Board-Certified Periodontist
Clinical Professor
Departments of Periodontics and Implant
Dentistry, Oral Surgery
New York University College of Dentistry
New York, NY, USA

**Dr. Pam Maragliano-Muniz, BSDH,
DMD, FACP**
Board-Certified Prosthodontist
Private Practice – Salem Dental Arts
Chief Editor, Dental Economics
Salem, MA, USA

Dr. Gerrarda O'Beirne, BDS, MSD
Board-Certified Periodontist
Private Practice Seattle Periodontics and
Implant Dentistry
Affiliate Assistant Professor
Department of Periodontics
School of Dentistry
University of Washington
Seattle, WA, USA

Dr. Luciana Safioti, DDS, MSD
Board-Certified Periodontist, Clinical
Assistant Professor
Department of Periodontics, School of
Dentistry, University of Washington
Seattle, WA, USA

Dr. Robert Schneider, DDS, MS
Emeritus Professor, University of Iowa
Hospitals and Clinics, Hospital Dentistry
Institute, Former Division Director
Maxillofacial Prosthodontics
Iowa City, IA, USA

About the Companion Website

This book is accompanied by a companion website:

www.wiley.com/go/wingrove/implant

The website includes:

- Dental instructor materials
- Review questions and answers
- Lesson plans
- Videos
- PowerPoint slides
- Skills evaluations
- Learning objectives

1 Implants 101: History, Implant Design, Parts, and Pieces

Understand as hygienists a tidal wave of ailing or failing implants may be imminent. It is imperative that hygienists are trained in identifying and treating peri-implant mucosal inflammation that could affect overall body health (1).
—G. Nogueira-Filho, DDS, MDent, PhD

Dental hygienists must be ready and be prepared to take on this next, very important challenge in our profession! The 21st century is an important and critical time to be a hygienist. During this exciting time in dentistry, we as hygienists have a critical role in implant therapy. As a hygienist, your role will be to access patients for healthy periodontium prior to placement of implants, to monitor the tissue surrounding the implants, and to maintain the implants through safe, effective implant maintenance. Current studies reveal that infections in the periodontium occur in more than 50% of implants placed (2).

Therefore, we as dental professionals will be faced with different dynamics, challenges, and complications.

As a hygienist, the history of implant dentistry makes you aware that implants are not new, but have been evolving for decades. Patients may have concerns that implants are so new that not enough research or development has been done for them to feel comfortable with the procedure. With your knowledge of the history, design, and research done on implants you will be better able to talk with your patients and address these concerns. A fundamental understanding of key terms and statistics associated with implant dentistry will also be a valuable tool to add to your verbal skills when talking with patients about tooth replacement.

History

Believe it or not, the history of dental implants dates back to 600 AD with the ancient Mayans. Dr. and Mrs. Wilson Popenoe found the lower mandible of a young Mayan woman in Honduras in 1931 (Figure 1.1). She was missing some of her lower teeth and they had been replaced with the earliest example of the first dental implants, made from pieces of shell, shaped to resemble teeth. Scientists believe that

Peri-Implant Therapy for the Dental Hygienist, Second Edition. Susan S. Wingrove.
© 2022 John Wiley & Sons, Inc. Published 2022 by John Wiley & Sons, Inc.
Companion website: www.wiley.com/go/wingrove/implant

these shells may have actually worked. Slots were made into the bone and the shells were pounded in like little wedges, without anesthesia!

Similar discoveries were made in Egypt, artifacts that date back to the 1700s. Ivory and the bones of animals were also sometimes used to replace missing teeth. It would be decades after these archeological discoveries before the modern world caught up with the Mayans' and Egyptians' dental technology.

In the late 18th and 19th centuries, the level of dental care went through many changes. Through the letters, journals, and

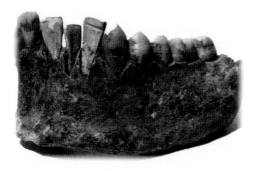

Figure 1.1 Discovery by Dr. and Mrs. Wilson Popenoe, Honduras, 1931. Reprinted with permission from Ring (20).

accounts left by our first president, George Washington, we have a well-documented case history of his lifelong dental problems and the level of dental care available at that time. George Washington started losing his teeth at the age of 24 and by 1789, the year that Washington took his oath of office, he had only one of his original teeth left (Figure 1.2).

Dr. John Greenwood made a set of dentures for Washington made of hippopotamus ivory and eight real human teeth attached by brass screws. The denture, which was anchored on the one remaining tooth in Washington's mouth, has a hole that fits snugly around the one tooth. Dr. Greenwood was noted to be quite ahead of his time in his dental practice, extracting teeth, and utilizing them in the manufacture of dentures, but he also experimented with implantation.

Unfortunately for Dr. Greenwood, the 18th century's lack of antibiotics and any understanding of germ theory or antisepsis doomed any such experiments to failure. He did make President George Washington several sets of dentures, none made out of wood as often referred to. They were made from gold, ivory, lead,

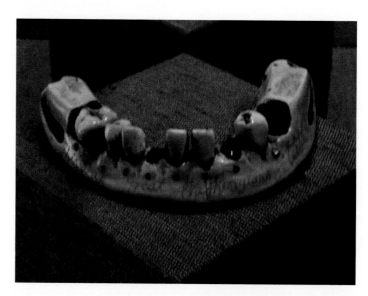

Figure 1.2 George Washington's lower denture. Courtesy of Rick Blanchette.

and human and animal teeth (horse and donkey teeth were common components), with springs to help them open and bolts to hold them together.

In the 18th century, researchers experimented with gold and other metal alloys including lead as implants. Dr. Maggiolo fabricated gold implants that were placed in sockets where teeth had recently been extracted and after a healing period attached a *donor* tooth. Dr. Harris, a physician, attempted the same procedure with a platinum post, both had poor results.

Dr. Edmunds in 1886 was the first in the United States to implant a porcelain crown mounted on a platinum disc and presented at the First District Dental Society of New York. Other metal alloys with porcelain crowns were experimented with, but these implants did not have a long-term success rate.

Dr. E.J. Greenfield, pioneer of the endosseous implant, provided many of the basic concepts of nascent field of implantology. He was known for his patented hollow-cylinder implants made of wire soldered with 24 karat gold. This hollow-basket design was a similar design that Straumann Implant Company from Switzerland adopted many years later. He presented his research and surgical technique in 1913, and although histological proof of bone-to-implant contact was not available at that time, he understood the clinical importance to what he called *primary stability or osseointegration*. His surgical techniques, stepwise use of drill diameters starting with round bur, were presented in 1913 and are still practiced today (3).

It was not until 1937 before the first relatively long-term implant success was noted. Dr. A.E. Strock used the metal alloy Vitallium®, placing a series of implants at Harvard University in animals and humans. He published a paper on the physiological effects of Vitallium in bone, with no postoperative complications or reactions noted, total toleration. These were the first relatively successful dental implants and certain types of implants are still cast in Vitallium today.

The turning point of implant dental history happened in the 1950s, when Professor Per-Ingvar Brånemark, an orthopedic surgeon, discovered that titanium components can bond irreversibly with living bone tissue. His team designed many studies on the healing effects of bone with one specific study on rabbits in which a titanium metal cylinder was screwed in a rabbit's thighbone. A several-month healing period and other experiments of the blood circulation in animals using a hollow titanium cylinder demonstrated that the titanium cylinder fused to the bone. Brånemark named this discovery osseointegration (the firm, direct, and lasting biological attachment of a metallic implant to vital bone with no intervening connective tissue) (Figure 1.3).

Brånemark's research and other colleagues from other disciplines evolved this theory of osseointegration along with the design of the *Brånemark titanium* screw

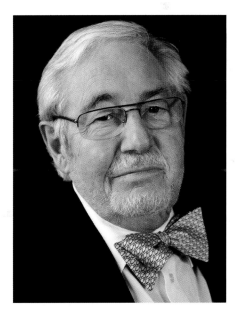

Figure 1.3 Professor Per-Ingvar Brånemark, an orthopedic surgeon. Courtesy of Nobel Biocare.

device with a number of specific surface treatments to enhance bioacceptance with bone. One of the key reasons that titanium was chosen by Brånemark is his relationship to Hans Emneus, an orthopedic surgeon, who studied different metals used for hip joint prostheses. His research indicated that a new metal, titanium, from Russia and used in nuclear industry, might be optimal. Brånemark used a sample from Russia and from there on, the best metal for implants has been pure titanium.

In 1964, commercial-grade pure titanium was accepted as the material of choice for dental implants. Other bodies of medicine (i.e., joint replacements) had recognized the fact that the body does not recognize titanium as a foreign material, which results in higher success rate and fewer rejections. Eventually, the use of commercial pure titanium evolved into the use of titanium alloys ($TiAl_6V_4$ being the most commonly used) due to experimentation and improved durability.

In 1981, Dr. Per-Ingvar Brånemark published his findings covering all the data on the animal and human clinical trials: success rate, concept, and the design of endosteal root-form titanium implants most commonly placed today. In an effort to gain international support and collaboration, based on patient care with sound biological and clinical principles Brånemark founded the Association of Brånemark Osseointegration Centers (ABOC).

Brånemark identified the edentulous patient as an amputee, an oral invalid, to whom we should pay total respect and rehabilitation ambitions. He was also instrumental in identifying the mouth as a much more important part of the human body than medicine and controlling agencies had previously recognized. He coined the term *osseoperception*, "the dentate mouth communicates with the brain, possibly improving not only daily function but also being an important factor in restitu-tion after intra-cranial vascular events" (P-I Brånemark, September 2005).

In the 21st century, technology and clinical awareness will take on more importance. The science and clinical advancements have made it possible for oral and maxillofacial surgeons, periodontists, and general dentists in the United States to double the number of implants performed per dentist between 1995 and 2002.

Dental implant history timeline

Ancient history: Mayans back in AD 600 had dental implants made from pieces of shell and ancient Egyptians used shells and ivory.

1700s: Lost teeth were often replaced with teeth from human donors. The process was mostly unsuccessful due to immune system reactions to the foreign material.

1800s: Researchers fabricated gold, platinum, and other metal alloys, including lead, into posts that were placed into the sockets of extracted teeth and donor teeth were attached after a healing period.

1886: Dr. Edmunds was the first in the United States to implant a porcelain crown mounted on a platinum disc and presented at the First District Dental Society of New York.

1913: Dr. E.J. Greenfield, pioneer of endosseous implant, provided many of the basic concepts of the nascent field of implantology. He was most known for his patented hollow-cylinder implants made of wires soldered with 24 karat gold and outlined surgical implant placement technique (Figure 1.4).

1939: Dr. A.E. Strock introduced the first biocompatible material, the metal alloy Vitallium, to place a series of implants at Harvard University in animals and humans. He is credited with the first relatively long-term successful dental implants.

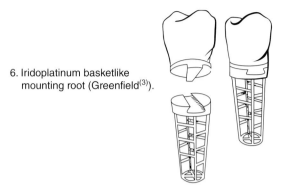

6. Iridoplatinum basketlike
mounting root (Greenfield[3]).

Figure 1.4 Dr. Greenfield's basket design. Greenfield (3).

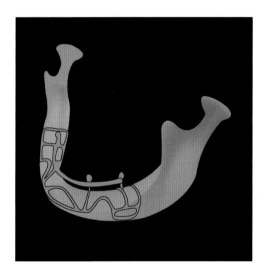

Figure 1.5 Dr. Dahl subperiosteal design.

1941: Dr. Gustav Dahl of Sweden is credited with the development of the **subperiosteal implant**, a metal framework that is surgically placed on top of the jawbone for completely edentulous patients (Figure 1.5).

1952: Professor Per-Ingvar Brånemark discovered that titanium components can bond irreversibly with living bone tissue and coined the term osseointegration.

1964: Commercial grade pure titanium, or commercial pure titanium, was accepted as material of choice for dental implants.

1967: Dr. Leonard Linkow of New York developed the blade implants and Doctors Ralph and Harold Roberts are also credited with the development of **endosteal implants** (Figure 1.6).

1968: Dr. Irwin Small developed the **transosteal dental implant** (Figure 1.7).

1969: Dr. Per-Ingvar Brånemark provided the proof of long-term success of titanium implants.

1981: Dr. Per-Ingvar Brånemark published his findings covering all the data on the animal and human clinical trials: success rate, concept, and the current design of **endosteal root-form titanium implants.**

1982: The Toronto Conference on Osseointegration in Clinical Dentistry created the first guidelines for what would be considered the standardization of successful implant dentistry.

1986: Implants received the endorsement of the American Dental Association (ADA).

1989: The Brånemark Osseointegration Center (BOC) in Gothenburg, Sweden, was founded. BOC's primary mission was to provide treatment for patients with severe oral, maxillofacial, and orthopedic impediments.

2002: An ADA survey showed that oral and maxillofacial surgeons, periodontists, and general dentists doubled the number of implants performed per dentist between 1995 and 2002.

Today: The Food and Drug Administration (FDA) regulates the oral and dental implants being placed, requiring implant companies to furnish data and controlled studies under medical devices to gain full approval.

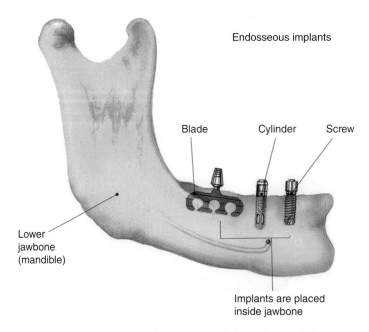

Endosseous implants

Blade   Cylinder   Screw

Lower
jawbone
(mandible)

Implants are placed
inside jawbone

Figure 1.6   Endosteal design. Juodzbalys and Wang (21).

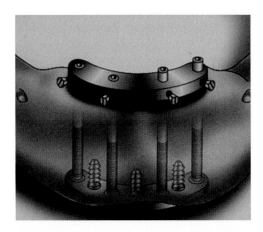

Figure 1.7   Transosteal design. Reprinted with permission from Zwemer (22) © 2008 Elsevier, Inc. All rights reserved.

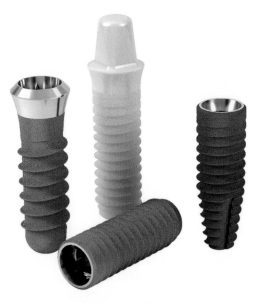

Figure 1.8 Titanium and ceramic (zirconia) implant examples. Courtesy of Straumann.

Implants

Over the past 30 years, research has validated the success of osseointegrated implants as a viable alternative to fixed or removable prosthetic restorations (Figure 1.8) (4). Implant placement in the premolar and molar are 95% successful and are considered the first choice in tooth-replacement options (5, 6). This is supported by the dental literature for many implant systems in every area of the mouth (7). According to Michael Tischler et al. (8, 9), because of "the amount of edentulism currently documented, it is essential for clinicians to incorporate dental implants into everyday practice." The American Association of Oral and Maxillofacial Surgeons report that 69% of adults between ages 35 and 44 years have lost at least one permanent tooth and 43% of adults over the age of 65 years old are missing six or more teeth due to tooth decay, periodontal disease, a failed root canal, or trauma (8, 9).

As hygienists, these changes have evolved into a new phase of maintenance care for our patients. Before we can understand the new protocols for our maintenance appointments, an understanding of the basics of implants and why most implants are made from titanium alloy is necessary. The choice of which type of implant to use will be in the hands of the surgeon, titanium or ceramic. Hygienists need an understanding of the component parts. The main component parts of an implant are the fixture (design, length, shape, diameter, and surface), transmucosal abutment, and the restoration/prosthesis.

Why is titanium metal used for dental implants? Titanium metal is chosen because of its biocompatibility (not rejected by the human body), formation of titanium dioxide (TiO_2) layer that prevents corrosion of the titanium implant. Other reasons that also make quite a remarkable list: it is strong, lightweight, corrosion resistant, nontoxic, nonferromagnetic, biocompatible, long lasting, and osseointegrative (joins to human bone), and its flexibility and elasticity are similar to that of human bone. Titanium alloy which is what the majority of dental implants are made from are mainly $TiAl_6V_4$ otherwise known as medical grade 5 and grade 23 for the greatest fracture resistance.

Another point to call the patient's attention to regarding titanium implants is the nonferromagnetic quality of titanium. *The benefit of being nonferromagnetic allows for patients with titanium implants to safely be examined with magnetic resonance imaging (MRIs) and national magnetic resource imaging (NMRIs).* One of the biggest benefits is the osseointegration of titanium and the human body, allowing for the patient's own natural bone to integrate and attach to an artificial device.

Titanium implants have a rough, smooth, and/or coated surfaces to speed up the osseointegration process (Figure 1.9). Types of treated surfaces are always evolving with the goal being to provide a biologically compatible surface to attract the bone to integrate to the implant. Some examples of surface treatments are hydroxyapatite (HA), the crystalline phase of calcium phosphate found naturally in bone mineral that is sprayed onto the implants, and titanium plasma sprayed (TPS), which simply means a heat/spray technique used in the industry to apply to the titanium implant surface. These coatings are sprayed on the implant body at the factory, placed in sterile container, and sealed. According to Vallecillo Capilla et al. (10), "long term success rates were outstanding for HA-coated implants and acceptable for TPS-coated implants after 5 years" (10).

Ceramic, zirconia-based implants, and abutments have emerged as a metal-free, tooth-like color, and light transmission especially preferred for aesthetic zone but

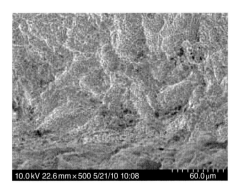

Figure 1.9 SEM titanium implant surface. Courtesy of PDT, Inc.

can be placed in other zones. Ceramic implants have no oxide layer, a nontoxic alternative, and treatment of choice for patients who want or need a metal-free option. (11) Zirconia implants are machined (ZrO_2m) or sandblasted (rough ZrO_2r). The ZrO_2r implants, have a rough surface and have shown in the literature to achieve a higher stability in bone (12) (Figure 1.10).

There is still some confusion on how ceramic, zirconia-based implants, are considered metal-free with zirconium in the composition. Zirconium is by definition the metallic form of the element Zr, a grayish-white transition metal. Zirconium dioxide (ZrO_2) by contrast is a white crystalline oxide of zirconium also called zirconoxide and is 100% ceramic material. Metals are highly reactive and atoms of metal elements such as zirconium collide with atoms of nonmetallic element like oxygen forming an ionic compound ZrO_2. This allows for changes in properties, such as the white color, minimal electrical conductivity, and relatively no reactive response.

When you compare titanium versus ceramics implants besides the metal and nonmetal differences, ceramic implants do not have an oxide layer in comparison to titanium that has an oxide layer that can be removed by multiple factors. While the surface coatings added to titanium implants is an advantage for osseointegration, it can have its own disadvantage if it is removed with the oxide layer due to mechanical or chemical means. More on this in Chapter 7, titanium dissolution particles that can lead to implant corrosion complications.

Implant design

Since there are multiple types of dental implant systems, hygienists need to be aware of the implant design, the patient presents with, in order to ensure safe and effective implant maintenance. The three main implant design types are transosteal, subperiosteal, and endosteal (endosseous) implants. They are classified according to their shape and how they interface with the bone.

Subperiosteal implants (Figure 1.11) are custom-casted framework of surgical grade metal or alloy that lies on top of the jawbone. They are surgically placed onto the ridge of an edentulous patient, similar to how a saddle is placed on a horse, and underneath the gum membrane.

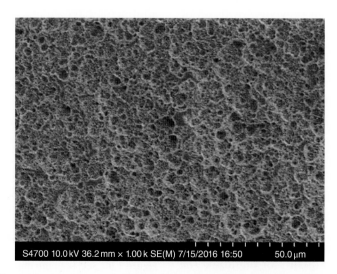

S4700 10.0 kV 36.2 mm × 1.00 k SE(M) 7/15/2016 16:50   50.0 µm

Figure 1.10   SEM ceramic (zirconia) implant surface. Courtesy of PDT, Inc.

This was a treatment option for patients when there was not enough bone to place an endosteal implant. Most of the implant structure, as illustrated in Figure 1.11, is covered with the original ridge tissue, so only the posts and bar are exposed above the gingiva. Subperiosteal implants come in different designs: unilateral, bilateral, and circumferential posterior only. A custom-designed superstructure denture or partial attaches to the posts for retention of this prosthesis. These implants were somewhat successful, but infection was common and it caused damage when they needed to be removed. Hygienists must be aware of this form of implants because they may encounter a patient with this form of implant design. Radiographs are going to be necessary to monitor this type of implants and it may be necessary to refer to a specialist if infection or pathology is observed.

A **transosteal** or **staple implant** (Figure 1.12) is an orthopedic device that is inserted through the inferior border of the mandible and is designed to function for an edentulous atrophic mandible. A titanium plate with five to seven parallel posts or dowels, two of which protrude through the mandible, function as abutments to attach a custom-designed overdenture. The discovery by Brånemark of osseointegration made rigidly designed fixed implant restorations possible to provide firm anchorage. The original design allowed for stress-directing attachments connected to transosteal pins to provide the stability for a removable overdenture. The implants for this procedure are costly and difficult to produce, so this procedure is not usually recommended. However, hygienists need to be aware of this design and monitor with radiographs. A referral to a specialist may be necessary if infection or pathology is observed.

Endosteal (within the bone) **implants** are generally made of titanium alloy and are designed to replace the root of one or more teeth. They are classified as **blade-** or **root-form**, cylindrical/press-fit or screw-threaded, and come in many different sizes, lengths, and shapes. The **blade-form**

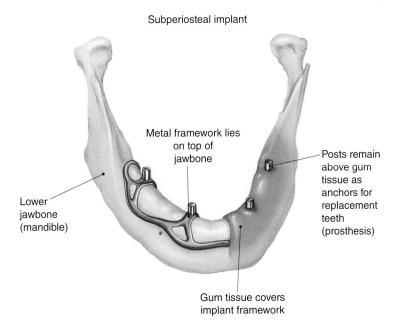

Subperiosteal implant

Metal framework lies on top of jawbone

Posts remain above gum tissue as anchors for replacement teeth (prosthesis)

Lower jawbone (mandible)

Gum tissue covers implant framework

Figure 1.11 Subperiosteal implant. Reprinted from Taylor and Laney (23), with permission from the author.

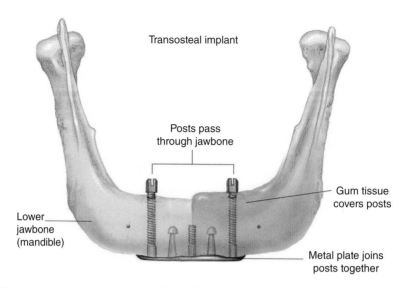

Transosteal implant

Posts pass
through jawbone

Gum tissue
covers posts

Lower
jawbone
(mandible)

Metal plate joins
posts together

Figure 1.12 Transosteal implant. Reprinted from Taylor and Laney (23), with permission from the author.

endosteal implant (Figure 1.13) is wide, flat metal plate or blade in cross section available in different heights and lengths, some with tapered sides. They may replace one to multiple teeth with a single blade and were used for narrow bones in maxillary or mandible, which had sufficient height to accommodate the implant placed. The blade-shaped implants (see Figure 1.13) were surgically placed into the bone, then posts were attached to the blade, and an individual crown or bridgework affixed on the posts after a healing period.

The **root-form implants** (Figure 1.14) mimic the shape of natural root, threaded, smooth, or rough surface, with or without coating. They are stepped, parallel, or tapered, with or without grooves or vents and designed to join with multiple components to retain prosthesis. They can replace one to multiple teeth, are placed directly into the bone, and can be used in maxillary or mandibular arches. The bone must be of sufficient height, width, and length to accommodate the implant(s) placed. These implants are referred to as cylinder or press-fit implants; screw-retained implants also referred to as threaded implants or a combination of the two.

They are available in different widths, varying from 3.2 to 7 mm, and are available

(a)

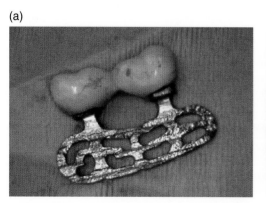

(b)

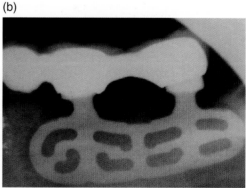

Figure 1.13 Blade-form implants. Courtesy of Dr. Frank Wingrove.

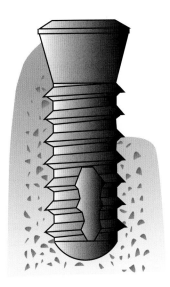

Figure 1.14 Endosteal root-form implants. Reprinted from Taylor and Laney (23), with permission from the author.

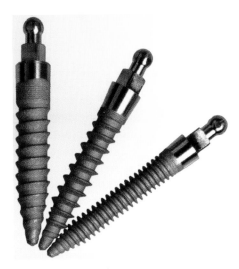

Figure 1.15 Mini dental implants. Courtesy of Glidewell.

in different lengths, varying from 10 to 18 mm. The width and length are decided by the dentist, depending on the width and the height of the bone, the type of bone, and the number of teeth to be replaced. An implant-supported abutment, often called a post, attaches to the surgically placed implant. Alternatively, one-piece root-form implants are also available that do not require placement of separate abutments. The two-stage root-form implants are placed in the bone, an abutment is attached to the implant, and the prosthesis is then placed. The final restoration or prosthesis is fabricated into a crown, bridge, or overdenture.

Looking to the future, we may see more endosteal implants made from ceramic (zirconia) or a combination of titanium and zirconia. Studies are being conducted due to its biocompatibility, tooth-like color, mechanical properties, and low plaque affinity. It has the potential to become the alternative to titanium as the alloy of choice. More long-term studies are being conducted on different rough surfaces with one-piece ceramic (zirconia) dental implants, which to date, have an average of 95% success rate after 5 years (13). More specialized types of endosteal implants,

to be aware of, are mini dental implants (MDIs) and zygoma implants.

MDIs (Figure 1.15) were introduced in the 1980s and accepted by the FDA as long-term implant devices by 1999. They are very narrow (1.8–2.9 mm), some as thin as toothpicks, and can be temporary anchoring devices (TAD) or permanent MDIs used to stabilize a lower overdenture. They are solid, not hollow like traditional implants, and are made in one piece that includes the abutment. In most cases, mini implants are used in the lower jaw to stabilize a lower denture. They can also be used for temporary implants, replacement of smaller diameter teeth such as lower incisors, or in cases where a traditional implant is too large in diameter. They are generally placed as a single-stage surgical process and are often loaded immediately.

Orthodontic implants/temporary anchoring devices (TADs)

TADs are titanium mini-screws, used primarily by orthodontists. They are screwed directly into the bone through the gingiva to facilitate tooth movement and to anchor an orthodontic appliance. Once treatment is complete, the clinician can remove the TAD without trauma or need for bone grafting.

TADs are placed in adolescents to adults and used on an average of 6–12 months. Primarily used for stabilization and to assist in tooth movement without stressing the surrounding teeth. Also, used to force eruption of impacted canines or misaligned teeth, or to stabilize an appliance (14).

Hygienist's role is to identify TAD patients, monitor, and treat to eliminate the biofilm and prevent soft tissue inflammation. Be aware, TAD implants may be located in the sulcus or palate of the orthodontic patients. Give patients the tools (i.e., sulcus or end tuft brushes), antimicrobial rinse, and other recommendations to eliminate the oral biofilm. Biofilm will accumulate on these TADs and can prevent the success of the orthodontic treatment as well as the overall oral hygiene of the patient. TADs are a tool in the toolbox for orthodontist to enable teeth to be moved in especially noncompliant patients with good oral hygiene as the KEY, see Chapter 8 for more recommendations on at-home-care.

Zygoma implants (Figure 1.16), also referred to as zygomatic implants, are longer than regular implants, initially developed by Brånemark in the 1980s. They are usually recommended to stabilize fixed full-arch final prosthesis in maxillary jaw, in cases where severe bone resorption is present in the maxilla. They are longer than regular dental implants; they extend up to 55 mm, compared with 10–15 mm. Zygomatic implants penetrate through the maxillary sinus and anchor in the very dense zygomatic bone. The head of the fixture normally emerges in a slightly palatal position in the second premolar/first molar area of the maxilla. The advantage to this choice of treatment is for patients with insufficient bone quality who may not be good candidates for traditional implant treatment or traditional dentures because of the high level of bone resorption. This can allow these patients durable, long-lasting, stable implant-supported fixed final prosthesis without additional bone grafting procedures.

There are many styles and types of dental implants that have been placed and are currently being placed on the market today. Their use is determined by the type of bone available and the prosthesis needed to accomplish the treatment. Implant systems have been developed by different manufactures with a variety of component parts, but there are primary components that are generally used.

Parts and pieces for implants

Today, the FDA regulates and requires data on all oral and dental implants being placed with controlled studies under medical devices to gain full approval. It is not

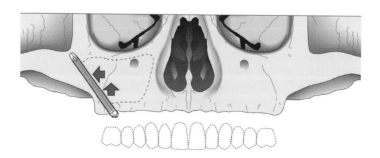

Figure 1.16 Zygoma implants. Courtesy of Nobel Biocare.

necessary for hygienists to know all the ins and outs of implant metals and designs, since the choice of implant to use will be in the hands of the surgeon. However, the biomechanics of implants or component parts of an implant are important to know and understand. The three main component parts of an implant are the implant body, with different designs, lengths, shapes, diameters, and surfaces; secondly, the abutment, which comes in many different types and materials, and even custom abutments are available, all screw directly into the implant to connect with the restoration/prosthesis. The final stage is the prosthesis; crown, bridge, fixed prosthesis, or removable overdenture (see Figure 1.17).

After the implant is placed into the bone, a cover screw or healing abutment (Figure 1.18) is placed directly into the implant to prevent bone and/or soft tissue from infiltrating the internal aspect of the implant during osseointegration. The healing abutment extends through the gingival tissue, forming the tissue contour/emergence profile to receive the final abutment and restoration (Figure 1.19).

At this time, well over half a million dental implants are being surgically placed annually. Implants are being properly planned and executed with success rates well over 90%. And yet, as rapidly as this

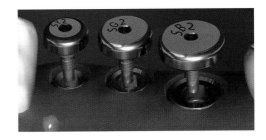

Figure 1.18   Examples of cover screws. Courtesy of BioHorizons.

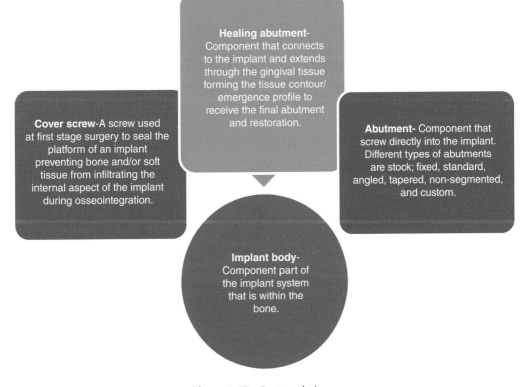

Healing abutment- Component that connects to the implant and extends through the gingival tissue forming the tissue contour/emergence profile to receive the final abutment and restoration.

Cover screw- A screw used at first stage surgery to seal the platform of an implant preventing bone and/or soft tissue from infiltrating the internal aspect of the implant during osseointegration.

Abutment- Component that screw directly into the implant. Different types of abutments are stock; fixed, standard, angled, tapered, non-segmented, and custom.

Implant body- Component part of the implant system that is within the bone.

Figure 1.17   Parts and pieces.

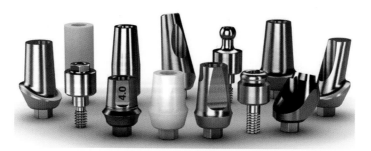

Figure 1.19 Examples of abutments. Courtesy of BioHorizons.

field of dentistry is growing, the majority of potential dental implant patients are unaware that this treatment exists. To address this, dental hygienist can take the lead and talk with his or her patients about tooth replacement and implant dentistry. As hygienists, we need to *plant the seeds* with our patients that the technology exists today to better their quality of life. The knowledge of key implantology terms will allow hygienists the opportunity to talk with their patients about implants and these quality of life issues. See the Appendix for more implant dentistry terminology.

Implant dentistry terminology

Connecting bar: System between two or more implants to be utilized for stability for implant prosthesis.

Dental implant: A biocompatible device placed in the bone to replace the root lost, preserve the bone level, and support the prosthesis.

Dental implant abutment: The component part that screws directly into the implant to retain the crown, bridge, and/or overdenture prosthesis in place.

Implant thread: The screw-like component part of the body of the endosteal, root-form implant.

Osseointegration: The firm, direct, and lasting biological attachment of an implant to vital bone with no intervening connective tissue.

Peri-implant diseases: Collective term for inflammatory lesions that may affect the peri-implant area, mucositis, and peri-implantitis.

Peri-implant mucositis: A pathological condition occurring in the tissue around dental implants, inflammation similar to gingivitis, reversible, caused by bacteria, biofilm, or residue. Manifests in the form of redness and inflammation, in the peri-mucosa, with no additional bone loss.

Peri-implantitis: A pathological condition occurring in tissue around dental implants, characterized by inflammation in the peri-mucosa and progressive loss of supporting bone that can be irreversible.

Periosteum: Fibrous vascular membrane that fits tightly on the outer surface of the bone.

Permucosal seal: The tissue seal that separates the connective tissues from the outside environment around a dental implant.

Prosthesis: The removable or nonremovable restoration that attaches to the implant to replace the teeth.

TADs: Titanium mini-screws used primarily by Orthodontists in the facilitation of moving teeth or anchoring an orthodontic appliance.

Summary

The 21st century is an important and critical time to be a hygienist! History has shown us that implants are not new and are definitely here to stay. An understanding of the evolution of implants, implant design, and the key terminology will allow you to talk to patients about the background of implantology. The relationship between periodontal health and diseases involving other organs and physiological systems (i.e., cardiovascular disease, preterm birth, diabetes, and respiratory disease) has been clearly documented (15–19). Hygienists need to be trained in the long-term prevention of peri-implant complications.

According to Dr. Nogueira-Filho et al., writing in 2010 (1), *"There is no reason to believe that mucosal inflammation affecting endosseous implant (i.e., peri-implant mucosal inflammation) would have fewer effects on general health than similar levels of inflammation affecting teeth (i.e., periodontitis, gingivitis)." Therefore, it is imperative that hygienists are trained in identifying and treating peri-implant mucosal inflammation that could affect overall body health.* The explosion of dental implants over the next decade will change the way we practice dental hygiene.

References

1. Nogueira-Filho G, Iacopino AM, Tenenbaum HC, Perio D Prognosis in implant dentistry: a system for classifying the degree of peri-implant mucosal inflammation. J Can Dent Assoc. 2010; 77: b8.
2. Froum SJ. My patient's implant is bleeding; what do I do? DentistryIQ, 2011.
3. Greenfield EJ Implantation of artificial crown and bridge abutments. Dent Cosmos. 1913; 55: 364–369, 430–439.
4. Research, Science and Therapy Committee of the American Academy Position paper dental implants in periodontal therapy. J Periodontol. 2000; 71: 1934–1942.
5. Simon RL Single implant-supported molar and premolar crowns: a ten-year retrospective clinical report. J Prosthet Dent. 2003; 90: 517–521.
6. Jivraj S, Chee W Treatment planning of implants in posterior quadrants. Br Dent J. 2006; 201: 13–23.
7. Lemmerman KJ, Lemmerman NE Osseointegrated dental implants in private practice: a long-term case series study. J Periodontol. 2005; 76: 310–319.
8. American Association of Oral and Maxillofacial Surgeons. Dental implants. 2011. aaoms.org/dental_implants.php. Accessed March 31, 2011.
9. Centers for Disease Control and Prevention, National Center for Chronic Disease Prevention and Health Promotion. Oral health resources. 2021. https://www.cdc.gov/oralhealth/basics/adult-oral-health/adult_older.htm
10. Vallecillo Capilla M, Romero Olid Mde N, Olmedo Gaya MV, Reyes Botella C, Zorrilla Romera C Cylindrical dental implants with hydroxyapatite- and titanium plasma spray-coated surfaces: 5-year results. J Oral Implantol. 2007; 33(2): 59–68.
11. Apratim A, Eachempati P, Krishnappa SKK, Singh V, Chhabra S, et al. Zirconia in dental implantology: a review. J Int Soc Prev Commun Dent. 2015; 5(3): 147–156.
12. Gahlert G, Gudehus T, Eichhorn S, Steinhauser E, Kniha H, Erhardt W Biomechanical and histomorphometric comparison between zirconia implants with varying surface textures and a titanium implant in the maxilla of miniature pigs. Clin Oral Implants Res. 2007; 18(5): 660–668.
13. Ozkurt Z, Kazazoqlu E Zirconia dental implants; a literature review. J Oral Implantol. 2011; 37(3): 367–376.
14. Hoste S, Vercruyssen M, Quirynen M, Willems G Risk factors and indications of orthodontic temporary anchorage devices: a literature review. Aust Orthod J. 2008; 24: 140–148.
15. Hein C Translating evidence of oral-systemic relationships into models of interprofessional collaboration. J Dent Hyg. 2009; 83(4): 188–189.
16. Hein C Scottsdale revisited: the role of dental practitioners in screening for undiagnosed diabetes and the medical co-management of patients with diabetes or those at risk for diabetes. Compend Contin Educ Dent. 2008; 29(9): 538–540, 542–544, 546–553.
17. Iacopino AM What is the role of inflammation in the relationship between periodontal disease and general health? J Can Dent Assoc. 2008; 74(8): 695.
18. Iacopino AM Practicing oral-systemic medicine: the need for interprofessional education. J Can Dent Assoc. 2008; 74(10): 866–867.
19. Iacopino AM Periodontitis and diabetes interrelationships: role of inflammation. Ann Periodontol. 2001; 6(1): 125–137.

20. Ring ME. Dentistry: An Illustrated History, 1st ed. St. Louis, MO: Mosby.
21. Juodzbalys G, Wang HL Guidelines for the identification of the mandibular vital structures: practical clinical applications of anatomy and radiological examination methods. J Oral Maxillofac Res. 2010; 1(2): e1.
22. Zwemer TJ. Mosby's Dental Dictionary, 2nd ed. St. Louis, MO: Mosby, 2008.
23. Taylor TD, Laney WR. Dental Implants: Are They for Me? 2nd ed. Carol Streams, IL: Quintessence, 1993.

2 Implant Therapy: Oral-Systemic Health, Medical History, and Risk Assessment

The terms oral health and general health should not be interpreted as separate entities. Oral health is integral to general health; this report provides important reminders that oral health means more than healthy teeth and that you cannot be healthy without oral health.

—Surgeon General Report, 2001

Over the past 30 years, implantology and periodontal medicine (periodontal and peri-implant disease) have changed the way we think about dentistry. Dental professionals have moved away from the examination for decayed or broken teeth to a comprehensive examination of the entire mouth and overall health of the patient. The traditional dentistry resolution for missing teeth was to fabricate a bridge, partial or full removable denture or do nothing. After 15 years of wearing a full denture, patients can suffer from gastrointestinal disorders from reduced ability to chew their food and this may lead to a shorter life expectancy (1). Partial denture wearers often experience the *domino* effect, losing the teeth that support the partial at a rate of 44% within 10 years (2). There are even romantic consequences for edentulous patients, as they can be reluctant to start new relationships. Some edentulous patients are categorized as oral invalids unable to wear their dentures without pain (3). Today, the optimal restorative options for replacing missing teeth are implants.

It is an exciting time to be in dentistry, with the increasing use of regeneration tissue/bone procedures, and implant dentistry. Implants rank second only to bleaching procedures as the most sought after treatment in dentistry. Hygienists play an important role, recommending, assessing, maintaining, and monitoring implants. Hygienists have 50–60 minutes with patients on a regular recare basis and hold the key to many of the relationships of our patients to the practice. Often, hygienists are asked; *"What should I do to replace this tooth?" and "What are my options?"*

Hygienists should learn all they can about regeneration and implant therapy. What these procedures can do to benefit

Peri-Implant Therapy for the Dental Hygienist, Second Edition. Susan S. Wingrove.
© 2022 John Wiley & Sons, Inc. Published 2022 by John Wiley & Sons, Inc.
Companion website: www.wiley.com/go/wingrove/implant

the lives of the patient for aesthetics and overall health. Keep in mind that many implant candidates are dental failures, periodontal disease patients, or patients with poor oral health habits. Hygienists can educate patients on implant options that can improve their oral health and might change the patient's life!

The best candidates for implants are your *existing patients of record*. You have patients with missing teeth, partials, dentures, and bridges that are failing. You already have a relationship and trust with these patients. If your office wants to do more implant dentistry a key source of prospective implant candidates are referrals from your existing satisfied implant patients. Do not be afraid to ask for referrals from your satisfied patients to encourage more like-minded patients to learn about their options for implant dentistry.

Patient selection for implants is based on a number of factors including oral-systemic health, medical history, risk assessment, and hygiene status. Patients who are immunosuppressed or taking anticoagulants, steroids, or IV bisphosphonates can be contraindicated for implant therapy or need to be evaluated on risk levels. Heavy smokers, poorly controlled diabetics, patients with previous poor bone-healing history, and patients with multiple systemic health problems should also be evaluated carefully. Any diseases that can directly affect the ability of osteoblasts to lay bone or interfere with wound healing of bony tissue are contraindicated for placement of implants or the dentist needs to evaluate the options with the patient's physician.

Uncontrolled diabetics and heavy smokers are at the top of the list of contraindicated patients due to the poor vascularization of the gingival tissues as well as higher risk for infection and slower healing time. However, a controlled diabetic is an ideal implant patient due to the added benefit of implant dentistry that the implants do not decay.

A smoker can also be a good candidate for implant therapy if he or she first attends a smoking cessation program and agrees to the risks associated with possible loss of the implant. Immunosuppressed patients, such as HIV-positive patients, who want to improve digestion can be considered for implants, but would need to be controlled and monitored.

Age, osteoporosis, and periodontal bone loss may also be an obstacle that can be hurdled. Periodontal maintenance patients who are compliant with home-care can be excellent candidates, but should be placed on 3-month recare for implant maintenance. The same bacteria that caused the periodontal disease will still be present in their oral cavity. If a patient enquires about having an implant, review all the options and let the patient know that the doctor will determine if he or she is a candidate for implant therapy.

An edentulous patient at any age can benefit from implant dentistry; there is no cutoff age. As a general rule, it is recommended that growth be completed prior to implant placement for children younger than 16 years of age, but younger children can be considered for implants on an individual case-by-case basis.

The hygienist is the ideal person to assist the dentist in the selection process to determine the patient's motivation, dexterity for home care necessary for the selected treatment and expectations of therapy outcome, as well as to identify patients with risk factors, habits, and conditions that place patients at a higher risk for implant failure. The hygienist can talk to the patients about their needs, expectations, and questions to share with the dentist. Due to the hourly schedule that most hygienist have, if a patient is interested in implant dentistry a separate appointment can be made with the dentist to have an implant consultation.

The patient's aesthetic and functional expectations have a direct correlation to the number of implants necessary, type of restoration to be used, time to heal, and how much the final cost of treatment will be. All of these factor into patient selection and need to be discussed with the patient prior to treatment.

A complex or larger treatment case will require a separate treatment conference and possible models or other diagnostics prior to the conference. Schedule the conference with the doctor and/or implant coordinator to walk the patient through the treatment options, time involved, and fees associated with the case. The doctor may also need to collaborate with the patient's physician prior to proceeding with implant therapy due to the systemic health factor.

Implant treatment planning is interdisciplinary and the hygienist needs to have an understanding of oral-systemic health, medical history, and risk factors to assist with the necessary diagnostics and questions/answers for the dentist to complete the best treatment plan for the patient.

Oral-systemic health link to overall health

It is now widely accepted and confirmed through research that there is an *oral systemic connection.* A link established between bacterial infections, oral bacterial biofilm, and cytokine release in periodontal tissues. The link between oral infection and certain systemic diseases has taken center stage, and inflammation is the key!

Who better to identify inflammation than hygienists who evaluate for potential periodontal disease on a daily basis? Periodontal disease is one of the major inflammatory diseases in the body. Dental professionals, therefore, hold a key role now, not only in the treatment of periodontal disease and peri-implant disease but also in comprehensive disease management.

Periodontal medicine is now the coined term that looks at the risk for certain systemic diseases that is increased by an oral infection (i.e., periodontal and peri-implant disease) from patients' inflammatory response to infection. To fully understand the severity of the problem, a basic knowledge of how bacteria from the periodontal or peri-implant sulcus gains access to the systemic circulation (i.e., blood stream) is important.

The bacterial biofilm comes in contact with ulcerated epithelium, which creates a pathway directly to the systemic circulation. Gram-negative bacteria, which are always present in the oral cavity, have access to the blood vessels, which allows the infection to reach other tissues and organs throughout the body. Periodontal and/or peri-implant disease act as a reservoir of pro-inflammatory mediators or modules that enhance the inflammatory response. They enter the systemic circulation and can induce and/or perpetuate systemic effects that can ultimately affect the overall health of the patient (see Figure 2.1).

There are four major diseases with proven links to periodontal disease and are by association considered risk factors for peri-implant disease: *cardiovascular/cerebrovascular disease, preterm birth/low birth weight, diabetes,* and *respiratory disease;* see Box 2.1.

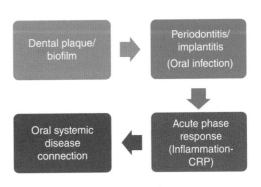

Figure 2.1 Inflammation process.

Box 2.1 Four major diseases linked with periodontal disease/risk factors for peri-implant disease.

Cardiovascular/Cerebrovascular (CV/CV) disease: A link between periodontal/peri-implant disease and cardiovascular disease/stroke has been established. Changes caused by infection and/or inflammation responses affect the build-up of plaque on the inner lining of the blood vessels supplying the heart (coronary arteries) or brain (carotid arteries) and atherosclerosis can occur (4, 5).

Preterm birth/low birth weight: Studies have proven a link between periodontal/peri-implant disease/infection and the risk of adverse pregnancy outcomes, including preterm birth and low-weight babies (6, 7). This is caused by the action of blood-borne oral bacteria or an increase in the blood levels on the inflammatory mediators that can cause early delivery.

Diabetes: Periodontitis/periimplantitis is a proven complication and all patients with diabetes should be evaluated for periodontal disease and monitored for signs of infections in the periodontium of implants. Good news, controlled diabetics show the same dental implant survival rate as patients without diabetes and it is now considered a predictable dental rehabilitation procedure for diabetics. (8)

Respiratory disease: Lung diseases, especially hospital-acquired pneumonia, are linked to poor dental health. Pulmonary pathogens in plaque are aspirated into the lungs increasing the risk of pneumonia and chronic obstructive pulmonary disease (COPD). This includes implant patients with implant supported removable overdentures, often the implants are overlooked in institutional care facilities without the necessary information on care of dental implants. Treatment for good oral health care can reduce the patient's risk of fever and fatal aspiration pneumonia (9–12).

Cardiovascular/cerebrovascular (CV/CV) disease

There is a documented association between inflammation, periodontal/peri-implant disease, infection, and the risk of cardiovascular/cerebrovascular (CV/CV) disease. The national survey of health conditions of the US population collected between 1988 and 1994 (NHANES III database) states; "the relationship between periodontal attachment loss and the risk of myocardial infarction was demonstrated." This data suggest a real and important influence of periodontitis on the risk of CV/CV disease. According to the American Academy of Periodontology (AAP) Mouth Body Connection, "Researchers have found that people, especially diabetics with periodontal disease are almost twice as likely to suffer from coronary artery disease" (4).

As dental professionals, we can provide treatment for periodontitis/implantitis that may help prevent the onset of and delay in the progression of CV/CV disease. Oral bacteria/biofilm can affect the heart by attaching to fatty plaques in the arteries and forming clots. These clots can cause obstructions that can lead to a heart attack. Infection and/or inflammation responses can also affect the buildup of biofilm on the inner lining of the blood vessels supplying the heart (coronary arteries) or brain (carotid arteries) that occurs in atherosclerosis (4, 5).

A growing number of research studies also support the contribution of periodontal/peri-implant infection to the inflammatory burden theorized to be both a direct action on blood vessel walls and by indirectly inducing the liver to produce cardiac reactive proteins (CRPs) through an acute-phase response (13). CRPs are produced by the liver in response to infection and inflammation, and are a specific systemic marker of vascular inflammation that appears to have a strong association with adverse vascular events; see Figure 2.1 (14).

CRPs are also referred to as hepatic plasma proteins or C-reactive proteins. They are found in trace amounts even in healthy people, however, if elevated levels of these proteins are found it can signify

Table 2.1 Levels of cardiac reactive proteins (CRPs).

Normal CRP	<1.0 mg/L
Intermediate CRP	1.0–2.9 mg/L
High CRP	>3.0 mg/L

serious inflammation in the body. CRP levels can go as high as 400–500 mg/L in seriously ill patients (see Table 2.1). Many different diseases and conditions can elevate CRP levels such as; periodontal disease, cardiovascular disease (CVD), trauma, surgery, burns, advanced malignancy, Alzheimer's disease, blood sugar disorders, smoking, and obesity.

Alzheimer's disease is being viewed as an inflammatory brain disorder due to studies that have shown that patients with high levels of CRPs were three times more likely to develop Alzheimer's disease. Tobacco also raises CRP levels and has a residual effect that remains in the body for years. Smoking causes oxidants to form and might accelerate the oxidation of low-density lipoproteins (LDLs) constituents, which causes arterial inflammation even in healthy individuals with normal LDL levels.

To detect and monitor inflammation, the CRP blood test is becoming a leading marker for systemic inflammation in the body. Intermediate to high levels of CRPs found in this specific blood test indicate an increase in inflammation somewhere in the body, are cause for concern, and the inflammation needs to be identified.

CRP testing is a significant tool for identification of patients at risk for CV/ CV, CVD, and prevention of CVD (15). Dental professionals are currently using high-sensitivity C-reactive protein (hs-CRP) testing in dental practices chairside. They are requesting the test from the patient's physician to identify and monitor patients at risk for acute coronary syndromes or periodontal/peri-implant disease.

Severe periodontal/peri-implant disease patients have more harmful bacteria in their bloodstreams than patients with moderate or no disease (Figure 2.1). The inflammatory process of periodontal/peri-implant disease increases CRP levels and when periodontal disease or peri-implant disease are treated, the CRP levels decrease and the hemoglobin A1c (HbA1c) levels improve (16, 17). HbA1c level is also an important marker in monitoring diabetes. Both CRP and LDL cholesterol level tests are minimally correlated, but CRP has been found in some studies to be a stronger predictor of future cardiovascular events than LDL cholesterol (14).

The bottom line is that CRPs are going to be an important link for dentistry. Inflammation is turning out to be the missing link for diagnosing and treating many systemic diseases. The key for dentistry is that periodontal disease and now peri-implant disease is one of the most prominent inflammatory diseases in the body. In medical journals, the recommendation is that the first stop for a patient with increased CRP levels is a screening by a dentist or specialist for periodontal/peri-implant disease or other oral infections. If the CRP levels remain elevated over 3.0 mg/L, a referral to the primary care physician is recommended for evaluation for systemic diseases. Educate your patients about pre-procedural health before treatment for optimal successful long-lasting results.

Preterm birth/low birth weight

There is a direct link between oral infections and premature births and low birth weight infant outcomes (6). Chronic infections such as periodontitis and implantitis can lead to an increased inflammatory response in pregnant mothers which, in turn, causes the production of higher levels of prostaglandins prematurely. The prostaglandins are produced naturally by the placenta to stimulate the birth of the baby, the end result being a low weight, and a prematurely birthed infant. In recent studies, researchers have also found that periodontal pathogens may travel from the oral cavity to the placenta to directly cause premature birth (7).

Periodontal therapy for pregnant mothers has few adverse side effects and is recommended during the second trimester to reduce the occurrence of preterm low birth weight infants. The AAP strongly recommends good dental care during pregnancy. Women may experience increased gingivitis or pregnancy gingivitis beginning in the second or third month of pregnancy that increases in severity up to the eighth month.

It is recommended to have an oral checkup with a dental professional with two dental prophylaxis visits: one in the first trimester and one in the third trimester. Studies demonstrate that periodontal therapy before 28 weeks of gestation can reduce the risk of preterm low birth weight infants in women with periodontitis.

Diabetes

Diabetes mellitus is a group of metabolic diseases recognized as a global epidemic by the World Health Organization (WHO) that affects over 8% of the adult population worldwide (18). Diabetes is defined by elevated levels of glucose in the bloodstream. Type 1 diabetes is absolute insulin deficiency and type 2 diabetes is a metabolic disorder with high blood glucose with insulin resistance and some insulin deficiency.

According to the latest 2017 World Workshop, Peri-implantitis Review, the evidence is; "inconclusive as to whether diabetes is a risk factor/indicator for peri-implantitis" (19). Recent studies showed evidence that a diabetic patient who completes dental implant therapy can masticate food, which will lead to improved nutrition and metabolic control (8). Diabetic patients do have an increased inflammatory response, are at risk for other complications, such as retinopathy, nephropathy, neuropathy, macrovascular disease, and poor wound healing. If they have poor metabolic control, successful periodontal and peri-implantitis therapy can greatly improve diabetics' metabolic control and tissue inflammation (20–26).

It is recommended prior to implant therapy, that the dentist request a HbA1c test/results of any diabetic patient and continue to monitor their diabetic implant patients. This test allows for the dentist to monitor the diabetic patient's blood sugar level to confirm that the patient's levels are staying within a controlled range. Dental professionals can now offer their diabetic patients HbA1c tests in-office. This allows the dentist the ability to monitor diabetic patients, identify and treat any signs of peri-implant inflammation early.

Good news for diabetic patients that current studies indicate that controlled diabetes show the same dental implant survival rate as patients without diabetes and it is now considered a predictable dental rehabilitation procedure for diabetics (8).

Respiratory disease

Respiratory disease or lung diseases, especially hospital-acquired pneumonia, are linked to poor dental health (9, 10). To define this link, pulmonary pathogens in plaque are aspirated into the lungs increasing the risk of pneumonia and chronic obstructive pulmonary disease (COPD) (9–12). At greatest risk because of this link are the elderly, especially those in nursing homes. Also, at risk are patients in the hospital, institutional patients, patients with NG tubes, and intubated patients.

Research suggests that bacteria/oral biofilm found in the mouth and throat can be drawn into the lower respiratory tract. These patients can all benefit from good oral hygiene with application of topical chemotherapeutic agents. This includes implant patients with implant-supported removable overdentures, often implants are overlooked in institutional care facilities without the necessary information on care of dental implants. Treatment for good oral health care can reduce the patient's risk of fever and fatal aspiration pneumonia.

Rheumatoid arthritis (27), osteoporosis (28), head and neck cancer, pancreatic cancer, kidney disease, and COPD (10, 11) are other proposed connections to periodontal disease that are still being studied. Oral systemic health also has an inferred relationship between periodontal disease and Alzheimer's (29–31). All these studies are based on the acute phase inflammatory response from periodontal disease or peri-implant disease that invokes a local and systemic immune response (32). As the oral-systemic diseases are further defined, dental professionals must consider the impact of periodontal disease and peri-implant disease (i.e., perimucositis or peri-implantitis) on the patient's overall health.

Chair-side testing kits are now commercially available as an important tool in the new paradigm of oral-systemic medicine without the need for an additional license or personnel, (see Box 2.2). Many patients do not get physicals on a routine basis. As health professionals, we can screen, monitor, and treat patients more comprehensively by offering chair-side testing. Medical billing can also help your practice offer more comprehensive testing, monitoring, and treatment plans with decreased out-of-pocket costs for the patient.

The entire team needs to be educated on any tests your office will be providing. Obtain brochures and establish a system to identify which patients need to be tested.

Patients with risk factors, heart disease, periodontal disease, and diabetes are prime candidates. For patient's treatment planning on implants or bone and tissue grafting procedures, a CRP, vitamin D, and if the patient is diabetic HbA1c testing. For diabetics, you can provide HbA1c tests at each maintenance visit or once yearly as a quality service to provide for these patients. If a patient has periodontal disease or heart disease a CRP and/or vitamin D test could be considered.

In the United States, 50–75% of all adults have a vitamin D deficiency which

---

Box 2.2   Chair-side tests for risk factors

■ **C-Reactive Protein (hs-CRP)**: Highly sensitive blood test to evaluate inflammation and to monitor whether inflammation is still present after treatment. Also available is the CRP plus HbA1c combination test. There are also chair-side tests being developed and can be ordered by a dentist at a blood testing lab.

■ **Diabetes Risk Assessment Test**: Hemoglobin A1c (HbA1c) is designed to screen for diabetes and fasting blood glucose. The HbA1c can be ordered by a dentist at a blood testing lab. There are also chair-side tests being developed but currently FDA has approved them only for those that already are diagnosed with diabetes.

■ **Perio-Metabolic Profile**: A comprehensive test for eight risk factors: total cholesterol, LDL, triglycerides, HDL, hs-CRP, HbA1c, and fasting insulin. To specifically detect for periodontal/peri-implant disease, heart disease, and diabetes. This profile can be ordered by a dentist at a blood testing lab.

■ **Vitamin D Test**: For detection of deficiency in vitamin D, an indicator of potential health risks of systemic diseases. A factor for linking innate and adaptive immunity connected with low-density lipoprotein cholesterol which can slow implant osseointegration and increase risk of graft infections. This test can be ordered by a dentist at a blood testing lab.

is associated with dental treatment complications such as healing after implant or soft tissue surgeries (33). It is also an indicator of potential health risks of systemic diseases including heart disease, strokes, diabetes, and even cancer.

For implant dentistry, the Vitamin D test can also be a key factor for linking innate and adaptive immunity. Together with excess LDL, cholesterol (dyslipidemia) can cause slower bone metabolism and a decrease in dental implant osseointegration. Therefore, a deficiency in vitamin D can slow implant osseointegration and increase the risk of graft infection (34). The recommended daily intake of vitamin D is now, 600–800 IU daily to meet nutritional needs, increased from 400 IU per day. Research in a double-blind, randomized clinical trial in Calgary, Canada by Dr. Laureen Burt showed that individuals taking 10,000 IU a day had lower bone mineral densities and increased bone resorption compared to individuals taking 400 IU per day (35).

Vitamin D testing and recommendation of supplements are now a consideration before and after implant placement for patients with poor wound healing in previous dental surgeries and in coordination with their medical physicians.

It is important to remember when discussing oral health and risk factors with your patients that having an infection in the oral cavity does not mean the patient is now going to suffer a heart attack or stroke. Rather, these systemic disorders are considered as complex diseases with multiple risk factors contributing to the patient's overall health risk. As dental professionals, we need to provide comprehensive care for our patients for their overall health which may postpone the risk for certain systemic diseases (36). Stay up to date on all the latest research coming out the oral-systemic connection to provide optimal care for your patients.

Medical history/risk assessment

Risk assessment questions are a vital part of a comprehensive medical history and implant treatment plan. Health risk factors include uncontrolled diabetes, history of poor wound healing, and any diagnoses of systemic diseases. Risk factors, such as age, gender, obesity, smoking, functional habits, oral health (biofilm), and socioeconomic status are also important. If these factors are combined it could make any implant treatment case more complicated and a risk for a successful case outcome.

One standard risk assessment often used with patients is offered through the Academy of Periodontology (AAP). Twelve questions on age, gender, oral health (bleeding gums, loose teeth, recession, missing teeth), smoking or tobacco use, habits (frequency of dental visits, flossing, brushing), oral-systemic diseases (including periodontal disease), and genetics are used to determine a risk score. Etiology risk factors include all the risk factors mentioned on the AAP Risk Assessment in addition to caries rate and occlusion (bruxism), to be taken into consideration in determining whether a patient is a good candidate for implant therapy. If a patient has a high caries rate, he or she is actually at low risk for implant therapy. For example, a controlled diabetic patient would benefit with implant therapy because the implants would not decay.

Occlusal issues such as bruxism make implant therapy a higher risk due to the possibility of overloading the implants with occlusal forces, which could lead to bone loss or implant failure. Treatment to correct bruxism and fabrication of an occlusal guard can greatly increase the success rate of implant therapy for these patients.

For a periodontal disease patient, the evidence from both longitudinal and cross-sectional studies shows that a history of periodontal disease is a higher risk factor and indicator of peri-implantitis (19). A clear indicator that prior to placing an implant, strong consideration should be made to bring the patient into a stable periodontal condition, is the key. Once a periodontal patient, always a periodontal patient, and these patients should be kept on a more frequent recare maintenance schedule. All the factors that caused this patient to have periodontal disease are still present.

Smokers, once considered high risk, according to the 2017 AAP/EFP World Workshop to develop new classifications and conditions stated; "there is currently no conclusive evidence that smoking constitutes a risk factor or indicator for peri-implantitis" (19). Studies vary widely on this topic, but the results of smoking as a risk factor can be related to other risk factors like previous periodontal disease. Many experts believe biofilm accumulation, smoking, and radiation are the top three risks factors for peri-mucositis. Patients who quit smoking or underwent a smoking cessation program can however improve their overall health and therefore greatly increase the success rate for implant therapy. Patients who have had radiation therapy, pathological conditions in the bone, active periodontal disease, and/or acute infections are contraindicated for implant therapy. These contraindications can be reversed with treatment at a slightly lower success rate. See the Appendix for resources on inflammation and organizations that offer risk assessments and are up-to-date on research on peri-implant therapy risk factors.

Bisphosphonates, BRONJ/BON, ARONJ, MRONJ

What does the hygienist need to know about the nomenclature of bisphosphonate-related osteonecrosis of the jaw (BRONJ), medication-related osteonecrosis of the jaw (MRONJ)? Patients who are immunosuppressed or are taking anticoagulants, steroids, or bisphosphonates medications can be contraindicated for implant therapy. These patients can be at risk for osteonecrosis of the jaw (37).

The American Dental Association Council on Scientific Affairs wrote an executive summary published in 2011 outlining recommendation and listing the current antiresorptive agents with current dosages and indications (38). The report based on the literature and expertise of the scientific panel states; "the risk of developing antiresorptive agent induced osteonecrosis of the jaw (ARONJ) in a patient who does not have cancer appears to be low". The research available to date shows that the benefits of antiresorptive therapy outweigh the low risk of developing osteonecrosis of the jaw (38).

Dental Professionals do need to be aware of the latest research on MRONJ. Any medical condition or medication which inhibits cell mitosis or metabolism could affect the success of implants. The hygienist needs to be aware of patients taking antiresorptive therapy for not only the risk for implant therapy, but also tooth extractions or other dental surgical invasive bone procedures. Bisphosphonates are most common medication related to complications with osteonecrosis of the jaw and localized death of bone tissue, abbreviated BON or BRONJ. Also referred to as antiresorptive agent induced osteonecrosis of the jaw (ARONJ) Bisphosphonate are given in two forms; oral mainly for osteopenia and osteoporosis and IV mainly for cancer-related conditions.

BON diagnoses are 94% associated with intravenous (IV) administration of bisphosphonates and only 6% of cases from taking bisphosphonates orally (37). Cases of osteoporosis in the United States in 2020, increased to 14 million and over 47 million cases of low bone mass in the over 50 years old population. One in two Americans over the age of 50 is expected to have or develop osteoporosis of the hip and other sites in the skeleton according to the bone health and osteoporosis report by the surgeon general (39).

Since 2004, oral and maxillofacial surgeons and manufactures are aware of the link of bisphosphonates IV and oral preparations to nonhealing exposed bone or BON. For practical knowledge, a MRONJ patient is a patient who is currently or have previously taken antiresorptive or antiangiogenic agents. They have exposed bone in the maxillofacial region that persists for more than 8 weeks and no history of radiation therapy to be considered to have MRONJ (40).

Doctors prescribe bisphosphonates in oral or IV form for osteoporosis (low or decreasing bone mass patient at risk for bone fractures) and cancers that are associated with the bone. Bisphosphonates in IV form are mainly prescribed for cancer patients to decrease pain, bone fractures, and in some cases to decrease spread of cancers to the bone.

What this means for hygienists is that you should assist the dentist to identify these patients. Patients need to be informed that BON is a risk associated with implant surgery for patients who have taken or are currently taking bisphosphonates. Make sure that questions on anticoagulants, steroids, and/or bisphosphonates are included on your medical history form. *"Have you taken or are you taking anticoagulants? Steroids?"* *"Are you presently taking or have you in the past taken bisphosphonate drugs? Oral or IV?"* These are critical questions to have answered before a patient has oral, periodontal, periapical (endodontic) surgery, and/or implants placed (40). Take good record notes on what your patient explains about how long and which form of bisphosphonates they are currently taking or have taken, *note in the patient record.*

Bisphosphonates are a class of drugs used to treat osteoporosis and some tumors associated with cancer. They are prescribed for women after menopause, men with thinning bone (Paget's disease) caused by steroid treatment, and other bone problems associated with cancer. Bisphosphonates work by inhibiting osteoclast (bone cells) activity that removes bone tissue and induces bone cells to die. Therefore, if bisphosphonates inhibit the death of bone cells, osteoclasts will be able to continue to increase or maintain bone mass. Bone mass is maintained by a balance between bone cell destruction and bone cell generation, referred to as osteoblast activity. The jaw, with a greater blood supply than other bones, is more susceptible to high concentrations of bisphosphonates. In some patients, taking bisphosphonates can cause an abnormal imbalance of osteoblast activity that can result in infection and/or in osteonecrosis of the jaw (necrosis of the jaw).

The American Association of Oral and Maxillofacial Surgeons set the following criteria to diagnose BRONJ/BON in their updated 2009 BRONJ position paper (see Table 2.2). They concluded that "both the potency of and the length of exposure to bisphosphonates are linked to the risk of developing bisphosphonate-associated osteonecrosis of the jaw" (41). Patients receiving intravenous bisphosphonate therapy are more likely to develop BON than are those receiving oral therapy. Also, prolonged use of over 2 years and combined with smoking or diabetes, puts a patient at an increased risk of BON.

Table 2.2 Criteria to diagnose bisphosphonate-related osteonecrosis of the jaw.

1. Patient presents with an area of exposed, necrotic bone in the jaw that persists for 8 weeks or longer.
2. Patient has had no radiation therapy to the head or neck.
3. Patient must be taking or have taken bisphosphonate oral or IV medication.

To assess risk level for patients to develop BON (osteonecrosis) before the patient has an implant placed, the dentist/implant surgeon can prescribe a serum CTx (C-telopeptides) blood test. It evaluates CTx levels based on the C-telopeptides, fragments of collagen that are released during bone remodeling and turnover (see Table 2.3) (42).

The American Dental Association also put together a panel of experts on BON to make recommendations for treatment of patients taking or have taken oral bisphosphonates. A significant study, with over 700,000 cases, was completed and published in the 2008 Journal of Oral Maxillary Surgeons, titled "Bisphosphonate Use and the Risk of Adverse Jaw Outcomes." *It concluded that patients taking or who have taken oral bisphosphonates "can be a candidate for implant therapy", but need to be evaluated on an individual basis* (43). Patients taking or who have taken intravenous bisphosphonates can be contraindicated for implant placement. It is recommended that patients complete any oral surgery (i.e., tooth extraction), implant placement, periapical surgery, or periodontal surgery prior to starting bisphosphonate therapy, if possible.

Prior to starting any surgical treatment, a comprehensive exam including a very thorough medication history is essential. The patient also needs to be informed of any risks verbally and through written instruction, including risk of BON, and should sign a witness informed consent form.

Table 2.3 Risk assessment for osteonecrosis.

CTx Level (pg/mL)	Risk Level
• 300–600 (normal)	None
• 150–299	None to Minimal
• 101–149	Moderate
• <100	High

Xerostomia

The elderly population is increasing, living longer, and over 90% of adults 65 years or older are taking one or more medications that can cause xerostomia (dry mouth). Xerostomia is not limited to the elderly. A high percentage of younger people take antidepressants or other medications that have the side effect of dry mouth. Xerostomia can be caused by medications and is often increased by smoking or drinking alcohol.

Radiation therapy can also cause a reduction in saliva due to damaging the salivary glands from radiation treatments for head and neck cancer. Saliva production is necessary to help bathe the teeth, it prevents decay and makes it easier to talk, swallow, taste, and digest food. The systemic diseases associated with xerostomia are Sjogren's syndrome (SS), sarcoidosis, and amyloidosis, all of which are inflammatory diseases.

Implant therapy has been shown to have a high implant survival rate for patient with SS with low marginal bone loss or biological complications (44, 45). As hygienists, we can help these patients with good home care recommendations specifically designed for dry mouth. Multiple products are being developed specifically for xerostomia.

Hygienists, we can help dry mouth patients with xerostomia by recommending products that provide much-needed moisturizing relief. Neutral pH products with xylitol are ideal to prevent higher than the other patients' risk for decay and periodontal/peri-implant disease. Oral biofilm for dry mouth patient can lead to a higher gingival inflammation index and implant treatment has shown to be a good treatment choice for this population. Implants have the least amount of host response, as long as they remain healthy. They do not decay and have the highest success rate of any type of restorative procedure we provide in dentistry.

Oral biofilm drives periodontal inflammation starting with gingivitis/mucositis and progressing to periodontitis/implantitis. The 2017 AAP/EFP World Workshop to develop new classifications and conditions stated; "there is definitely evidence that if a patient does not control the plaque/oral biofilm and does not present for regular implant maintenance, poor biofilm control is a risk factor for peri-implantitis" (19). *Once infection is in the oral cavity it is a direct link to the bloodstream and can affect the overall health of your patient.* The process can be reversed if caught early, before infection has caused a loss of bone. If it is not caught in a timely manner it can also progress into oral-systemic diseases that can affect the heart, the lungs, and pregnancy.

Medical history/risk assessment forms

Periodontal medicine and implant therapy add a new dimension to how we look at medical history questions and develop our treatment and maintenance protocols. Dental professionals need to pay close attention to the medical history form with respect to what drugs, vitamins, and/or over-the-counter medications the patient is taking on a regular basis. Also, identify any risk factors that could interfere with successful implant therapy.

It is important to carefully read, review, and walk through the patient's medical history with the patient at every implant maintenance or restorative *appointment*. It is also important to record if the patient is in the care of a physician at the present time and for what medical condition. This could have an impact on the overall health of the implant, maintenance requirements, and/or the proposed treatment plan. If the patient has uncontrolled diabetes, for example, it increases the risk of peri-

implantitis and ultimately may result in implant failure.

How often have you asked a patient, "Are there any changes in your medical history?" and received the *"no changes"* comment, then, in the process of the patient's maintenance appointment, the patient mentions he or she has just had a stent or a pacemaker placed? The written medical history is important, but you must **ask specific questions, go down the list, listen, and be observant.** Previous periodontitis and poor wound healing following dental surgical treatments are identifiable for dental professionals and can help identify oral systemic risk factors.

Summary

Dentistry is changing with the dawn of periodontal medicine. Over 90% of adults over 55 and more than 70% of adults aged 35–44 are affected by periodontal disease (46). Peri-implant mucositis can occur around 43% of implants and peri-implantitis 22%, on an average of 5–10 years after implant placement (47). Patient selection, more important than ever to ensure implant success, involves a thorough medical history as well as comprehensive oral health and risk assessment. Well-informed and well-read physicians are now recognizing the benefits to interdisciplinary care with dentists. Many physicians and surgeons are now requiring written confirmation from dental professionals that the patient's oral health is stable and free of any infections prior to cardiac or joint replacement surgeries. Physicians are recommending their patients' good oral health and regular in-office dental prophylaxis appointments for overall health. Implant dentistry is truly interdisciplinary, requiring close collaboration between the dentist, hygienist, and the patient's physician for successful peri-implant therapy.

References

1. Feldman RS, Kapur KK, Alman JE, et al. Aging and mastication changes in performance and in the swallowing threshold with natural dentition. J Am Geriatric Soc. 1980; 28: 97–103.

2. Aquilino SA, Shugars DA, Bader ID, et al. Ten-year survival rates of teeth adjacent to treated and untreated posterior bounded edentulous spaces. J Prosthet Dent. 2001; 85: 455–460.

3. Humphries GM, Healey T, Howell RA, et al. The psychological impact of implant-retained mandibular prostheses: a cross-sectional study. Int J Oral Maxillofac Implants. 1995; 10: 437–444.

4. Beck JD, Elter JR, Heiss G, Couper D, Mauriello SM, Offenbacher S Relationship of periodontal disease to carotid artery intima-media wall thickness: the atherosclerosis risk in communities (ARIC) study. Arterioscler Thromb Vasc Biol. 2001; 21: 1816–1822.

5. Desvarieux M, Demmer RT, Rundek T, et al. Relationship between periodontal disease, tooth loss, and carotid artery plaque: the Oral Infections and Vascular Disease Epidemiology Study (INVEST). Stroke. 2003; 34: 2120–2125.

6. Scannapieco FA, Bush RM, Paju S Periodontal disease as a risk factor for adverse pregnancy outcomes; a systemic review. Ann Periodontol. 2003; 8: 70–78.

7. Han YW, Redline RW, Li M, et al. Fusobacterium nucleatum induces premature and term stillbirth in pregnant mice; implication of oral bacteria in preterm birth. Infect Immun. 2004; 72: 2272–2279.

8. Naujokat H, Kunzendorf B, Wiltfang J Dental implants and diabetes mellitus- a systematic review. Inter J of Implant Dent. 2016; 2: 5.

9. Scannapieco FA, Papandonatos GD, Dunford RG Association between oral conditions and respiratory disease in a national sample survey population. Ann Periodontol. 1998; 3: 251–256.

10. Azarpazhooh A, Leake JL Systematic review of the association between respiratory diseases and oral health. J Periodontol. 2006; 77: 1465–1482.

11. Garcia RI, Nunn ME, Vokonas PS Epidemiologic associations between periodontal disease and chronic obstructive pulmonary disease. Ann Periodontol. 2001; 6: 71–77.

12. Terpenning MS The relationship between infections and chronic respiratory diseases: an overview. Ann Periodontol. 2001; 6: 66–70.

13. Rose LR, Mealey BL, Genco RJ, et al. Periodontics: Medicine, Surgery, and Implants. St. Louis, MO: CV Mosby, 2004: 848.

14. Noack B, Genco RJ, Trevisan M, et al. Periodontal infections contribute to elevated systemic C-reactive protein level. J Periodontol. 2001; 72: 1221–1227.

15. Ridker PM, Rifai N, Rose L, et al. Comparison of C-reactive protein and low-density lipoprotein, cholesterol levels in the prediction of first cardiovascular events. N Engl J Med. 2002; 347(20): 1557–1565.

16. Persson GR, Mancl LA, Martin J, et al. Assessing periodontal disease risk: a comparison of clinicians' assessment versus a computerized tool. J Am Dent Assoc. 2003; 134: 575–582.

17. Rohlfing CL, Wiedmeyer HM, Little RR, et al. Defining the relationship between plasma glucose and HbA(1c): analysis of glucose profiles and HbA(1c) in the Diabetes Control and Complications Trial. Diabetes Care. 2002; 25: 275–278.

18. Diabetes Fact sheet N 312. World Health Organization. August 2011.

19. Schwarz F, Derks J, Monje A, Wang H Peri-implantitis 2017 world workshop. J Periodontol. 2018; 89(Suppl 1): S267–S290.

20. Nishimua F, Takahshi K, Kunhara M, et al. Periodontal disease as a complication of diabetes mellitus. Ann Periodontal. 1998; 3: 20–29.

21. Ryan ME, Carnu A, Kramer A The influence of diabetes on the periodontal tissues. J Am Dent Assoc. 2003; 134: 345–405.

22. Mealey BL, Oates TW For the American Academy of Periodontology: diabetes mellitus and periodontal diseases. J Periodontol. 2006; 77: 1289–1303.

23. Nelson RG, Shlossman M, Budding LM, et al. Periodontal disease and NIDDM in Pima Indians. Diabetes Care. 1990; 13: 836–840.

24. Diabetes and periodontal diseases [position paper] Committee on Research, Science and Therapy. American Academy of Periodontology. J Periodontol. 2000; 71: 664–678.

25. Liu R, Bal HS, Desta T, et al. Diabetes enhances periodontal bone loss through enhanced resorption and diminished bone formation. J Dent Res. 2006; 85: 510–514.

26. Taylor GW Bidirectional interrelationships between diabetes and periodontal diseases: an epidemiologic perspective. Ann Periodontol. 2001; 6: 99–112.

27. Mercado FB, Marshall RI, Bartold PM Interrelationships between rheumatoid arthritis and periodontal disease: a review. J Clin Periodontol. 2003; 30: 761–772.

28. Persson RE, Hollender LG, Powell LV, et al. Assessment of periodontal conditions and systemic disease in older subjects. I. Focus on osteoporosis. J Clin Periodontol. 2002; 29: 796–802.

29. Kondo K, Niino M, Shido K A case-control study of Alzheimer's disease in Japan: significance of lifestyles. Dementia. 1994; 5: 314–326.

30. Gatz M, Mortimer JA, Fratiglioni L, et al. Potentially modifiable risk factors for dementia in identical twins. Alzheimers Dementia. 2006; 2: 110–117.

31. Stein PS, Scheff S, Dawson DR III Alzheimer's disease and periodontal disease: mechanisms underlying a potential bi-directional relationship. Grand Rounds Oral-Sys Med. 2006; 1: 14–24.

32. Azuma M Fundamental mechanisms of host immune responses to infection. J Periodontal Res. 2006; 41: 361–373.

33. Ginde AA, Liu MC, Camargo CA Demographic differences and trends of vitamin D insufficiency in the US population, 1988-2004. Arch Intern Med. 2009; 169(6): 626–632.

34. Choukroun J, Khoury G, Khoury F, et al. Two neglected biologic risk factors in bone grafting and implantology: high low-density lipoprotein cholesterol and low serum vitamin D. J Oral Implantol. 2014; 40(1): 110–114.

35. Burt LA, Billington EO, Rose MS, Raymond DA, Hanley DA, Boyd SK Effect of high-dose vitamin D supplementation on volumetric bone density and bone strength:a randomized clinical trial. *JAMA*. 2019; 322(8): 736–745. https://doi.org/10.1001/jama.2019.11889.

36. Lamster IB, Lalla E Periodontal medicine: changing the face of dental care. Dimens Dent Hyg. 2004; 2(4): 10–14.

37. Osteoporosis medications and your dental health. Pamphlet W418, American Dental Association/National Osteoporosis Foundation, 2008.

38. AAOMS Updates Medication-Related Osteonecrosis of the Jaw 2014 Update of 2009 Position Paper by Special Committee.

39. National Osteoporosis Foundation. America's bone health: The state of osteoporosis and low bone mass in our nation. Washington (DC): National Osteoporosis Foundation; 2002./Bone Health and Osteoporosis: A Report of the Surgeon General. https://www.ncbi.nlm.nih.gov/books/NBK45515

40. Nase JB, Suzuki JB Osteonecrosis of the jaw and oral bisphosphonate treatment. J Am Dent Assoc. 2006; 137(8): 1115–1119.

41. Medical News Today AAOMS Updates BRONJ Position Paper January 23, 2009.

42. Misch CE. Contemporary Implant Dentistry, Vol. 456, 2nd ed. St Louis, MO: Mosby, 1999.

43. Cartsos VM, Zhu S, Zavras AI Bisphosphonate use and risk of adverse jaw outcomes. J Am Dent Assoc. 2008; 139(1): 23–30.

44. McDonald E, Marino C Dry mouth: diagnosing and treating its multiple causes. Geriatrics. 1991; 46: 61–63.

45. Almeida D, Vianna K, Arriaga P, Moraschini V Dental implants in Sjogren's syndrome patients: a systematic review. PLoS One. 2017; 12(12): e0189507.

46. Berglundh T, Lindhe J, Lang NP, et al. Mucositis and peri-implantitis. In: *Clinical Periodontology and Implant Dentistry*. 4th ed. Copenhagen: Blackwell Publishing/Munksgaard, 2003.

47. Lee CT, Huang YW, Zhu L, Weltman R Prevalences of peri-implantitis and peri-implant mucositis: systematic review and meta-analysis. J Dent. 2017; 62: 1–12.

3 What Lies Beneath the Surface? Natural Teeth, Bone, and Implant Surgery

As dental hygienists we sculpt root anatomy while being blindfolded. The goal is not to alter the root surface, but to uncover the pre-existing root anatomy which lies beneath.

—Catherine Fairfield, RDH

As hygienists, uncovering the underlying anatomy is critical to understanding how to access, monitor, and maintain implants. Being able to visualize the physical characteristics of natural roots and implants, as well as the differences between different types of bone and tissue surrounding implants, will allow hygienists to effectively maintain implants. As well as, a fundamental knowledge of the biomechanics and component parts of an implant and the many varied restorative options.

Natural teeth versus implants

The physical differences between natural teeth and implants are often compared to the roots of teeth. Replacing the root of a tooth helps to maintain the bone in the maxillary and inferior dental arch. There are differences that start with the surface of a natural tooth (i.e., cementum) and the implant surface of titanium alloy or ceramic (zirconia), rough, porous, or smooth. No cementum or periodontal ligament (PDL) are the main differences. Both natural teeth and implants have a sulcus, junctional epithelium, supracrestal fibers, and bone. The supracrestal fibers are different. In natural teeth, they are in a pattern of attachment and implants with an adherence. The natural teeth are held in, primarily, with the tissue attachment and the PDL and implants mainly by bone. Figure 3.1 shows how the implant attaches to bone.

Peri-Implant Therapy for the Dental Hygienist, Second Edition. Susan S. Wingrove.
© 2022 John Wiley & Sons, Inc. Published 2022 by John Wiley & Sons, Inc.
Companion website: www.wiley.com/go/wingrove/implant

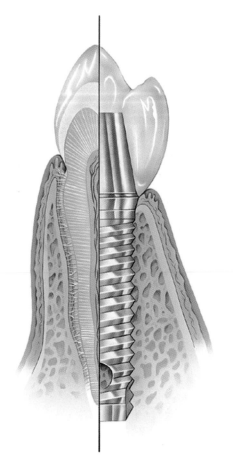

Figure 3.1 How an implant attaches to bone. Courtesy of Keystone Dental.

One of the key physical differences between a natural tooth/root and an implant is that implants are not susceptible to decay. This is one reason implants are a very good restorative choice for patients with controlled diabetes, xerostomia, or autoimmune disease patients. Xerostomia patients who suffer from decreased saliva go from an increase in decay to broken teeth and eventually dentures without much success. If an implant is placed when the first tooth is lost, this cycle can be broken and the quality of life for these patients greatly improved. Autoimmune diseases (i.e., AIDS, asthma, arthritis, or lupus) where the patient's immune system is not functioning properly can be helped by

implant therapy which does not rely on the host response to stay healthy.

The mobility of a natural tooth can cause a loss of attachment, periodontal disease, or trauma that can be reversed. The natural tooth can also test positive or negative for mobility due to periodontal disease or occlusion. Implant mobility is caused by occlusion, trauma, or infection, but with a much more negative result, often the loss of osseointegration which means the loss of the implant. Since an implant is held in by the bone with no periodontal ligament (PDL), such as a cement post in the ground, if it becomes mobile there is a good chance the implant will fail. The good news is that in most cases it can be replaced with a new implant.

The attachment of the tissue that surrounds the natural tooth and implants is where the bigger differences lie. The attachment of the gingival tissues to the neck of the implant is distinct from the attachment to natural teeth. Both the natural tooth and the implant have junctional epithelium (hemidesmosomes and basal lamina) and sulcular epithelium but implants have no evidence of Sharpey's fibers between an implant or implant abutment and bone.

The junctional epithelium of a natural tooth attaches to the tooth coronal to the bone up to 2 mm and has a sulcular epithelium of 2–7 mm with a definite connective tissue attachment. The implant has only an adhesion attachment of connective tissue with a junctional epithelium up to 1.5 mm. It runs parallel and circular to the fixture with a sulcular epithelium of 0.5–1.0 mm, but these do not insert into the implant surface. Making this attachment much more fragile and susceptible to damage by trauma and/or infection. This tissue–implant interface is known as the *perimucosal seal*. The perimucosal seal is the tissue barrier that prevents microorganisms and other inflammatory agents from the oral cavity from entering the tissues that surround the implant. It contains the

Table 3.1 Comparison between natural dentition/tissue and dental implants.

Structure	Natural Dentition	Implant
Attachment	Cementum, periodontal ligament, and bone	Bone (osseointegration)
Tissue: junctional epithelium, sulcular epithelium and connective tissue (CT)	**Junctional epithelium:** Attaches to the tooth coronal to the bone up to 2 mm **Sulcular epithelium:** 0.2–0.7 mm **CT:** Has attachment	**Junctional epithelium:** Run parallel and circular to the fixture up to 1.5 mm, do not attach **Sulcular epithelium:** 0.5–1.0 mm **CT:** Adhesion, no attachment
Vascularity and bleeding on probing (BOP)	**Vascularity:** Greater **BOP:** Reliable Supraperiosteal and periodontal ligament	**Vascularity:** Less **BOP:** Less reliable Periosteal only
Decay	Decay is possible	Do not decay
Infection	Yes, gingivitis and periodontitis	Yes, mucositis and peri-implantitis
Mobility	Yes, caused by loss of attachment, periodontal disease, or trauma. Reversible	Yes, caused by peri-implant disease, occlusion, or trauma. Not reversible

sulcular epithelium, and its presence is important for the longevity and success of the implants (see Table 3.1).

Bone: it is all about the bone!

In implant dentistry, the most important factor is bone: quality, quantity, and density influence successful outcomes. The volume density of bone matrix in cortical (outer layer) bone is approximately 80–90 and 20–25% in cancellous (inner layer) bone (1, 2). Bone is composed of cortical and cancellous bone, and intertwined between these two parts is a lattice network of trabecular that is the reservoir for active bone metabolism (see Figure 3.2). The bone structure is continuously repairing and remodeling to keep its form and function.

Dental hygienists need to have a clear understanding of bone quality and density. Be able to explain this to patient in terms of how much time will it take for the patient to complete his or her implant treatment.

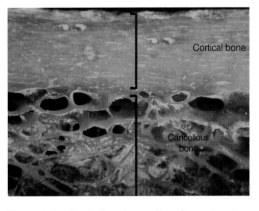

Figure 3.2 Cortical and cancellous bone. Courtesy of Keystone Dental.

To help the patient understand the expense associated with possible added procedures to have the necessary bone for successful treatment results. Research clearly states that *the strength of the bone is directly related to the density of the bone* (3, 4). Also, *the quality and density is directly related to the type of implant* the dental professional will choose to place, the healing time needed for the

Table 3.2 Bone classification (5).

Bone Type	Example
Type One Very compact, dense cortical bone 3–4 months of healing time Compares to oak/hard maple	Type 1 Bone **Anterior mandible**
Type Two Porous, compact cortical bone 4–6 months of healing Compares to spruce/white pine	Type 2 Bone **Posterior mandible**
Type Three Coarse, trabecularless cortical bone Usually a 6-month healing time Compares to balsa wood	Type 3 Bone **Anterior maxilla**
Type Four Fine, trabecularminimal cortical bone 6–8 months of healing time Compares to Styrofoam	Type 4 Bone **Posterior maxilla**

Figures courtesy of Keystone Dental.

patient, and success rate for the implant. Actual healing times may vary based on the patient's ability to remodel bone and his or her overall health.

For learning purposes and for a visual image to present bone types of the oral cavity to a patients, (see Table 3.2). Bone classifications are identified in four distinct bone types: *woven, lamellar, bundle, and composite*. Woven bone is rapidly replaced by mature, stress-bearing bone. Lamellar bone is the main component of mature cortical and trabecular bone. Bundle bone generally is found adjacent to the PDL with characteristics of ligaments and tendon attachments. Composite bone is a variation of fine cancellous compaction (osteons) or coarse cancellous compaction (whorling bone) (6). The literature points out that there are different surgical protocols for different bone types that affect healing and treatment planning (4–10). There are exceptions to the rule in location and type of bone for patients, but for an initial conversation with the patient, this classification is ideal.

Four classifications of bone

The hygienist needs a fundamental understanding of each type of bone and to be able to relate to the patient a tactile sense of the density of the bone in relation to where the implant will be placed (5). Each bone type can be compared to a type of wood to help the patient understand, visualize, and be able to relate to the surgeon's recommendation for healing time.

The bone is classified according to structure, composition, density, and volume with four types of bone referred to as types 1–4 or D1–D4 (the reference is the same; only the terminology is different). To further define this, the types are as follows:

1. **Type One Bone** is found in the anterior mandible, composed of dense cortical bone that has minimal trabecular spaces, making it the densest type of bone. The healing time is approximately 3–4 months. This varies based on multiple factors and is generally monitored by the surgeon. This bone density is compared to oak or hard maple wood.
2. **Type Two Bone**, generally found in the posterior mandible, is described as porous cortical or course trabecular. The cortical bone density is found in the superior and inferior borders and the trabecular in the center of the posterior mandible. The healing time is approximately 4–6 months based on amount of cortical bone present and monitored by surgeon. This bone density is compared to spruce wood or white pine.
3. **Type Three Bone**, found primarily in the anterior maxilla, is less dense crestal cortical bone than type one or type two while the remaining bone is quite trabecular. This translates into a more fragile type of bone, sometimes requiring more healing time and in which progressive loading of implants may be treatment planned. Progressive loading is the gradual increase in the application of load or forces on the final restoration and ultimately the implant monitored by the surgeon. The bone density is compared to balsa wood and healing time is approximately 6 months.
4. **Type Four Bone** is found in the posterior maxilla, consisting of minimal crestal cortical bone thickness with the remainder being very trabecular. This means this is the poorest quality of bone, with the highest implant failure rate, and for which progressive loading is strongly considered. Healing time is approximately 6–8 months and the bone density is compared to Styrofoam.

> **Hygienist Tip:**
>
> What the location, density, and quality of bone means to patients: "When and how fast can I get my implant/restoration?" Hygienists learn how to answer the most frequently asked questions and have the discussion with patients on WHY it is worth the wait for implants, it's all about the bone!

Frequently asked questions

Why is bone density or type so important?
The type of bone is critical in implant therapy. It is directly related to implant placement, implant selection, and the length of healing time for osseointegration.

A hygienist must know this for treatment planning and to be able to explain to the patient the different *types or densities* of bone in relation to healing time and restoration selection options.

What is the tooth relationship to type of bone?
Basel bone forms with or without teeth or implants. Alveolar bone forms because of teeth and residual bone is alveolar bone that has been resorbed.

What happens if teeth are lost and not replaced?

If teeth are lost and not replaced, atrophy and bone loss becomes apparent to facial aesthetics. This is commonly recognized as premature aging, increased wrinkles, jowl development, and loss of function.

Bone loss overview

Emphasize these points with patients when having the conversation on why bone is important. The width of bone decreases 25% in the first year after a tooth is lost or extracted and the bone height decreases 4 mm in the first year (11, 12). In the first 2–3 years after an extraction, 40–60% of the ridge width can be lost (13) and the overall bone can continue to be resorbed 0.5–1% yearly for the patient's life (14).

When there are missing teeth involved, bone and tissue degrade over time, losing their function. If a tooth is extracted and left to heal on its own, it will repair, but with tissue regenerating faster than bone causing a sunk-in effect, (see Figure 3.3).

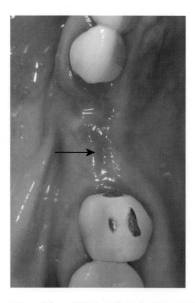

Figure 3.3 Ridge width lost (bone) with traditional extraction, no socket preservation. Courtesy of Dr. Kevin Frawley.

Resorption and remodeling of the alveolar bone occurs after teeth are lost due to periodontal disease, trauma, or tooth extraction (15, 16). If regenerative procedures such as socket preservation are done at the time of extraction, the bone will regenerate and keep its structure.

What happens if bone loss continues? As the jawbone continues to resorb or melt away, the patient returns for relines on his or her dentures to keep them in place and to accommodate for the remodeling of the jawbone. If this bone loss detoriates to severe levels, the patient may not even be able to wear dentures because the destruction of the jaw bone puts pressure on the nerve bundle with the denture, causing the patient pain, (see Figure 3.4).

To prevent bone loss and maintain the bone in the jaw for both natural teeth and implants, the bone needs to be stimulated. The teeth transmit force to the surrounding bone every time they come together in occlusion. Implants can maintain this by stimulation to the bone when occluded on. Also, by being placed into the bone like the roots of a natural tooth they can even increase bone density and preserves facial structure.

Hygienist Tip:

Learn how to explain this concept to patients with an understanding of Wolff's Law, developed by Julius Wolff in the 19th century (see Box 3.1). He states that *"bone in a healthy person or animal will adapt to the loads it is placed under"* (17).

After implant placement, the implant is loaded by placing a restoration or prosthesis. The bone will then remodel itself and become stronger (see Box 3.1). The converse is true that if the loading on the bone decreases due to loss of an existing tooth, the bone will weaken due to lack of stimulus for the remodeling that is required to maintain bone mass (18), (see Figure 3.5). *Bone needs to be stimulated!*

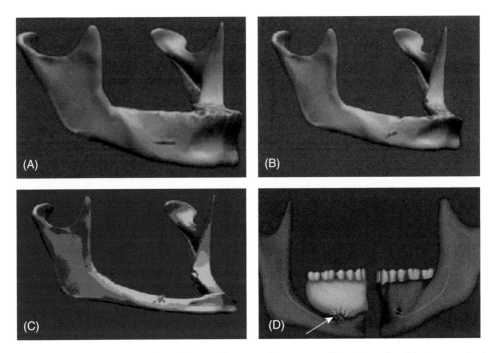

Figure 3.4 *What happens when bone loss continues?* Patient eventually will not be able to wear denture. Courtesy of Keystone Dental.

Box 3.1   Wolff's Law

Keys Points of Wolff's Law
■ Bone must be stimulated to be maintained.
■ Teeth transmit force to surrounding bone when in occlusion.
■ Lack of stimulation or occlusion results in bone loss or resorption.
■ An implant best replicates a natural tooth by replacing the root and crown.
■ Implants maintain and increase bone density, preserving facial structure.

Bone regeneration

Techniques and products are also available today to regenerate lost bone and tissue. To understand the principles of regenerative tissue engineered products and how they can promote healing, hygienists need to refer back to their sciences (i.e., histology), to their knowledge of how the cells work.

It starts with an understanding of the principles behind regeneration and

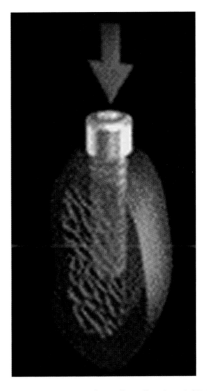

Figure 3.5 Bone needs to be stimulated (Wolff's Law). Courtesy of Keystone Dental.

Table 3.3 The principles behind regeneration.

Type of Healing	Definition	Example
Osteogenesis *(cells)*	Osteogenic materials that contain living cells within the graft that contribute to bone formation and remodeling.	Autografts Autloglous and allogeneic stem cell materials
Osteoinduction *(signals)*	Osteoinductive graft materials contain signaling growth factors and/or biologics that stimulate the chemotaxis, differentiation, and division of cells for that then form new tissues in regeneration.	Allograft materials (contain BMP) Autlologous blood concentrates (PRP, PRF) Enamel matrix derivatives (EMD) Recombinant Human Platelet-rich growth factor (rhPRGF) Recombinant Human Bone Morphogenic Protein (rhBMP) Recombinant Human Fibroblast Growth Factor (rhFGF)
Osteoconduction *(scaffolds)*	Osteogenic materials that serve as an inert scaffold that allows angiogenesis and guides native cell population of the graft material.	Autografts, Allografts Xenografts
	Space maintenance and occlusion of soft tissue cells can be achieved through the use of cell-occlusive membranes to separate graft materials from overlying soft tissues.	Alloplasts

osseointegration of implants into the bone. To grasp the full picture, refer to Table 3.3 to understand how bone remodels. Outlined are the types of healing that you need for regeneration. *Osteogenesis (cells)*, the osteogenic materials that contain living cells within the graft that contribute to bone formation and remodeling. *Osteoinduction (signals),* the grafting materials that contain signaling growth factors and/or biologics that stimulate the chemotaxis, differentiation, and division of cells form new regenerative tissues. *Osteoconduction (scaffolds),* are osteogenic materials that serve as an inert scaffold that allows angiogenesis and guides native cell population of the graft material. Space maintenance and occlusion of soft tissue cells can be achieved through the use of cell-occlusive membranes to separate graft materials from overlying soft tissues.

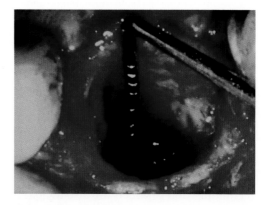

Figure 3.6 Blood clot is essential to healing. Courtesy of Dr. Kevin Frawley.

There are a number of steps to bone regeneration starting with the blood clot, essential to the healing process, (see Figure 3.6). Granulation tissue is formed, blood vessels migrating through the defect, and the precursor cells migrate to the site from the marrow spaces of the adjacent bone. The regenerative procedure and/or product can be added to help the body perform this task more effectively for optimal results.

The normal wound healing sequence is hemostasis and inflammation, followed by proliferation of the cells, and finally maturation and remodeling. So, you have bleeding in the inflammatory stage, then connective tissue regenerates (proliferation), and finally bone remodels. *If regenerative procedures and products are not used, the body generally heals with secondary intent in the form of scar tissue or scarring.*

The bone quality and quantity needs to be adequate or placement of an implant is not possible. Bone augmentation procedures are used with bioabsorbable (do not need to be removed) or nonresorbable (have to be removed) barrier membranes and bone grafting products or bone substitutes to enhance regeneration (19, 20). The regenerative products include mineralized/demineralized cadaver bone particulates, membranes, and growth factors; examples of these are listed, (see Figure 3.7 and Table 3.3).

Bone grafts are used to correct a defect and are categorized in four types: autografts, allografts, xenografts, and alloplasts. They can be used alone or in combination based on the osteogenic, osteoinductive, or osteoconductive principles (21); (see Table 3.3). Autografts are derived from patient's own bone from a donor site to the area to be grafted. Allografts are bone harvested from same species (i.e., human cadaver bone). The main concern of allografts is the risk of disease transmission, but this is all but eliminated with the current processes used to sterilize the cadaver bone (22, 23).

The use of xenografts goes back, as far as, 1889 and refers to bone grafts derived from another species (i.e., from an animal:

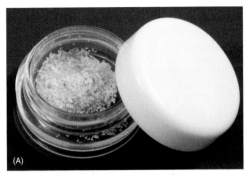

(A)

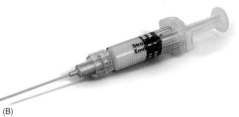

(B)

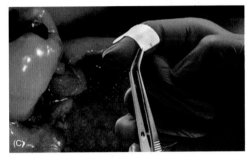

(C)

Figure 3.7 Examples of regenerative products. (A) Osteogenesis cells, OSSIF-i™ Particulate Allograft Bone Particulate Surgical Esthetics. (B) Osteoinductive growth factor, Straumann® Emdogain® Enamel Matrix Derivative. (C) Osteoconduction scaffold, GUIDOR Alloplast Bioresorbable Matrix Barrier.

bovine [cow], and equine [horse]). They are biocompatible, osteoconductive, and resorb over time *replaced with the patient's own natural bone* (24–26). Alloplasts are synthetic bone derivatives, are osteoconductive, but are not osteogenic or osteoinductive.

The use of bone particulates (autograft) is the gold standard for treatment of implant-related bone defects (21, 27). Allografts with the use of bone particulates derived from the same species (human donor bone) are used in forms of putty, gel, and collagen sponges. They also have a high success rate, eliminating the need for the morbidity associated with the donor site and many times eliminate the need for a second surgery (27). For more information on bone grafting options (see Chapter 4).

The growth factors and/ or biologics on the market are Allograft materials that contain blood morphogenic protein (BMP). Autologous blood concentrates; platelet-rich plasma (PRP) that is derived from the patient's whole human blood and processed through gradient density centrifugation. Platelet-rich fibrin (PRF) is also derived from the patient's whole human blood, centrifuged and then isolated proteins from the blood plasma are used to spray onto the implant body to accelerate osseointegration.

Also available are; Enamel matrix derivatives (EMD), a unique mixture of natural proteins. Once applied, these proteins form a matrix that can induce biological processes and may stimulate certain cells involved in the healing action of soft and hard tissues (28), (i.e., Emdogain® by Straumann). As well as, embryonic stem cells that are derived from early stage embryos and amniotic stem cells from donated placenta-derived products. These stem cell biologics are able to differentiate into various tissue types such as skin and bone with very promising study results (21, 27). Recombinant Human Platelet-rich growth factor (rhPRGF), Recombinant Human Bone Morphogenic Protein (rhBMP), and Recombinant Human Fibroblast Growth Factor (rhFGF) are also examples of osteoinductive growth factors (see Table 3.3).

Regenerative procedures

Regenerative procedures are often referred to as *guided bone regeneration* (GBR) or *guided tissue regeneration* (GTR). These procedures use the regenerative products especially the membranes that are designed to keep the unwanted cells out by creating a barrier, protecting the blood clot to allow for regeneration. The most common GBR procedures include socket preservation, implant defects (dehiscence or fenestration), and sinus and ridge bone augmentation.

Socket preservation procedure involves placing graft particulates and/or a scaffold in a tooth socket done at the time of extraction to preserve the alveolar ridge. If socket preservation is not done, the bone resorbs and is lost, as well as the alveolar ridge does not retain its original shape. Socket preservation is often done to prepare for an implant to be placed, however, it should be done after every extraction to preserve the bone and maintains the facial bone structure for the patient (see Figure 3.8).

If an implant treatment is planned to be placed, it is ideal to do a bone augmentation procedure at the time of extraction. A bone augmentation can be done at a later date, but at a much higher cost to the patient as well as with an additional surgical procedure. The key point to understand is that socket preservation differs for ridge augmentation; socket preservation is done before the bone structure is lost at the time of extraction and ridge augmentation is a procedure to bring back the lost bone and rebuild the ridge height and width. Socket preservation following tooth extraction is now becoming a standard of care. As a hygienist, record on the patient's record if the patient declines socket preservation, be sure to record it as an option presented to the patient at time of treatment planning an extraction, including any wisdom teeth extractions.

Implant defects (dehiscence or fenestration) are defined as the *gap* between the socket wall of less than 2mm and the implant. A dehiscence is a defect that extends to the bone crest. A fenestration is a defect that does not extend to the bone crest, leaving an isolated buccal or lingual area of an implant exposed to the oral

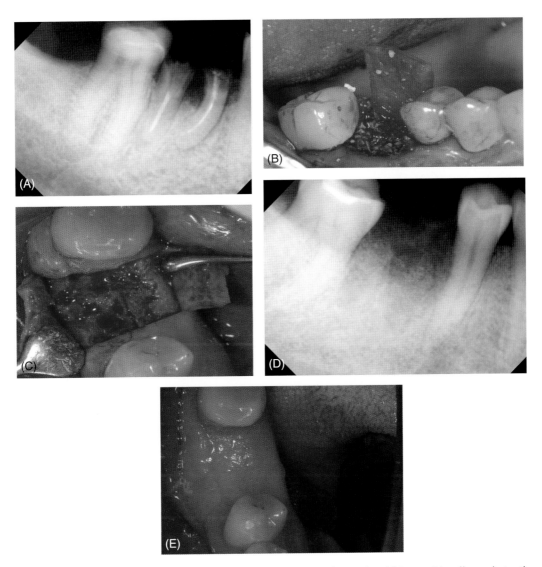

Figure 3.8 Example Socket preservation case. Courtesy of Dr. Kevin Frawley. (A) Pre-op PA radiograph, tooth extracted. (B) Allograft bone graft membrane and growth factor placed, then sutured closed. (C) 3-month evaluation, new bone and ridge width preserved. (D) 3-month post-op radiograph, not bone. (E) 5 weeks post-op: healing tissue.

cavity. A GBR/GTR procedure may be necessary to secure the implant for successful results.

Ridge and sinus augmentation are procedures to regenerate the lost bone or correct a bony defect for both function and aesthetics. For a ridge augmentation procedure to be successful both the width and height of the bone need to be regenerated due to bone resorption (see example in Figure 3.9). *Sinus grafts/lifts* are bone augmentation of the antral floor with autogenous bone and bone graft materials to allow the clinician the quality and quantity of bone necessary to place the implant and are considered very predictable and successful (29). A less invasive technique for a sinus graft is referred to as the osteotome technique used by many clinicians in which the sinus floor is elevated with

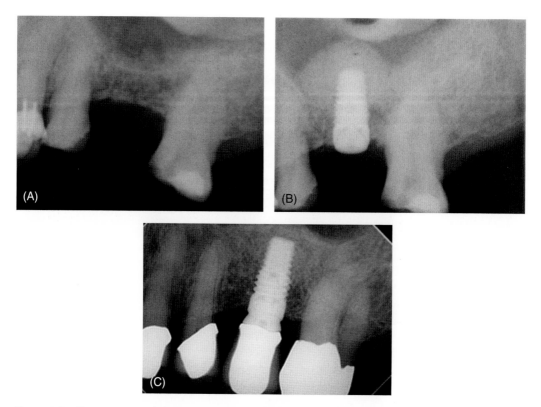

Figure 3.9 Sinus augmentation. Courtesy of Dr. Kevin Frawley. (A) Pre-op PA radiograph. (B) Implant placed with osteotome sinus lift and allograft. (C) Restored after osseointegration.

specific designed osteotomes, eliminating the need for the trap door access (30, 31). To achieve successful results with these procedures, regenerative products are used along with specific surgical techniques; for more on all these adjunctive procedures (see Chapter 4 adjunctive procedures).

Procedures to prevent bone resorption

Some clinicians will use progressive loading or platform switching to prevent bone resorption in implant therapy. *Progressive loading* is a procedure of a gradual increase in the application of load on a prosthesis and thus to a dental implant. Platform switching refers to using a small diameter abutment on a larger diameter implant.

The progressive loading technique is used to gradually add load or force to the implant to give the body time to acclimate to the increased force. Provisionals (temporary restorations) are used in a series with the progressive loading technique to gradually allow the occlusal forces to come in contact with the implant.

The objective of *platform switching* is to move the microgap away from the bone, therefore encouraging the bone level to remain the same, creating no shrinkage. In theory, the location of the microgap between the implant and the abutment will also have an influence on the resulting height of the bone level, similar to the correct biological width around natural teeth (32–35). By moving the abutment attachment from the implant shoulder, the implication is that it will also shield against possible irritants. The resulting bone stays. It limits the biologic width reformation with the ledge of the implant platform sealing the underlying bone. This isolates it and increases support for the soft tissues.

Post-regenerative procedures home care

Hygienists need to prepare their patients for home care following regenerative procedures, (see Chapter 8 and Box 8.1 Post-Regenerative Procedures Home Care Protocol). It is imperative that the patient keep the graft site area and the oral cavity clean. The dentist or surgeon may prescribe a prescription antibiotic and/or a prescription mouth rinse. The surgeon may also recommend to not brush or floss the area for a specific time, using only the prescribed mouth rinse. Encourage your patients to follow the surgeon's recommendations and call your office with any questions.

Implant surgery

It is important for you as a hygienist to have a clinical knowledge of the implant surgeries to support your patients. Observe an implant surgery or ask your local implant company representative to visit your office for a team meeting to walk the entire team through the process. This will help you gain an understanding of implant surgery and be able to talk to your patients about what to expect with implant placement.

Dental implant surgery can be performed in a hospital or at dental specialist's or general dentist's office. A clean and sterile environment is necessary to assure a higher success rate. Once the sterile field has been established, protocols need to be in place for presurgical patient, pre-op patient (at time of surgery), and post-op patient (see Table 3.4).

The implant surgeon prepares the implant site by removing just enough bone (osteotomy) and using specially designed drills that gradually widen the diameter to the size of the designated implant. Copious amounts of water are used in creating the osteotomy

Table 3.4 Example of patient protocols for implant surgery.

Pre-surgical patient protocol	• Consult with implant surgeon • Sign surgical consent forms • Receive prescriptions for antibiotics, inflammation, sedation, and/or medication for discomfort following surgical procedure as prescribed by surgeon • Receive presurgical instructions (i.e., no food or drink after 12:00 A.M. day prior to surgery)
Pre-op patient protocol	• Patient should arrive at surgery location with caregiver to drive patient home and receive post-op instructions • Review with patient any presurgical medications they have taken and options for prescriptions postsurgery that are available • Blood is drawn if using patients own blood for a PRP growth factor • IV is started if prescribed • Topical and initial anaesthetic given • Intra and external oral scrub completed • Patient reclined, eyewear or towel over patient's eyes and sterile drapes applied
Post-op patient protocol	• Patient slowly brought to seated position • Record patient's vitals • Remove sterile drapes; cleanse patient's face, place gauze and ice • Post-op instructions given to patient and caregiver, ***verbal and written*** • Post-op evaluation appointment confirmed and if possible, time to phone patient later that day • Release patient to caregiver/driver

to prevent overheating. If the bone cells die from overheating of the site, the bone may never integrate with the implant (36).

The implant is then placed into the bone by threading or tapping it into the osteotomy site. Over a period of several months, the implant will osseointegrate with a direct and lasting biological attachment of the implant to vital bone with no intervening connective tissue. The implant may remain covered for a healing period of 4–9 months depending on the surgeon's recommendations. The prosthetic options are a crown, a bridge, or a fixed or removable prosthesis (36).

Endosteal dental implant surgery

Endosteal implants can be placed as a one- or two-stage procedure (see Figure 3.10). The *two-stage implant procedure*, starting

with the first surgery (stage one): a hole is drilled into the bone according to the size of the implant, which prepares the site for placement of the dental implant and/or graft. The implant is placed by threading or tapping into the bone, a healing screw is placed in the implant until the healing is complete and an abutment is inserted in at stage two. Once the healing screw is in place, the gum tissue is sutured over the implant and the implant remains under gum tissue for 2–6 months until the implant is properly fused with the bone (osseointegrated), not exposed to the oral cavity. Since the implant is not exposed to the oral cavity until stage two, instruct the patient to follow postsurgical instructions from the surgeon until the surgeon has completed their post-op evaluation. After that is complete, instruct the patient to use an antimicrobial rinse twice daily and remove the biofilm twice daily from the adjacent teeth

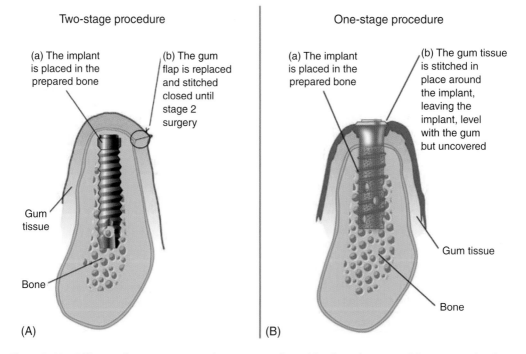

Figure 3.10 Difference between a two- and one-stage endosteal implant placement. (A). Two-stage implants: implant heals under the tissue not exposed to the oral cavity and margin of the crown will be located on the abutment. (B) One-stage implant: exposed to the oral cavity and the margin of the crown will be located on the implant.

until the implant has osseointegrated in stage two.

Stage two, after osseointegration is verified, a small incision is made to expose the implant, called an *uncover procedure*, and the healing screw is removed. An abutment is placed, a radiograph is taken to verify that the abutment is seated correctly and the dentist takes an impression and sends it to the laboratory. A temporary restoration or prosthesis may be fabricated to be attached to the implant(s) while the restoration is being fabricated at the laboratory.

When the restoration is complete from the laboratory, the patient returns to have the final restoration placed. The restoration is cemented or screwed into place and another radiograph is taken to be sure the restoration is seated correctly; occlusion is verified and the treatment is complete.

The **one-stage** *endosteal implant procedure*, is basically the same as the two-step procedure, (see Figures 3.10B and 3.11), with a few differences. The implant is placed at the tissue level, the margin of the crown is located on the implant, and the implant is exposed to the oral cavity from day one. Important to start biofilm-focused care when the surgeon has completed their post-op evaluation. Brush around the healing abutment, use a rubber tip stimulator, and rinse twice daily with antimicrobial rinse, (see Chapter 8 for more details on postsurgical and pre-restorative home care protocols).

After the healing period, there is no need for an uncover procedure with a one-stage procedure. For the tissue level implant, the dentist will remove the healing abutment and place a final abutment, take an impression to send to the laboratory to complete

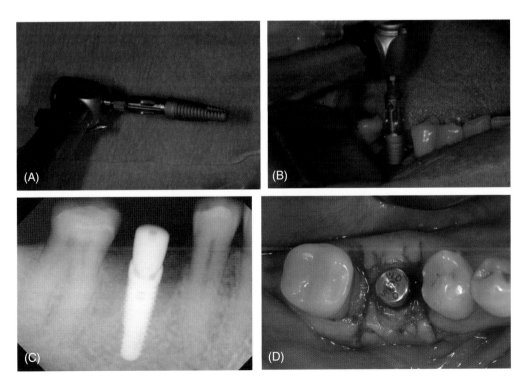

Figure 3.11 Example of a one-stage implant placement. Courtesy of Dr. Kevin Frawley. (A) Implant is taken out of sterilized case, placed on implant placement drill. (B) Implant is attached; implant torqued into place. (C) Post-op PA radiograph. (D) Healing abutment in place and final restoration will be placed at 6 months.

the final restoration. The dentist may or may not fabricate a temporary restoration and place on the abutment. If a Chairside Economical Restoration of Esthetic Ceramics (CEREC) final restoration is made, it can be seated that day. At the restoration seating appointment, the dentist removes the temporary restoration if placed and seats the final restoration. A radiograph is taken to verify the restoration seated correctly, occlusion is verified, and the treatment is complete.

For a *one-piece implant placement,* the implant and abutment are all one piece (see Chapter 1, Figure 1.8 of ceramic one piece implant as an example), the dentist follows the same steps for restoration as the one-stage procedure previously outlined. Since the abutment is in place (all one piece), a temporary restoration is often temporarily cemented on the abutment, *out of occlusion,* to give the patient the appearance of a natural tooth while the implant is osseointegrating. Similar to the tissue level implant, the one-piece implant is exposed to the oral cavity from day one.

It is important for the patient to start biofilm-focused at-home oral hygiene care when the surgeon has completed their post-op evaluation. Brush around the abutment/temporary restoration, use a rubber tip stimulator, and rinse twice daily with antimicrobial rinse. Once healing is complete, the temporary restoration is removed, an impression is taken and sent to the laboratory for fabrication of the final restoration. The temporary restoration is placed back on the abutment. At the restoration seating appointment, the dentist removes the temporary restoration and places the final restoration, take a radiograph to verify the restoration is seated correctly; occlusion is verified and the treatment is complete.

The restorative dentist, prosthodontist, and/or surgeon are ultimately responsible for whether a one- or two-stage procedure is used, the type of implant system, drill protocol, and final restorative solution. As a hygienist, your role is to prepare the patient for any at-home oral hygiene care recommendation following the implant placement. For a patient with a two-stage procedure the patient only needs to use an antimicrobial rinse twice daily and remove the biofilm twice daily from the adjacent teeth. Prepare the patient for the one-stage procedure implants with soft toothbrush or sulcus brush, rubber tip stimulator and antimicrobial rinse to use once the surgeon has completed the healing post-op visits, (see Chapter 8 for specifics on at- home oral hygiene care).

Post-surgery implant home care

Provide your patients with home care instructions to use after implant surgery. The dentist or surgeon may prescribe a prescription antibiotic and/or a prescription mouth rinse. The surgeon may also recommend to not brush or floss the area for a specific time, using only the prescribed mouth rinse. Encourage your patients to follow the surgeon's recommendations and call your office with any questions (see Chapter 8 for more details on postsurgical and pre-restorative at-home oral hygiene protocols).

Specialized implant placement

Subperiosteal dental implant placement

A subperiosteal dental implant procedure is not used routinely, however, it is used by some clinicians for patients who do not have adequate bone to place endosteal implants. Since a subperiosteal dental implant sits on top of bone instead of going into bone, the subperiosteal implant requires less bone to be successful. Subperiosteal dental implants are placed under the periosteum, the tissue that

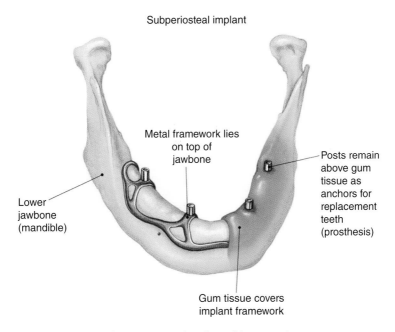

Figure 3.12   Subperiosteal framework.

covers the bone like a tightly fit blanket. The implant is placed on top of the jaw bone, like a saddle, on the day of insertion, not within the alveolar bone. A subperiosteal dental implant covers much of the lower jaw and a modern subperiosteal dental implant has three feet, one on each side and one in the front (see Figure 3.12).

Years ago, all subperiosteal dental implant required two surgical procedures. In stage one, an incision was made along the patient's edentulous ridge to expose the ridge and an impression was made, which was then sent to the laboratory for the implant to be fabricated. A second surgery was needed a month later to re-expose the ridge and seat the subperiosteal dental implant.

Today with computerized tomography (CAT) scan equipment and the computer software, a CAT scan can be taken and a precise model made of the patient jawbone. The laboratory will fabricate the custom-fit subperiosteal implant, making it possible for the patient to only have one surgery, the one to surgically insert the subperiosteal dental implant. If a CAT scan is not used, the two surgeries are performed with the impression being sent to the lab and a second surgery to place the subperiosteal implant. Subperiosteal dental implant surgery has mainly been replaced by the regenerative adjunctive procedures and products available to regenerate the bone and make it possible to place endosteal implants.

Transosteal dental implants placement

Transosteal dental implants are rarely placed today. They are also for patients with very limited bone, requiring two metal rods to be surgically placed below the chin, through the jaw bone, until the desired length is reached so the lower prosthesis can be attached. Only a viable option for the lower jaw, an extensive surgery and a hospitalization with general anesthesia is necessary. Transosteal dental implant surgery has been replaced by the regenerative adjunctive procedures and products available to regenerate the bone and make it possible to place endosteal implants (see example in Figure 3.13).

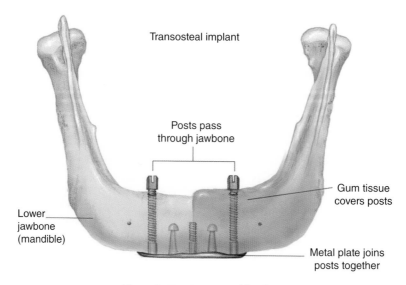

Transosteal implant

Posts pass
through jawbone

Gum tissue
covers posts

Lower
jawbone
(mandible)

Metal plate joins
posts together

Figure 3.13 Transosteal implant.

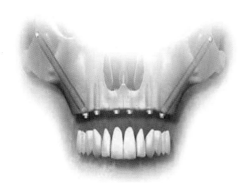

Figure 3.14 Zygomatic dental implants. Courtesy of Nobel Biocare.

Zygomatic dental implants

Zygomatic implants are used to stabilize an implant supported fixed final prosthesis, for patients with severe bone loss of the maxillary arch (see example Figure 3.14). The procedure for placement of zygomatic dental implants is generally performed in two stages and can be less invasive than that to place traditional dental implants. During the first stage, the implant posts are fitted in the cheekbones, through the use of computer scans that help guide the implant along the correct path of insertion, through the sinuses. A few days later, a temporary

acrylic bridge can be attached to the zygoma dental implants. The bite of the bridge is then checked and adjusted accordingly.

Over the next few months, the bone in the cheek then grows around the zygoma dental implants until it effectively fuses with them (osseointegrates). After the surgeon has verified that the healing is complete, the restorative dentist or prosthodontist attaches the final prosthesis.

Implant supported fixed final prosthesis dental implant procedure

A procedure, originally trademarked by Nobel Biocare as All-on-4™, was developed for fully edentulous patients with at least four implants, sometimes more, to support immediate load full-arch prosthesis. The procedure, now known as implant supported fixed final prothesis or hybrid, has several different names by each individual implant company. The patient is edentulous, or the teeth are all removed and the arch prepared. The implants are placed and a provisional prosthesis is fixed in place. The patient heals for approximately

6 months. When all the implants have osseointegrated, a final prosthesis is delivered (see Mastering the Arch in Chapter 9).

The uniqueness of the All-on-4™, the first fixed full arch prosthesis procedure to use angled posterior implants, allows for a minimal number of implants to be placed and no bone grafting procedure is necessary. Patients can expect improved support of a full arch final prosthesis, with minimal bone, and no cantilevers. Studies have confirmed this concept as a viable option with 92–100% survival rate (37–41), (see Figure 3.15).

Implant treatment plans for these procedures can be complex and confusing to the patient. Hygienists have an opportunity to ease these fears and prepare patients on what to expect at the time of implant surgery. Flip charts and visuals are available to show patients and walk your patient through the procedure by providing an overview of implant surgical procedures in general terms. Hygienists, you do not need to know everything about the procedures, just enough to help your patients feel more comfortable or arrange a consultation on implant options with the dentist. Team up as an office, with a surgical practice to provide patients with a postsurgical home care protocol to follow that both the surgeon and the restorative dentist have approved.

Multiple implant companies have developed systems for fixed full arch prosthesis edentulous solutions (i.e., Examples BioHorizons TeethXpress®, Neoss®4+, Nobel Biocare All-on-4™, and Straumann® Pro Arch). Not all surgeons perform these surgical procedures in the same way, although having a basic understanding helps to alleviate patients' concerns. Hygienists, do stress the importance of following the surgeon's pre- and postoperative instructions. Provide your patients with home care products and instructions to use after the surgeon has released the

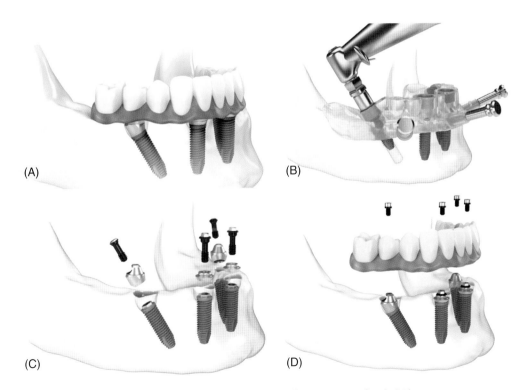

(A)

(B)

(C)

(D)

Figures 3.15 All-on-4™ step-by-step overview. Courtesy of Nobel Biocare.

patient to resume at-home oral care (see Chapter 8 for more information and home-care protocols).

Summary

Understanding natural teeth, implants, and maintaining bone is essential to providing optimal implant maintenance. Talk to patients about WHY bone is so important and WHY implants are the long-term treatment of choice for teeth replacement! It is critical for hygienists to understand all the facets of implant therapy, as well as all that regeneration dentistry, nowadays, has to offer. To be able to have a conversation with your patient on the types or density of bone will provide the patient with an answer for the most frequently asked question; "When can I get my teeth?" Follow that up with why it is worth the wait and stay up to date on the ever-changing field of information of implant and regeneration dentistry.

Understanding what lies beneath will enhance the clinical and verbal skills of hygienists to provide optimal implant maintenance.

References

1. Dental implants in periodontal therapy position paper. J Periodontol. 2000; 71: 1934–1942.
2. Thomsen JS, Ebbesen EN, Mosekilde L Relationships between stat histomorphometry and bone strength measurements in human iliac crest bone biopsies. Bone. 1998; 22: 153–163.
3. Aukhil L, Simpson DM, Suggs C, Pettersson E In vivo differentiation of progenitor cells of the periodontal ligament: an experimental study using physical barriers. J Clin Periodontol. 1986; 13: 862–868.
4. Misch CE, Qu M, Bidez MW Mechanical properties of trabecular bone in the human mandible: implications of dental implant treatment planning and surgical placement. J Oral Maxillofac Surg. 1999; 57: 11700–11706.
5. Misch CE. Contemporary Implant Dentistry, 3rd ed. St Louis, MO: Mosby, 2008: 134–135.
6. Roberts WE, Turley PK, Brezniak N, Fielder PJ Bone physiology and metabolism. J Calif Dent Assoc. 1987; 15(10): 54–61.
7. Esposito M, Hirsh JM, Lekholm U, et al. Biological factors contributing to failures of osseointegrated oral implants, (II) Etiopathogenesis. Eur J Oral Sci. 1998; 106: 721–764.
8. Morris HF, Ochi S, Crum P, et al. AJCRG, Part 1: a 6-year multicentered, multidisciplinary clinical study of a new and innovative implant design. J Oral Implantol. 2004; 30: 125–133.
9. Hermann I, Lekholm U, Holm S, et al. Evaluation of patient and implant characteristics as potential prognostic factors for oral implant failures. Int J Oral Maxillofac Implants. 2005; 20: 220–230.
10. Weng D, Jacobson Z, Tarnow D, et al. A prospective multicenter clinical trial of 3i machined surface implants results after 6 years of follow up. Int J Oral Maxillofac Implants. 2003; 18: 417–423.
11. Carlsson GE, Pearsson G Morphologic changes of the mandible after extraction and wearing of dentures: a longitudinal, clinical, and x-ray cephalometric study covering 5 years. Odontol Revy. 1967; 18: 27–54.
12. Misch CE What you don't know can hurt you (and your patients). Dent Today. 2000; 19: 70–73.
13. Misch CE. Contemporary Implant Dentistry, 2nd ed. St Louis, MO: Mosby, 1999: 455–464.
14. Christensen GJ Ridge preservation: why not? J Am Dent Assoc. 1996; 127: 669–670.
15. Atwood DA Post extraction changes in the adult mandible as illustrated by microradiographs of mid-sagittal sections and serial cephalometric toentgenographs. J Prosthet Dent. 1963; 13: 810.
16. Atwood D Some clinical factors related to rate of resorption of residual ridges. J Prosthet Dent. 1962; 12: 441–450.
17. Wolff J. The Law of Bone Remodeling. New York: Springer, 1986 (translation of the German 1892 edition).
18. Heller MO, Taylor WR, Aslanidis N, Duda GN The classic: on the inner architecture of bones and its importance for bone growth. Clin Orthop Relat Res. 2010; 468(4): 1056–1065.
19. Hermann JS, Buser D Guided bone regeneration for dental implants. Curr Opin Periodontol. 1996; 3: 168–177.
20. Hämmerle CH, Karring T Guided bone regeneration at oral implant sites. Periodontol. 1998; 17: 151–175.

21. Tolman DE Reconstructive procedures with endosseous implants in grafted bone: a review of the literature. Int J Oral Maxillofac Implants. 1995; 10: 275–294.
22. Buck BE, Resnick L, Shah SM, et al. Human immunodeficiency virus cultured from bone. Implications for transplantation. Clin Orthop. 1990; 251: 249–253.
23. Mellonig JT, Prewett AB, Moyer MP HIV inactivation in a bone allograft. J Periodontol. 1992; 63: 979–983.
24. Thaller SR, Hoyt J, Borjeson K, et al. Reconstruction of calvarial defects with anorganic bovine bone mineral (Bio-Oss) in a rabbit model. J Caniofac Surg. 1993; 4: 79–84.
25. Wallace SS, Froum SJ, Tarnow DP Histologic evaluation of a sinus elevation procedure: a clinical report. Int J Periodontics Restorative Dent. 1996; 16: 46–51.
26. McAllister BS, Margolin MD, Cogan AG, et al. Eighteen-month radiographic and histologic evaluation of sinus grafting with anorganic bovine bone in the chimpanzee. Int J Oral Maxillofac Implants. 1999; 14: 361–368.
27. McEwen W Infrahuman bone grafting and reimplantation of bone. Ann Surg. 1909; 50: 959–968.
28. Miron RJ, Sculean A, Cochrane DL, et al. Twenty years of enamel matrix derivative: the past, the present and the future. J Clin Periodontol. 2016; 43(8): 668–683.
29. Jensen OT, Shulman LB, Block MS, Iacono VJ Report of the sinus consensus conference of 1996. Int J Oral Maxillofac Implants. 1998; 13: 11–45.
30. Bragger U, Gerber C, Joss A, et al. Patterns of tissue remodeling after placement of ITI dental implants using an osteotome technique: a longitudinal radio-graphic case cohort study. Clin Oral Implants Res. 2004; 15: 158–166.
31. Fugazzotto PA, de Paoli S Sinus floor augmentation at the time of maxillary molar extraction: success and failure rates of 137 implants in function for up to three years. J Periodontol. 2002; 24: 177–183.
32. Berglundh T, Lindhe J, Ericsson I, Marinello CP, Liljenberg B, Thomsen P The soft tissue barrier at implants and teeth. Clin Oral Implants Res. 1991; 2: 81–90.
33. Berglundh T, Lindhe J Dimension of the peri-implant mucosa: biological width revisited. J Clin Periodontol. 1996; 23: 971–973.
34. Cochran DL, Hermann JS, Schenk RK, Higginbottom FL, Buser D Biologic width around titanium implants: a histometric analysis of the implantogingival junction around unloaded and loaded nonsubmerged implants in the canine mandible. J Periodontol. 1997; 68: 186–198.
35. Hermann JS, Cochran DL, Nummikoski PV, Buser D Crestal bone changes around titanium implants: a radiographic evaluation of unloaded nonsubmerged and submerged implants in the canine mandible. J Periodontol. 1997; 68: 1117–1130.
36. Misch CE. Contemporary Implant Dentistry, 3rd ed. St. Louis, MO: Mosby, 2008: 457.
37. Malo P, Rangert B, de Araujo Nobre M "All-on-Four" immediate function concept with Brånemark system implants for completely edentulous mandibles: a retrospective clinical study. Clin Implant Dent Relat Res. 2003; 5(Suppl 1): 2–9 88–94.
38. Malo P, Rangert B, de Araujo NM, Petersson U, Wigren S A pilot study of complete edentulous rehabilitation with immediate function using a new implant design; case series. Clin Implant Dent Relat Res. 2006; 8(4): 223–232.
39. Malo P, de Araujo NM, Lopes A The use of computer-guided flapless implant surgery and 4 implants placed in immediate function to support fixed denture preliminary results after a mean follow-up period of 13 months. J Prosthet Dept. 2007; 97(Suppl): 26–34.
40. Pomares C A retrospective clinical study of edentulous patient rehabilitated according to the all-on-four or the all-on-six immediate function concept. Eur J Oral Implantol. 2009; 2(1): 55–60.
41. Testori T, Del Fabbro M, Capelli M, Zuffeti F, Francetti L, Weinstein RL Immediate occlusal loading of tilted implants for the rehabilitation of the atrophic edentulous maxilla; 1 year interim results of a multicenter prospective study. Clin Oral Implants Res. 2008; 19(3): 227–232.

4 Setting the Stage: Adjunctive Surgical Procedures, Restorative Options, and Treatment Planning

With contributions by Dr. Robert Horowitz, Dr. Robert Schneider, and Dr. Maria L. Geisinger

Take the necessary steps to gain an understanding of adjunctive procedures, the surgical/restorative options for implants, and what evaluation steps are needed to develop a comprehensive implant treatment plan.

A new frontier of implant dentistry is interdisciplinary, with coordination of therapy: hygienists, auxiliaries, dentists, lab technicians, and specialists all working together to provide regeneration dentistry! The restorative dentist is the *quarterback of the team* and the hygienist plays the key role of helping to identify the wants and needs of the patient for replacing hopeless or missing teeth with implants. The specialist is usually the member who has the extra training in either the surgical aspects or advanced restorative techniques that are very often necessary in more challenging cases.

Hygienists can take the lead to evaluate necessary adjunctive procedures and to discuss wants, needs, and restorative options with the patients. Treatment planning is essential and most of all the patient's questions, financial concerns, and final expectations must all be addressed prior to the first surgical procedure. Talk with your patients on what to expect from implant therapy.

To place implants, you need a proper foundation of bone. Gingival tissue follows the biologic type and anatomy of the bone. To achieve optimal treatment results, the dentist needs to *set the stage* with tissue and bone in mind for long-term success. Implant dentistry and regenerative adjunct procedures are no longer, something for the future, they are a predictable and effective way to assure successful implant dentistry.

Adjunctive surgical procedures

Contributed by Robert Horowitz, DDS

Adjunctive procedures in implant dentistry are on both the surgical and restorative sides. To have an ideal, aesthetic, implant-supported restoration, the implant must be placed in as ideal a location as possible. There needs to be sufficient alveolar bone to support the gingival margin and papillae that will frame the proximal surfaces of the implant-supported fixed restoration. An optimal volume of bone is required to obtain sufficient osseointegrated support for facilitation of occlusion and force transfer from the restoration to the alveolar bone. To achieve these simple goals, there are a multitude of surgical and restorative options to obtain the necessary osseointegrated support or retention for the planned prosthetic device.

Surgical therapy

Implant dentistry begins with a tooth that has to be extracted or a site where it has been extracted. Improper extraction socket therapy is a major concern related to either the inability to place implants at all or functional and/or aesthetic issues related to the resulting implant-restorative complex. Case reports, studies, and meta-analysis papers have all reinforced what is seen clinically on a daily basis.

When a tooth is extracted, if no socket preservation or augmentation strategies are performed, there is concomitant loss of both hard and soft tissue. More than 45 years ago; Pietrokovski, Massler, and their coworkers performed a dried skull study (1) that verified *where teeth had been lost on the patients, plus identified there was bone loss*. The resulting alveolar ridge had collapsed from both the buccal side and occlusally. What bone remained in the alveolar ridge was shorter and more lingually located than when the teeth had been present.

When multiple teeth were extracted, the resulting bone loss was magnified. Leaving the socket with no graft material does lead to a *fill with vital alveolar bone* as described by Amler in the 1960s (2). This was one of a number of papers that validated the conclusion that leaving a blood clot to heal in an undisturbed manner will leave vital bone suitable for osseointegration in the area. However, if we follow the work by Massler and others, this may not leave sufficient bone nor in the ideal location to either place a dental implant or a conventional prosthetic replacement for the missing tooth or teeth.

Critical in extraction therapy, is the removal of the affected tooth with minimal destruction to either the alveolar bone or surrounding gingival tissues. The group of techniques incorporated into the achievement of this goal is known as *atraumatic extraction* (3). As the periodontal ligament (PDL) is what holds the nonankylosed tooth in place, that component of the periodontal apparatus must be stretched and broken to get out the root or roots with maximal preservation of the structures adjacent to the tooth. It is the surgeon's responsibility to have the appropriate instrumentation required to remove the tooth and root, leaving the bone and gingival region as intact as possible. The first instrument utilized in this process is the periotome.

The periotome (see Figure 4.1) is a single- or double-ended instrument that is *inserted manually* or with a mallet in the PDL space. The goal is to widen the potential space of the PDL into a wider area that can accept larger instruments. In some cases, the tooth or root can be extracted using only this type of instrument.

Other teeth require more *aggressive* instrumentation to remove them. Multi-rooted teeth are sectioned so that individual roots can be removed. Fewer macro and micro fractures will affect the facial and

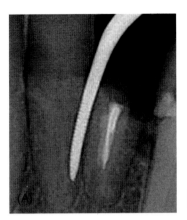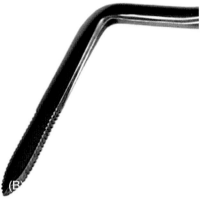

Figure 4.1 Example of serrated periotome. Courtesy of PDT, Inc.

lingual plates of bone when single roots can be taken out of the jaw. Piezosurgery (4) and high-speed rotary instruments can be used when teeth are severely broken down and/or have no mobility.

Depending on the cross-sectional form and longitudinal shape of each root, many can be rotated to increase their individual mobility, facilitating atraumatic removal. As Fickl and coworkers have shown in animal studies (5), surgical access at the time of extraction increases volumetric bone loss. While bone grafting reduced the site collapse, the material used in their study did not prevent it entirely.

Socket preservation

Extraction socket preservation is essential to minimize the amount of bone and gingival loss following tooth removal. Studies in animals and humans have documented a multitude of strategies that have been attempted over the years to achieve certain goals. Our patients want the fewest number of procedures in which maximal results can be obtained. It is up to the dentists who are treating the patient to come up with their objectives for each and every individual site.

There are short- and long-term goals to be realized after a tooth is removed. We wish the patient to be free from dental disease and discomfort as quickly as possible. The maximal volume of bone and keratinized tissue should be preserved to support or aesthetically frame the final prosthesis inserted in the site. *True regeneration of vital bone with keratinized tissue in the area is the ideal result.*

Many classes of bone replacement graft materials and barriers have been used while trying to improve the simplicity and predictability of reaching our socket preservation goals. Analysis of the results of these procedures has to be framed in light of the desired outcomes. Case reports, human and animal controlled studies, and meta-analyses have all been done to assist the surgeon in choosing the materials he/she will use to place in and/or over the socket immediately after tooth extraction.

Barriers and grafts of varied types have been used with significantly different clinical and histologic outcomes. Combinations are chosen depending on the endpoint desired by the site and surgical/restorative team to be working on the patient. A number of these materials will be described here for illustrative purposes.

A barrier membrane is inserted over an untreated or grafted socket. The goals are to protect the graft or for blood clot and enhancement of guided bone regeneration by preventing migration of epithelium or connective tissue into the area.

Bone replacement grafts can be synthetic, can come from an animal, another donor human, or the same patient. Once they are placed in the body, they can remain for a short time, long time, or may never be removed. These materials can have some or no mineral content and can degrade quickly, slowly, or not at all. The specific formation or processing of the material will determine the amount of and time of resorbability, which can affect the amount of vital bone formation. It is the formation of vital bone that is critical for osseointegration, as osteocytes must be present in the grafted or treated site to enable bone-to-implant contact. That light microscopic contact with vital bone will enable force transfer from the prosthesis to the jaw and ensure stability of the bone–implant interface over time.

For proper physiology, the bone must resorb and remodel as occlusal stresses are transferred through it. Having osteoclasts acting on the vital bone and any residual graft material is important for this process to maintain homeostasis in the site. An analysis of the time of resorption/replacement of the graft has to be weighed against the amount of bone formation desired and volume preservation expected. All of this has to fit into the discussions with the patient as to when, after extraction, an implant should be placed and then safely, predictably loaded with a prosthetic device.

Graft and/or barrier protection of the socket

As aforementioned studies have taught us, leaving a socket untreated will enable it to fill with vital bone. That is at the cost of 35% or greater loss of height on the facial and up to 50% of the width, primarily from the facial as well. There are concerns if graft particles are placed alone in an extraction socket. Particle loss or infection can lead to loss of the preservation and/or increase attempted. *With no barrier to keep out the quicker migrating epithelial or connective tissue cells, there is potential for more connective tissue encapsulation of the graft particles and less vital bone formation* (Figure 4.2).

Tal and coworkers (6) described this in a socket preservation study. They grafted extraction sockets in humans with anorganic bovine bone mineral (ABBM). After extraction and flap elevation, sockets were debrided and filled to ideal contour with ABBM. Nine months later, the areas were exposed for placement of implants. The buccal plate resorption (in all but three cases where none was evident) ranged from 2 to 12 mm, with an average of 5.64 mm. There was almost 20% resorption of the buccal bony walls. Some of the cases exhibited lingual or palatal resorption of between 3 and 6 mm, as well as the significant buccal bone loss. Cores of material were retrieved at the time of implant placement from the central portion of the sockets. Apically, there was up to 60% vital bone, compared with only 16% coronally. Clinically, the ABBM particles were evident at the crest in all cases. Histologically, there was 30% residual graft present throughout the cores.

The authors concluded that resorption of the graft material was extremely slow from this data. They also stated that; *"the ultimate bone substitute should induce/conduct new bone formation and eventually completely resorb and be replaced by bone."* Other authors (7), similarly agreed with the conclusion that ABBM did not contribute to bone formation in an extraction socket and did not advise the use of this material to enhance vital bone-to-implant contact.

Removable barriers can work well when primary closure is obtained and maintained over them. In a dog model, Stavropoulos (8) studied grafted defects that had barrier protection. Two different types of resorbable barriers were tested in intra-alveolar defects that were created in healed sites. Both of the resorbable barriers led to vital bone formation underneath them.

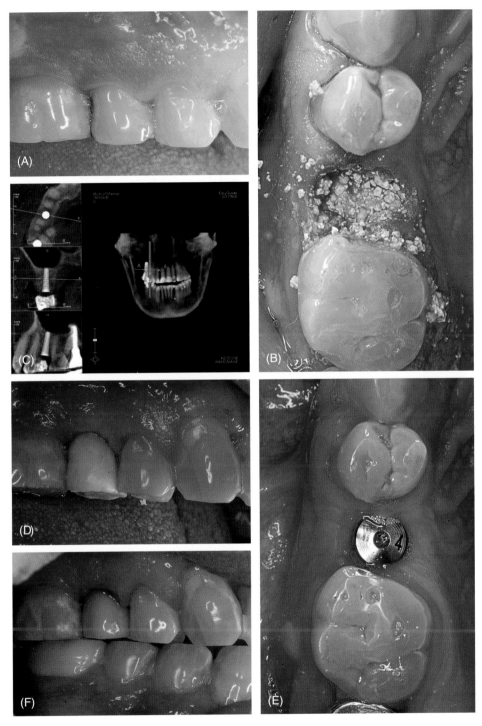

Figure 4.2 Socket preservation case. Courtesy of Dr. Robert Horowitz. (A) Initial tooth and abscess. (B) Socket grafted with barrier by MIS. (C) Cone beam scan implant planned. (D) Screw-retained provisional crown. (E) Implant placed and site healed. (F) Final restoration.

Retrievable barriers alone have been used successfully in a number of studies. There are significant differences between dense and expanded polytetrafluorethylene (PFTE) barriers. Studies such as those by Becker (9), Zitzmann (10), and others have shown bone loss with exposed expanded PTFE (ePTFE) barriers. The same occurrence is not true with the dense PTFE barriers. Building on the research of others, in 2005 Horowitz (11) published a series of cases showing the use of a dense polytetrafluoroethylene (dPTFE) barrier alone for socket volume preservation and bone regeneration. Atraumatic extractions were performed with no or minimal flap elevation. After debridement of the socket, no graft was placed; the volume was allowed to fill with a blood clot and covered with the barrier.

Clinically, though width measurements were not given, a significant percentage of the width of the original socket was preserved. Histologically, as no graft was placed in the socket, there was no residual material that could potentially interfere with osseointegration of the implant inserted into the healed area. Vital bone was formed throughout the core to the region where the barrier was placed. Despite an average vital bone percentage of 28%, there were very thick and dense trabeculae at the apical portion of the socket with a more cancellous nature coronally.

Expanding on this study, Hoffmann and coworkers (12) treated patients in a similar manner and evaluated 276 sockets. No graft material was placed in the socket under the barrier membrane. As in the other studies, primary closure was not obtained due to the design of the material. It is removed approximately 3 weeks postoperatively or when one edge of the barrier becomes exposed.

A small percentage of the sockets was evaluated histologically after 12 months of healing. They appeared full of vital bone and having a consistent preservation of socket volume. These and other studies confirmed Amler's original work (2), stating that a blood clot left undisturbed in an extraction socket will predictably form bone in a 3-month time frame. Adding a dense PTFE barrier to the treatment protocol increased the amount of the original socket volume that was preserved. In the absence of both graft material and the need for flap surgery, the extraction socket was preserved in volume and regenerated and filled with vital bone. This is an ideal result from both the patient's and surgeon's standpoint. Only one surgical visit is required, with maximal physical and biologic results in terms of bone preservation and keratinized tissue augmentation.

Bone graft materials are categorized depending on their source. *Autogenous* bone is retrieved from the same patient, usually in a different site. Intraorally, cortical shavings are taken from the ramus. *Cancellous* bone is removed from osteotomies or using trephines from anywhere in the mouth. Monocortical blocks and corticocancellous blocks that are primarily used for ridge augmentation are removed from the anterior mandible or the ramus. Extraoral donor sites from which a patient's own bone can be removed include the calvarium, iliac crest, and tibia.

Allograft or donor bone is processed from another member of the same species and can come in any of the four forms. The material can be retrieved from either a cancellous or cortical location and can either be obtained as either mineralized or demineralized freeze-dried bone graft substitute.

Xenograft is retrieved from a member of another species and is processed in a steam or sintered manner to remove some, most, or all of the proteins. The primary sources of these materials are cows, pigs, and horses. These materials have been shown in some studies (6) to be practically nonresorbable and act primarily as a scaffold on which new bone is deposited.

Alloplastic materials are synthetic in nature. These are calcium-containing *salts* in the families of hydroxyapatite, calcium sulfate, or tricalcium phosphate (TCP). Particle size, three-dimensional (3-D) structure, and chemical composition all play a role in the resorption or dissolution rate of the graft material.

Earlier in this chapter, studies on xenografts were mentioned, indicating they were not ideal to use where regeneration is desired in extraction socket therapy (6). That paper reinforced what had been shown in other papers in that resorption of anorganic bovine bone was not clinically nor histologically seen in the time frame ideal for placement of dental implants. Similar results were seen in a paper by Carmagnola in 2003 (13). In 21 patients, 31 sockets were grafted with either anorganic bovine bone, covered with a resorbable barrier, or left untreated. Timing for reentry and histologic specimen retrieval was not standardized. The sockets that were covered with the resorbable barrier had, at approximately 4 months postoperatively, 52% vital bone. There was a very high standard of deviation of 16%, leading to the conclusion that results were not consistent.

Where the sockets were untreated, reentry was performed between 1 and 15 years postoperatively with a resulting 56% vital bone, with almost a 20% standard deviation in results. The poorest histologic result was when ABBM was inserted into the socket at the time of extraction. The remaining ABBM particles were 21% with only 8% vital bone about 7 months after extraction. This is significantly less vital bone than shown by Horowitz (11), where a dPTFE barrier was used over no graft material, only a blood clot.

A clinical case report looked at the healing of sockets filled with demineralized, freeze-dried bone compared with autogenous bone in extraction sockets (14). Becker and his colleagues saw more vital bone formation when autogenous bone was used.

Increasing the amount of vital bone formed around allograft particles has been shown by Sottosanti (15) and others with the addition of 20% calcium sulfate to the mixture. In their randomized, controlled clinical trial on two types of graft and barrier protection of extraction sockets, in 24 patients, clinical and histologic analysis was taken of ABBM covered with a resorbable barrier or demineralized, freeze-dried bone allograft mixed with calcium sulfate in putty and covered with a calcium sulfate barrier (16). There was similar ridge width preservation for both groups and slightly better height maintained with the ABBM and barrier.

The differences in vital bone formation were significant. In the ABBM-treated sites, there was only 26% vital bone compared with 61% in the sites grafted with demineralized freeze-dried bone allograft (DFDBA) and calcium sulfate. Additionally, in the allograft-treated sites, there was only 3% residual graft material compared with 16% remaining bovine bone material. This study demonstrated that the use of an allograft combined with calcium sulfate led to significant preservation of socket volume with a high percentage of regeneration of alveolar bone in the socket, significantly more than when ABBM was placed. For long-term success, having more vital bone should give better osseointegration and may resist peri-implant disease.

In addition to the works by Pecora and others from Italy, there is a recent paper documenting the clinical and biologic advantages of a new calcium sulfate graft material. Mazor et al. (17), showed clinical preservation of volume after extraction of a severely infected mandibular molar tooth. The site was grafted with this new formulation of a calcium sulfate hydrated in sterile saline and covered with a dense PTFE barrier. The barrier was removed in a nonsurgical manner 3 weeks postoperatively. Two-dimensional radiographs and the cone beam volumetric tomography confirmed a similar radiation density in the grafted site and the adjacent bone 4 months after the extraction at the time of implant placement.

Histologically, the area was filled with densely woven bone that amounted to 47% of the volume of the analyzed specimen. There was no residual graft material at that time. Furthermore, a 10-month post-placement radiograph demonstrated full preservation of the regenerated alveolar bone at the crest. All of those are ideal results to achieve in such a short time period.

The research group comprising of Horowitz et al. (18), evaluated a pure phase β TCP for use in extraction socket grafting. After atraumatic extraction, sockets were carefully debrided and grafted with a pure phase β TCP whetted in the patient's own blood from the socket. The site was filled to contour with the graft material and covered with a barrier. When the barrier was collagen, primary closure was obtained. In the cases that were covered with a dPTFE barrier, there was no attempt at primary closure. There were no infections postoperatively and all 30 sites healed well. Approximately 6 months after grafting, the sites were reentered for placement of dental implants. All implants have been successful to date. The average width of alveolar ridge preservation in the buccolingual dimension was 87.6% with these methods. If the larger particle size graft was considered, 92% of the original alveolar width was preserved. One key to the long-term success rate with this material may be its complete resorption and replacement with vital bone.

Alveolar ridge and maxillary sinus augmentation

Despite the significant amount of literature dedicated to extraction socket preservation, many patients still present to the surgeon or restorative dentist with insufficient hard tissue and/or keratinized gingiva to support an aesthetic restoration. There are numerous surgical procedures that have been documented to assist patients who have a debilitated ridge. Some of these will be described in more detail.

Certain surgical approaches require sophisticated radiographic analysis and tremendous experience to obtain a high degree of success and predictability. Lateral nerve reposition, harvesting autogenous bone blocks from extraoral locations, and avoiding sinus grafting with pterygoid and zygomatic implants fall into that category. Prior to entering any alveolar augmentation, the patient must have a full prosthetic workup including a wax-up of the ideal restoration on articulated diagnostic casts. Then, a cone beam scan is taken with a radio-opaque stent showing in all dimensions where the final tooth position is going to occur for ideal function and aesthetics. Planning software then shows ideal implant locations and where bone volume should be for proper support.

Deficient ridges can be enhanced with the addition of autogenous bone blocks harvested from either the mandibular ramus or the anterior mandible between the mental foramina. After careful recipient site preparation, Pikos has published numerous articles and lectured internationally on these techniques (19, 20). Though it is a predictable way to gain width and/or height in the deficient alveolar ridge, there are potential neurologic and other sequelae from this type of procedure.

Similarly, a thin ridge can be split with saws, piezosurgery (4), or burs to enable crestal expansion. This type of procedure has less risk of bleeding and numbness, but there are other issues. There are discussions as to whether it is better to perform this type of procedure in one visit with simultaneous placement of implants, or in two steps.

Allograft putties and block grafts can be added to these procedures to replace the more aggressive surgeries. Either the need for a donor site or risk of segment loss can be eliminated by taking material that is properly processed to enhance biologic activity while eliminating the chance of disease transmission. Toscano and coworkers (21), documented the success of an osteoinductive allograft putty for increasing alveolar ridge width.

A decorticated alveolar base was prepared in the deficient site. The putty was prepared and placed on the bone and contoured to shape. The graft was stabilized by screws and/or the barrier placed over it. After allowing 4–9 months for the site to heal in an undisturbed manner, the sites were re-entered for implant placement. There was a gain in horizontal ridge width of 3–6 mm for an average of 3.5 mm. The authors concluded that this was an effective means of increasing the buccolingual width of the alveolus. As there are decreased postoperative sequelae using a bone replacement graft not taken from the same patient, there is a very high acceptance rate for this type of therapy. Histologic validation of the formation of vital bone ideal for osseointegration has been published in this and other papers (see Figure 4.3).

Sinus augmentation

Maxillary posterior tooth extraction is usually followed by loss of crestal alveolar bone. Simultaneously, the sinus often pneumatized, as there is no root structure to preserve the apical cortex of bone. These two processes can significantly reduce the opportunity to place a dental implant of ideal dimensions. Dr. Ziv Mazor has been involved in sinus grafting research for many years and his papers have included a range of techniques and graft materials used for the successful placement of appropriately sized dental implants in these challenging areas.

As an introduction to the case (see Figure 4.4), the initial presentation was tooth #14 missing with mesial drift of tooth #14 narrowing the interdental space. A full thickness flap is elevated, showing the buccal plate over the pneumatized maxillary sinus. After making the osteotomy through the buccal plate, the Schneiderian membrane is elevated with a Mazor curette. The site is filled with a pure phase β tri-calcium phosphate bone replacement graft material (i.e., Cerasorb M). The site is then covered with a barrier stabilized with a titanium tack. Six months after grafting, the site is reentered. The barrier has resorbed and an intact buccal plate is present. An implant is placed to support a cement-retained restoration in an area where there will be shallow sulcus depth. The final restoration, 4 years after loading, shows excellent tissue health.

Research now shows there are a wide variety of bioactive materials being added to the armamentarium of the Periodontist. These include growth factors, bone grafts, barriers, and accessory devices. Most bone replacement grafts are *passive* in nature and are osseoconductive scaffolds. Very few have been shown to be able to induce new bone formation.

Over 50 years ago, Dr. Urist demonstrated that extracted teeth contained bone morphogenetic protein, the most potent growth factor utilized in osseous surgery. A novel method of preparing extracted teeth to formulate two discreet particle sizes of ground dentin (i.e., Kometabio Smart Dentin Grinder). This material is used to graft extraction sockets with the smaller particles being resorbed more quickly, releasing growth factors during that time. At a cellular level, they change macrophages from *Type 1*, that removes inflammatory and diseased components to *Type 2* which participates in bone formation. Research papers, book chapters from

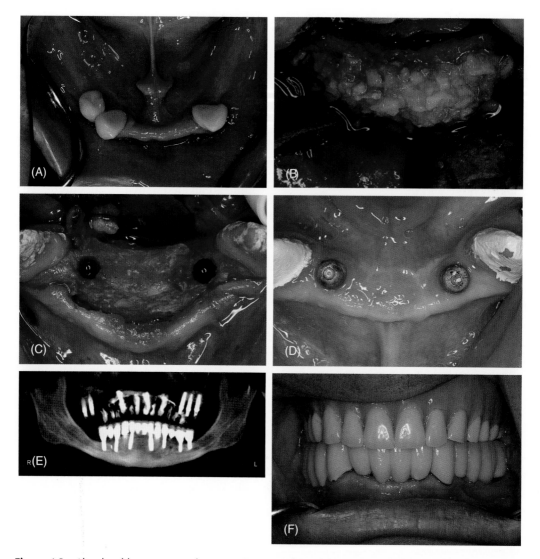

Figure 4.3 Alveolar ridge augmentation case. Courtesy of Dr. Robert Horowitz. (A) Initial occlusal view of deficient ridge. (B) Allograft putty in Site. (C) Ridge after augmentation. (D) Implants placed and site healed. (E) Panorex. (F) Facial view of final restoration.

centers in the United States, Israel, and Europe have shown bone preservation at the time of extraction at the same, or better volume than other grafts (22). Histologically, the bone is dense, vital, and ideal for implant placement (23). Research shows the benefit of this material for combined extraction and periodontal defects.

Microvibration, is also being utilized as an accelerator for orthodontic therapy. In medicine, similar types of therapy have been shown to increase bone healing and bone density. This device has shown to be an aid to repair surgically deficient bone sites after peri-implant bone loss (24).

Platelet derived growth factor (rh PDGF bb) have also returned to the dental arena. Initially utilized for periodontal treatment, treated sites demonstrated *root coverage and fill* of periodontal defects. The same areas also showed true periodontal regeneration with new PDL and alveolar bone (25). Other studies have shown alveolar ridge augmentation and

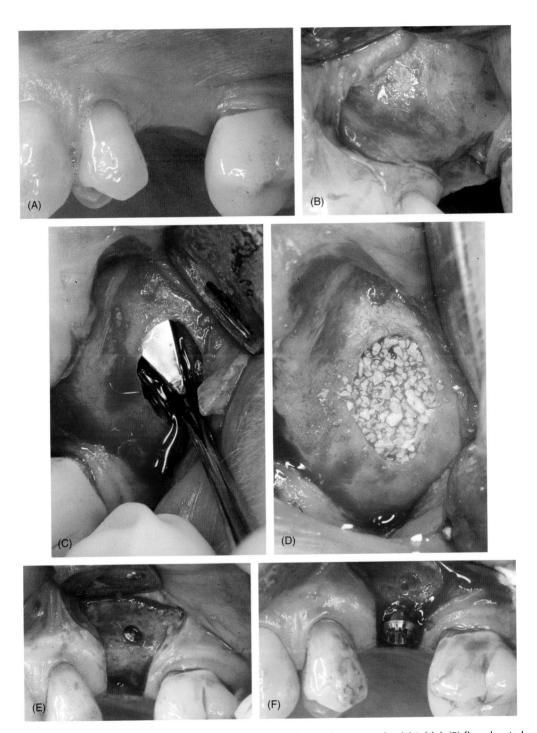

Figure 4.4 Maxillary sinus augmentation case. Courtesy of Dr. Robert Horowitz. (A) Initial, (B) flap elevated, (C) membrane elevation, (D) grafted, (E) re-entry at 6 months, and (F) implant placement.

regeneration of deficient facial plates of bone (26). Altogether, novel materials, techniques, and returning materials can improve the predictability to save teeth and optimize the success rates of dental implant therapy.

Summary

Hygienists and all team members should be aware of what regenerative procedures are now available. Socket preservation, nongrafted- or nonbarrier-treated extraction sockets, lose bone, even if immediate implants are placed. Alveolar ridge preservation and augmentation strategies are predictable from a clinical and biologic standpoint as long as the appropriate techniques and biomaterials are undertaken. *All clinical and office team members need to be on the same page to help the patient understand why adjunctive procedures are essential for overall implant treatment success.*

Restorative options

Contributed by Robert Schneider DDS, MS

Many clinicians feel that, due to the substantial success rate, implants should be considered as a definitive choice for tooth-replacement alternatives (27).

Dental implants have provided our profession with many functional and aesthetic options for replacing missing teeth. The options depend on the number of teeth missing, bone, patient preference (i.e., removable or nonremovable), and cost. The ideal option for a single tooth is an implant with a crown that will look, feel, and function like a natural tooth. Restorative options can be categorized into; fixed cement-retained, fixed removable screw-retained implants (restorations / final full-arch prosthesis), removable tissue-supported attachment-retained, or removable bar-supported attachment-retained (see Table 4.1).

Implant-supported removable tissue-supported or bar-supported attachment-retained overdentures are now becoming mainstream as an entry-level, cost-effective option for edentulous patients (see Figure 4.5). Two to four implants on the lower and four to six on the upper with a removable overdenture can offer patients the benefit of stability, comfort, and increased quality of life. The use of multiple mini-implants to provide immediate support of a provisional overdenture at the time of placement is also becoming increasingly popular.

The implant-supported fixed final prosthesis is also an option with the palate-free upper prosthesis that not only allows the patient to taste but also provides enhanced aesthetic appearance. Often the hygienists hold the key relationship with the patient and can have an informal conversation with the patient to help identify the best restorative option for tooth replacement. The hygienist knows what the patient's occupation is, what the patient likes to do for entertainment, and, most important of all is the patient's oral hygiene.

For instance, the implant-supported maxillary fixed final prosthesis option with no upper palate could be the answer if a patient is a wine specialist either for work or leisure. This option makes it possible for the patient to be able to taste and appreciate the wine, versus a traditional denture with a full palate for retention, where everything the patient eats or drinks tastes like plastic (see Figure 4.6). *The choice of prosthesis becomes a lifestyle choice and not just a choice to repair what was lost.*

Hygienists, learn all you can on the restorative options (Table 4.1), to be able to talk with your patients on what to expect when the implant is placed. For more on having a conversation with your patient on the risks, benefits, and alternatives to replacing missing teeth, refer to Chapter 5.

Fixed cement or screw-retained restorations (crowns or bridges) implant options

Why implants? According to the American Academy of Implant Dentistry, "*Implants with attached crowns are the preferred method for treating tooth loss because they function the*

Table 4.1 Comparison of restorative options and advantages.

Restorative Options	Advantages
Fixed cement-retained 	■ Nonremovable by patient ■ Single or multiple teeth ■ Abutment like a prepared tooth for a crown ■ Permanent or temporary cement-retained or screw-retained
Fixed removable screw-retained implants (restorations/final full-arch prosthesis) 	■ Nonremovable by patient ■ Crown and prosthesis removable by dental professional as needed ■ Abutment screws attach restoration directly to implant ■ Predictable retrievability as needed
Removable tissue-supported attachment-retained 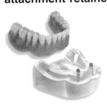	■ Overdenture (prosthesis) removable by the patient ■ Replaces an entire arch of teeth and replicates soft tissue ■ Economical with as few as two to three implants ■ Increases stability and function, but does not eliminate all movement of the overdenture ■ Male attachment secured into implant, female portion secured into denture (i.e., Locator, ball [OD] attachments) ■ Prosthesis (overdenture) is removable by patient for daily cleaning and implants ■ Minimizes bone deterioration in the area of the implants, relines may be needed over time
Removable bar-supported attachment-retained 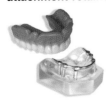	■ Overdenture removable by the patient ■ Replaces an entire arch and replicates soft tissue ■ Two to eight implants connected with a metal bar (bars may be fabricated utilizing CAD-CAM technology) ■ May have greater stability and less to no movement of denture based upon the number of implants (compared to tissue-retained) ■ Male attachment secured into implant, female portion secured into denture (i.e., Locator, ball [OD] attachments) and clips attach denture to bar for more retention ■ Helps to minimize bone loss/resorption ■ No palate, restores taste sensation (four implants minimum) ■ Prosthesis (overdenture) is removable by patient for daily cleaning and implants ■ Bar can be removed by dental professional as needed

Images courtesy of Salvin Dental Specialties; models are available as patient educational tools.

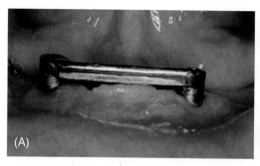 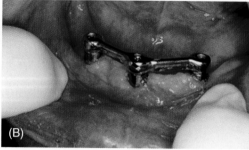

Figures 4.5 Examples of bar-supported attachment-retained overdenture cases. Courtesy of Dr. Robert Schneider. (A) Ball attachment. (B) Locator attachment.

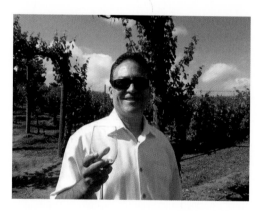

Figure 4.6 Lifestyle choice of enjoying a glass of wine. Courtesy of Carla Frey.

same as natural teeth and help preserve the jaw structure by preventing atrophy from bone loss."

Bridgework and dentures address the cosmetic problem of missing teeth, but do not prevent bone loss. Implants maintain proper chewing function and exert appropriate, natural forces on the jawbone to keep it functional and healthy. There is a growing consensus that dental implants are the most successful, long-term, and preferred option for replacing missing or compromised teeth. Patients will benefit from a more nutritious diet, better physical health, and natural facial appearance, as these all enhance patients' overall sense of wellness and self-confidence.

The principal reason single implants are the best option for tooth replacement is that they look, feel, and act like natural teeth. The missing tooth is replaced by a surgically placed implant and in some cases can be loaded with a provisional or permanent crown the same day. The traditional way to restore a single implant is with a cement-retained or screw-retained crown, appear very similar to traditional crowns on natural teeth (see Figure 4.7).

When speaking with a patient who may have already had a crown, he or she can relate to the ease of the restoration process. An impression is made and sent to the lab to be fabricated. Patients need to be aware that there is an increased cost for the restoration due to the parts and pieces necessary for the lab and restorative process, which does vary from a traditional crown. The patient will then return to the dentist's office in 2–3 weeks for permanent placement of the restoration on the implant or Chairside Economical Restoration of Esthetic Ceramics (CEREC) implant abutments/crown solutions can be fabricated in-office and made available sooner. A full arch of dentition can be replaced with either a fixed or removable prosthesis.

Options for the edentulous arch

For an edentulous arch, multiple treatment options are available; research shows that traditional denture patients use their dentures 80% of the time the first year, 60% in 4 years, 40% in 5 years, and only 20% in

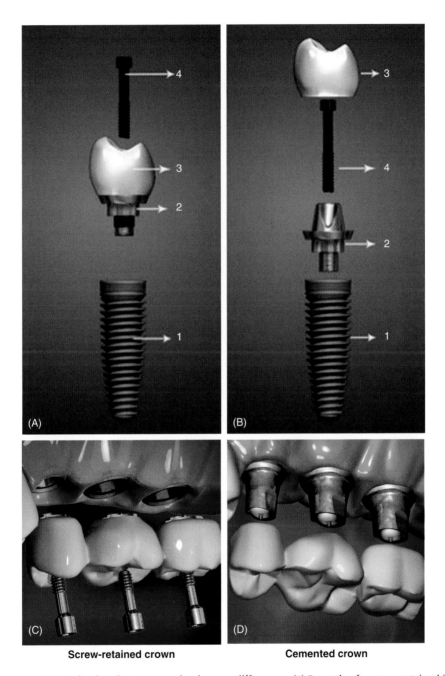

Figure 4.7 Screw-retained and cement-retained crown differences. (A) Example of a screw-retained implant crown. (1) Implant fixture: integrated in bone and soft-tissue adherence. (2) Anti-rotational portion: this will allow the crown to be secured to the implant. (3) Crown portion: 2 and 3 are part of the same unit; they are fixed together. (4) Implant crown screw: this screw will secure the crown (2 and 3) to the implant fixture. (B) Example of a cement-retained implant crown. (1) Implant fixture: integrated in bone and soft-tissue adherence. (2) Implant abutment: notice the most apical portion has an anti-rotational feature. (3) Abutment screw: the screw will secure the implant abutment to the implant fixture. (4) Implant crown: the crown will be secured onto the implant with the use of dental cement. (C) Screw-retained crown (D) cement-retained crown. Panels A and B reprinted with permission from Dr. Boris Pulec. Courtesy of BioHorizons.

10 years (28). The advantages implant-supported full-arch fixed and removal prostheses are; function, comfort, increased stability, better taste of food, and more natural appearance. Patients also report an increased self-esteem and confidence with the choice of implant-supported full-arch prosthesis over traditional dentures. The healing time varies with bone quality, tissue health, and overall health of the patient, refer to Chapter 3.

The patient's aesthetic and functional expectations have a direct correlation to the number of appointments necessary. What aesthetic adjunctive procedures may be needed, if a provisional restoration or prosthesis is requested, and the time frame for the completed treatment. Provisionals are used in implant dentistry not only for aesthetics, but to ease the implant into sustaining the full occlusal forces (i.e., progressive loading). Provisionals are natural-looking temporary restorations (i.e., crown or bridge) or temporary dentures that can be worn by the patient at different stages of treatment to provide the patient with natural-looking teeth for aesthetics and function.

If a provisional restoration or prosthesis is necessary, this can be planned for in advance, but may require more appointments and expense for the patient. Communicate to and reassure the patient that the process for implant therapy is necessary for a successful, long-lasting result.

More than 36 million Americans are edentulous (no teeth) and 12 million are edentulous in one arch according to the American College of Prosthodontists (29). A removable lower overdenture supported by two to four implants is the most popular edentulous tooth replacement option and is now considered *standard of care* in many parts of the world for lower edentulous patients (30). Other prosthesis restorative options include implants attached to a Hadar clip bar system that supports a removable overdenture and attachments that attach to the implants (i.e., ball or Locator attachments) that support an overdenture, or implants-supported fixed final prosthesis that is not removable by patient. What this means for the patient is smaller and more comfortable options, most with a palate, compared with a traditional tissue-retained full denture.

Removable tissue-supported attachment-retained overdenture option

This prosthesis is a full-arch prosthesis, retained by two to four implants to provide the patient with improved stability and retention of their complete dentures (see Figure 4.8). The overdenture is held in place by various implant attachments (i.e., Locator caps or O-rings) to afford the patient more comfort and improved chewing ability. The overdenture is removable by the patient for cleaning, but the attachments are only removed by the dental professional as needed. *Tissue-supported overdenture means the implants are not connected with a bar;* they are free-standing and the functional loads from chewing can be transferred to the edentulous ridge. Typically, there is still a need for relines.

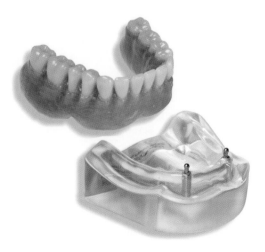

Figure 4.8 Ball implant, O-ring attachment, and lower overdenture example. Courtesy of Salvin Dental Specialties.

Movement of the overdenture during function will be based upon the number of implants placed and the types of attachments used.

Removable bar-supported attachment-retained overdenture

This prosthesis is a full-arch prosthesis, retained by two to six implants to provide the patient with improved stability and retention of his or her complete dentures. A metal bar (i.e., Miller or Hader) is attached to the implants (see Figure 4.9). The overdenture is attached to the bar by clips and overdenture is held in place also by various implant attachments (i.e., Locator caps or O-rings). This affords the patient more comfort and improved chewing ability.

The Removable full-arch bar-supported attachment-retained prosthesis has a bar that connects the implants for additional retention and is not removable by the patient, but the overdenture prosthesis that attaches is removable for cleaning. The overdenture prosthesis is supported by the bar to resist lateral displacement and based upon the number of implants and the type of attachment. The bar may also support the functional loads generated from chewing as opposed to the forces being distributed to the edentulous ridges with a tissue-supported attachment-retained overdenture. One bar supported option is the milled bar overdenture.

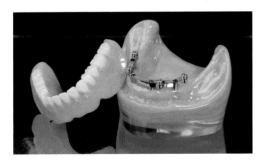

Figure 4.9 Milled bar-supported attachment-retained removable overdenture example. Courtesy of Glidewell.

Implant-supported fixed full-arch final prosthesis

A fixed full-arch final prosthesis, sometimes referred to as a hybrid (see Figure 4.10), is retained by abutment screws into the implants to provide replacement teeth in the edentulous arch *(i.e., All-on-4, Pro Arch, Neoss4+, TeethXpress)*. An implant-supported fixed full-arch, screw-retained final prosthesis provides the patient with the most aesthetic and stable option. Six to eight implants are placed in the upper jaw and five to six implants in the lower jaw to support the restorations that are nonremovable by the patient but can be removed by a dental professional if needed.

This option is considered the most natural looking option for the patient, over the removable overdenture option. The understructure for the crowns and pontics are cast as one piece. Patients will like the *palate-free option benefit* of being better able to taste their food instead of plastic, the comfort, and the aesthetic appearance. It has the added benefit of being nonremovable by the patient, but removable by the dental professional for evaluation of the implants, abutments, and for implant maintenance.

All-on-4

The All-on-4 is a trademarked treatment concept for edentulous arches developed by Nobel Biocare (see Figure 4.11). This procedure was the first implant-supported fixed full-arch option and *uses angled posterior implants* allowing for minimal number

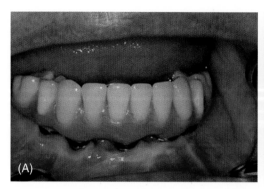
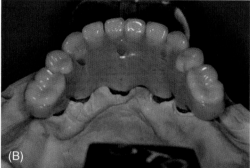

Figure 4.10 Fixed-removable screw-retained hybrid final prosthesis in patient's mouth and presented from the lab. Courtesy of Dr. Robert Schneider.

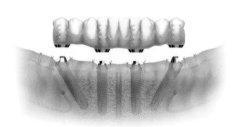

Figure 4.11 All-on-4 example. Courtesy of Nobel Biocare®.

of implants plus no bone grafting procedures. Patients can benefit from this procedure with immediate implant-supported prosthesis the same day. A provisional prosthesis is screwed onto the implants immediately after surgery. There are multiple fixed immediate solutions for edentulous patients. The restorative dentist and implant surgeon will treatment plan using the implant manufacturer they feel offers the patient the best results.

Specialty options pontic designs, cases by Robert Schneider, DDS, MS

A pontic is an artificial tooth to fill the space created within a dental arch by a missing tooth. It is attached to the abutment retainers (teeth or implants) by connectors (solder joints) (31). The condition pertaining to an edentulous space requires detailed attention to pontic design if the space is to be restored and maintained by appropriate hygiene in an acceptable manner (see Figure 4.12). Generally, the criteria for pontics described in Box 4.1 should be met to ensure proper oral hygiene access and maintenance (32).

Types of pontics most frequently utilized
Ridge Lap: This is an undesirable shape for a pontic. The large concave gingival contour makes the removal of plaque and calculus difficult and likely impossible. Soft-tissue inflammation is often associated with this type of pontic.

Modified Ridge Lap: This is the most popular type of design. It provides good aesthetics with a convex contour toward the tissues and is much easier to clean.

Ovate: Developed in the 1980s, this design has a convex *bullet* shape and is easier to clean. A drawback is that in scalloped periodontium, it is sometimes very difficult to get floss to pass under this design without damaging the soft tissues, especially in patients with a thin biotype of periodontium (33).

Pontic materials
Historically, most authors feel that glazed porcelain is the material of choice for pontics against the edentulous ridge, however, many other investigators have shown there

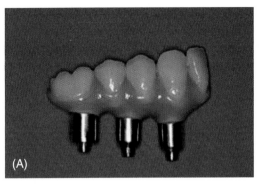
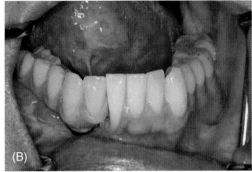

Figure 4.12   Gunshot case. Courtesy of Dr. Robert Schneider.

Box 4.1   Criteria for pontics

■ The tissue surface of the pontic area should be convex for easy cleaning.
■ Pontics should seldom, if ever, put pressure on the underlying tissues.
■ The pontic and connectors must be of adequate bulk to withstand occlusal forces but not impinge on the interproximal tissues.
■ Pontics should be aesthetic where indicated and restore masticatory function.

---

is no clinical or histologic difference in the response of the mucosa to pontics properly fabricated of cast gold, acrylic resin, or glazed porcelain (33, 34). Today, many clinicians are utilizing zirconium restorations for most of their routine fixed implant restorations. However, currently there is no long-term histologic data to prove this material is superior. The consensus is that the soft tissues tolerate highly polished or glazed zirconia well.

Maintenance criteria for pontics

All pontic tissue surfaces should be *convex and not concave* to allow for ease of cleansability by the patient and the hygienist. The embrasures in the posterior of the arch should be open for hygiene access. While the embrasures in the maxillary and occasionally the mandibular anterior are under the influence of aesthetics and phonetics and are usually more closed than is opti-

mally desirable in the posterior, they must also be designed in such a manner as to afford optimal access and cleanse ability.

Summary

Tooth restoration becomes a lifestyle choice and not just a choice to repair what was lost. Hygienists need the knowledge of the features and benefits of all the different restorative options to have a conversation with their patients on the advantages to implant dentistry. A maxillary full upper traditional denture versus no palate implant-retained prosthesis can help or omit gagging, aesthetic bone retention, and improve chewing and taste.

Also, hygienists should be able to identify the specialized pontics that are convex or concave. The convex are going to allow for the patient and the hygienist ease of cleansibility, so a hygienist should be aware of the concave pontics and monitor these more closely at implant maintenance appointments.

Hygienists, include in your conversations with your patients the differences between implant tooth replacements and natural teeth. Highlight that one implant can replace multiple teeth in some locations and still maintain the space, function, and bone. For fully edentulous patients, explain all the advantages of implant-supported fixed or removable prosthesis for function, comfort, increased stability, improved self-esteem, and confidence that make it the primary choice. For more on having a conversation with your patient on the risks, benefits, and alternatives to replacing missing teeth, refer to Chapter 5.

Treatment planning for long-term implant success

Contributed by Maria L. Geisinger, DDS, MS

It has been well established that careful treatment planning to identify risk factors and establish ideal conditions for implant placement is critical to success for dental implant therapy (35–37). To ensure that the patient is set up for success, initial examination and interdisciplinary treatment planning is critical to success. A dental hygienist has a key role in the initial treatment planning in gathering important medical and dental history and assessing the current oral condition of the patient a well as identifying potential tooth replacement options for missing and/or hopeless teeth.

In order to *set the stage* and *create an environment* for optimal treatment outcomes, adjunctive procedures and careful treatment planning are a critical component to establish health and place implants in ideal positions for the necessary restorative care. Dental hygienists are often the first point of contact for a patient who might benefit from dental implant therapy and can begin the process of assessing patient desires, examining the current oral condition, and discussing treatment options, including the risks and benefits of various therapies, with patients. It is important to understand patients' individual desires and their expectations as well as address concerns, including financial and time commitments, prior to initiation of any treatment. A frank discussion with patients about implant therapies and what

they may entail is important to allow patients to truly provide informed consent for implant treatment.

As an integral part of the dental implant treatment team, dental hygienists provide preventative care for peri-implant diseases and are well equipped to discuss with patients the rationale for restorative and surgical care that is recommended during the course of implant therapy. Understanding the treatment planning steps and the procedures performed during implant therapy is key to be able to provide this critical information to patients.

Treatment planning introduction

Dental implants should be restoratively driven and biologically executed. In order to achieve high levels of success, risk factors for both biologic and prosthetic/mechanical risk factors should be identified in the initial patient evaluation. While longitudinal survival rates of osseointegrated dental implants range between 90% and 95% (38–40), these numbers represent implants that are present and in function, but may not fully capture rates of peri-implant disease and/or health. It is estimated that rates of peri-implantitis range from 10% to 47% (41–43) and rates of peri-implant mucositis have been observed in up to 65% of subjects with dental implants (44). It has also been demonstrated that the incidence of peri-implant diseases may be increased based upon specific risk factors (43, 45, 46).

Given the high prevalence of peri-implant diseases, preventative measures should be addressed in the treatment planning process, including identification of patient-related risk factors, long-term maintenance, and meticulous oral home care. Peri-implant diseases are initiated by accumulation of dental plaque biofilm and exposure to such biofilm leads to inflammatory changes in tissues surrounding the implants (41, 44, 47, 48). This bacterial primary etiology, therefore (45), dental implant at initial placement and the elimination of niches for bacterial accumulation (49). It has been noted that once inflammation has been established it is very difficult to eliminate through noninvasive means (50, 51). After implant placement, regular maintenance and monitoring allows for early identification of disease and significantly reduces the presence of dysbiotic peri-implant microbiota (mucositis and peri-implantitis that demonstrate different subgingival biofilm composition) (52).

Dental implant complications: risk factors and prevention

Biologic complications

Biologic complications, peri-implant mucositis and peri-implantitis, have been associated with systemic diseases, medications, anatomical and site-specific factors, smoking status, periodontal disease history, adherence to peri-implant maintenance and plaque control, and peri-implant soft-tissue quality and quantity (35, 37, 47, 48). To identify individuals at an increased risk for biologic complications of implant therapy, a thorough review of medical and dental history as well as a comprehensive oral examination is necessary. In particular, establishment of periodontal health prior to dental implant placement is critical to long-term reduction of biologic complications in patients receiving dental implants. It is well established that a history of periodontitis is a risk factor for peri-implantitis (47, 48, 52, 53). Findings suggest that bacteria associated with periodontal disease and peri-implant diseases are similar (54–56). Colonization with these bacterial species occurs within the first 28 days after implant exposure to the oral environment (55) and bacteria can be transferred from distant reservoirs, such as periodontal pockets at teeth elsewhere within a patient's mouth (57).

Furthermore, during treatment planning, assessment of the local site for implant placement is a critical step. Anatomic variations at sites throughout the oral cavity may influence overall implant success. These anatomic variations may also have myriad underlying causes, including as sequelae of resorptive processes after extraction or trauma, resultant hard and soft tissue loss due to periodontitis or peri-implantitis, growth and development, and other factors (58). Generally, the maxillary alveolar bone is less dense than the mandible, particularly in the posterior maxilla, and implants that are placed in these areas may have decreased primary stability and overall success rates (59, 60).

While these clinical scenarios are generally not associated with peri-implantitis, implant placement in a suboptimal position to avoid anatomical structures or inadequate bone volume may lead to either off-axis forces or increased plaque retention, which may predispose an implant to peri-implant mucositis or peri-implantitis. Lastly, a careful dental history to assess previous procedures at the proposed implant site is critically important. Placement of implants at sites where a previous implant has failed has demonstrated lower survival rates than reported for implant placement at a naïve site (61). Retreated sites have reported cumulative survival rates of 86.3% (61), which while this represents an overall decrease in survival, may still be acceptable, particularly if a modifiable risk factor can be identified and addressed.

Prosthetic complications

Prosthetic complications include six general categories of technical or mechanical failures: loosening of screws, screw fracture, fracture of framework, fracture of abutment, chipping/fracture of veneering material, and decementation (62). Overall, prosthetic/occlusal risk factors in the absence of inflammation are not thought to increase the risk of peri-implantitis, but these factors may modify disease progression if inflammation is present. Factors that may increase the risk for prosthetic complications include prosthesis design and occlusal overload, retained cement, and history of parafunctional habits. It is also important to note that prosthetic complications may be associated with industrial components (i.e., implant and/or abutment fracture) and those associated with customized components (i.e., restorative porcelain veneer fracture, restoration debonding) (63).

Assessment of risk factors for implant complications prior to implant placement may inform maintenance intervals and/or drive surgical and restorative choices to create the lowest risk environment for development of such complications (52).

Adjunctive surgical procedures overview

Implant site preparation procedures
To establish ideal function and aesthetics, implant site preparation procedures are often required. Bone volume in a position that allows for ideal prosthetic restoration is critical to creating a functional occlusion and establishing a healthy and cleansable implant environment. To achieve these goals, careful treatment planning and evaluation is required and selection of surgical and restorative treatments that allow for optimal outcomes is necessary.

Initial clinical and radiographic evaluation
Initial evaluation, including a comprehensive oral examination is necessary to establish baseline diagnoses and develop a treatment plan. Additionally, in patients who are missing teeth, digital and/or analog impressions to create a prosthetic

wax-up is critical. This wax-up can then be used to create a radiographic guide and to facilitate capture of radiographic images, in particular 3-D cone beam computerized tomography (CBCT). Assessment of the underlying osseous architecture in the presence of the ideal positioning for the prosthesis allows for evaluation of underlying tissues and the potential for hard tissue augmentation prior to or simultaneous with dental implant placement. It is also important to note that some grafting procedures may require temporization techniques that avoid applying pressure to grafted areas or that shape soft tissues during the healing process. In this way, coordination of restorative and surgical care can result in optimal functional and aesthetic outcomes.

Tooth extraction: natural healing and ridge preservation
In patients who are planned for extraction and subsequent implant placement, it is important to consider how the extraction site will heal and what procedures may be performed to limit volumetric loss at the extraction site. Following tooth extraction, if no grafting is performed, bony resorption is observed with an average loss of 0.9 ± 1.6 mm vertical bone height and 2.7 ± 1.2 mm bucco-lingual ridge dimension (64). Furthermore, in areas with prominent roots, periodontal attachment loss, and/or dehiscences or fenestrations demonstrate more significant resorption (65, 66). It is anticipated that an undisturbed blood clot will result in healing beginning at the apical extent of the socket and histologic new bone formation (67). While this healing will result in new, vital bone formation, it may come at the cost of bone volume loss, which can result in an inability to place implants.

The progression of post-extraction healing is also dependent upon the presence of an intact socket, which may also be an important source of osteogenic material if ridge preservation grafting is performed (3, 65, 66). Because maintaining the socket architecture is so important to healing outcomes, minimally traumatic tooth extraction allows for more predictable healing. To accomplish minimally traumatic tooth extraction, flapless extraction techniques and utilization and delicate extraction instruments, such as periotomes (see Figure 4.1) and delicate elevators may be utilized. Furthermore, advanced technologies, like piezoelectric surgical instrumentation to section teeth or create targeted areas for purchase during extraction while preserving the surrounding hard and soft tissues (see Figure 4.13).

Ridge preservation procedures are designed to limit bone volume loss, but depending upon the bone replacement graft material used, may result in a decrease in the amount of new bone formation and an increase in the presence of residual bone particles at the time of implant placement. Ridge preservation involves placement of bone replacement grafts within the extraction socket to mitigate bone dimensional changes during the post-extraction healing period. While multiple systematic reviews have not found significant differences between ridge preservation grafting techniques or the materials used (67–70), buccal bone thickness > 1 mm was associated with improved healing outcomes (67). Furthermore, the use of barrier membranes in cases where bone fenestrations or large dehiscences are present have been shown to improve outcomes for ridge preservation procedures (70). It is important to note that other treatment options could include natural healing, delayed, early grafting after approximately 6–8 weeks of socket healing, immediate implant placement at the time of tooth extraction, or alveolar ridge preservation (71). The need of extraction socket preservation/augmentation immediately after tooth extraction should be determined by the aesthetic, functional, and risk-related viewpoint (71) (see Figure 4.2).

Bone replacement grafts

Bone replacement grafts are used throughout implant dentistry to serve as a scaffold and allow new bone formation at a desired site. These grafts are generally categorized by their source as (i) autogenous, (ii) allogeneic, (iii) xenograft, and (iv) alloplast. Autogenous bone is harvested from the patient receiving the bone graft and can come from an intraoral or extraoral source. While autogenous bone has the potential to contain osteoblasts and/or osteoblast progenitor cells, the use of autogenous bone can also be associated with increased intrasurgical time and increased morbidity at the donor site. Allogeneic bone is derived from a human tissue donor source and is processed so that cellular material is removed. It may be mineralized or demineralized and may contain cortical or cancellous bone or a mixture of both. Xenografts are bone replacement grafts from another species, generally bovine, porcine, or equine sources, and are treated with deproteination. Xenografts have been shown to

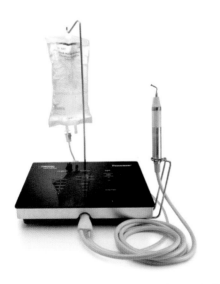

Figure 4.13 Example of a piezoelectric surgical unit. PIEZOSURGERY® touch by Mectron.

be volumetrically stable over long periods of time with very little resorption seen up to 9 years (72). Lastly, alloplastic materials are synthetic materials with anorganic mineral components such as hydroxyapatite or calcium sulfate. The choice of graft material should be based upon the procedure being performed and the requirements during the healing process.

Alveolar ridge augmentation

At sites where extractions have already occurred and post-extraction healing has resulted in inadequate bone volume for implant placement. In these cases, deficient ridges may be treated using vertical or lateral ridge augmentation procedures. While there are myriad techniques to increase bone width and height, the predictability of bone grafting in these cases may not be predictable in all clinical scenarios and some techniques may provide improved outcomes based upon the anatomic findings and patient-related conditions. In general, lateral ridge augmentation procedures are more predictable than vertical grafting procedures. All of these types of grafting rely on a *regional acceleratory phenomenon* (RAP), which leverages the wound healing capability after decortication and space maintenance to encourage new bone formation. Because of these underlying mechanisms, choosing graft and barrier materials which allow for volumetric stability and resorbtion at appropriate rates to encourage the healing at these sites. On average, lateral ridge augmentation procedures result in approximately 3.7 mm of bone gain (73) and vertical ridge augmentations result in approximately 4 mm of bone gain (74) (see Figure 4.3).

Sinus augmentation

Maxillary posterior tooth extraction can result in a relative expansion of the maxillary sinus resulting in inadequate bone height for implant placement in the posterior maxilla. In order to determine the ideal sinus augmentation treatment, quantification of the residual bone coronal to the maxillary sinus is critical and can be assessed using CBCT images. It should also be noted that sinus augmentation may be performed via a lateral or a vertical approach, depending upon the amount of bone augmentation needed. A lateral sinus augmentation can generally result in more bone gain when compared to a vertical approach (i.e., 8.5 mm versus 4.4 mm, respectively) (75). Lastly, simultaneous implant placement may be performed if adequate coronal bone height is present to stabilize the implant during the healing process (see example of sinus augmentation case, Figure 4.4).

Other treatment options at severely deficient sites

While the above grafting techniques may be sufficient in many cases, for sites with severely atrophic alveolar bone, more advanced techniques may be required. These may include the use of distraction osteogenesis, extraoral bone graft harvest, lateral nerve repositioning, and the use of zygomatic or pterygoid implants. All of these techniques require high levels of skill and familiarity with the individual treatment modalities as well as advanced prosthetic plans, including temporization plans.

Adjunctive soft-tissue grafting at dental implants

It has been proposed that the establishment of a circumferential seal of tightly packed collagen around the implant–oral cavity interface may improve long-term implant success and that this is better facilitated in the presence of keratinized mucosa (76). Implant survival rates have been shown to be equivalent for implants placed in keratinized and alveolar mucosa, but increased radiographic bone loss and higher levels of gingival inflammation are associated with a lack of keratinized mucosa (77, 78). Particularly in patients with other biologic risk factors, including increased oral biofilm accumulation and previous history of periodontitis, increased keratinized mucosa and increased mucosal thickness may be protective to allow for personal and professional oral biofilm removal (77–80). Based on this, adjunctive therapy is used to increase the band of keratinization around dental implants may improve implant outcomes and allow patients to better perform oral home care around dental implants (81, 82). Both free gingival grafts and connective tissue grafts have demonstrated increased postoperative gingival thickness and keratinization, which can improve long-term outcomes (83, 84).

Treatment planning overview

Setting the stage for patients starts with the end in mind. Are adjunctive tissue or bone regenerative procedures needed first before implant placement? What are the patient's wants for a final result?

Understanding a patient's desires and ultimate goals is critically important in developing a treatment plan that will be well accepted by the patient. It is also important to understand the feasibility of different treatment options and the individualized patient risk factors that should be considered for this case. Hygienists have the key role of building a relationship with the patient to help determine and clearly define what the patient wants included in their dental implant treatment plan. The hygienist often has the most direct relationship with the patient and can be the most aware of the patient's oral health and ability to do daily home care.

Understand the differences in quality of life for the patient of a tissue-supported denture, loose on the bone, or bar-retained implant(s)-supported overdenture that snaps in place. Or a fixed removable that is a thinner overdenture, removable only by a dental professional with the advantage of teeth and tissue plus stability.

The hygienist's influence and input are invaluable in the treatment process that goes far beyond the single unit restorations. Careful assessment of current levels of oral hygiene and patient dexterity can allow for determination of realistic future home care capabilities and can play a role in how well the restoration will be maintained. This insight can allow for selection of restorations that can be maintained healthy for years to come and may sway the decision making between fixed and removable implant-supported restorations. For example, when deciding between a bar overdenture versus the one supported by a locator, it is well established that the bar will need more visual and hand dexterity to keep clean and a patient's ability to maintain implant health is critical to long-term implant success.

To achieve case acceptance and a satisfied, happy patient you need to start with the end in mind. There are often many treatment options, ranges of expense, and time commitments to propose to the patient. The key is not to begin the treatment process until the final treatment plan and financial arrangements have been made, and, most importantly, the patient's questions have all been answered. This allows for truly informed consent and results in patients who are more committed to therapy.

Therefore, just as a builder does not start constructing a house until the architect has made the final plans, we should not begin implant therapy until a final treatment plan is formulated (85; see Box 4.2). A good rule to follow is to listen to the patient, understand what the patient wants and can afford, and agree on a treatment plan.

Box 4.2 Comprehensive treatment plan

■ Assess patient's chief complaint and expectations.
■ Understand patient's motivation and limitations.
■ Collect data to assess patient risk factors and overall oral health.
■ Present and explain treatment options, including adjunctive and restorative treatment options.
■ Discuss advantages and disadvantages of all treatment options.
■ Develop a final treatment plan that meets the patient's needs and expectations, allow patient to ask questions about the treatments, and document the consent discussion with a signed treatment plan and consent form.

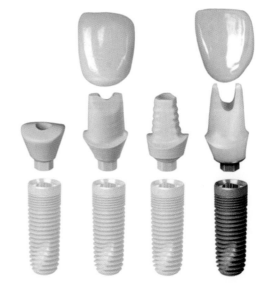

Figure 4.14 Custom CAD milled provisional components, abutment, and BruxZuir crown. Courtesy of Glidewell.

What can I expect to happen during the preliminary examination process?

It is important to inform the patient that implant dentistry is not a quick fix. The time and number of appointments will depend on the prosthesis and if any adjunctive procedures are needed before or after the implant is placed. The healing time will vary depending on the bone quality, tissue health, and the overall health of the patient. Implant success relies on the biology of hard and soft-tissue healing and these biological processes take time to achieve optimal results.

The patient's aesthetic and functional expectations also have a direct correlation to the number of appointments necessary. What aesthetic adjunctive procedures may be necessary? Is a provisional restoration or prosthesis requested? Is there a desired time frame for treatment completion?

Provisionals are natural-looking, temporary restorations (i.e., crown or bridge), temporary denture, or Essix retainer that can be worn by the patient at different stages of treatment for aesthetics and/or function (see Figure 4.14). If a provisional

restoration or prosthesis is requested by the patient, it can be planned in advance, but may require more appointments and expense for the patient.

Present all the options for tooth replacement, as well as costs and time frame considerations, and explain necessary adjunctive procedures that might be needed to regenerate the bone or tissue. Ask the patient what questions he or she has for the dentist prior to the dentist coming into the room for the exam. Patients are often more relaxed and have a closer relationship with their hygienist, which makes them more likely to talk freely. The hygienist can relay these questions, from the patient, to the dentist.

Once the patient has decided to have implant therapy, the dentist, hygienist, and assistant can gather the necessary diagnostic records. The hygienist can start with a visual assessment of tissue, asking questions such as, is it keratinized? Keratinized tissue is optimal for implant/tissue interface and will be less prone to peri-implantitis and peri-implant gingival recession after the implant is restored (86). A lack of keratinized and/or attached gingiva may indicate a need for adjunctive soft-tissue grafting prior to or in conjunction with implant therapy.

A comprehensive periodontal exam should occur, involving charting of existing dental oral health and with any pain or mobility recorded. Since periodontitis is a risk factor for peri-implant diseases, diagnosis of periodontal disease and treatment prior to implant therapy is critically important to overall success. Tooth mobility, occlusal trauma, malocclusion, and screening for oral pathology should be undertaken prior to developing a treatment plan and initiating care. Preoperative photographs need to be taken of the patient's full face, with a close up on just the smile, and of the proposed implant site. The implant site is documented for soft-tissue contours, adjacent teeth, and aesthetics.

The dentist and assistant start with a set of diagnostic casts to do a digital or prosthetic wax-up of the proposed implant treatment case. The surgeon may also want a surgical template (also referred to as a surgical guide) that is fabricated based on the diagnostic data to identify where each implant is to be placed. Other diagnostic records that will be needed are radiographs, bite records, and a shade of the patient's existing teeth for provisional and final restoration.

Having this information is valuable to the dentist to precisely plan the patient's implant case, from both the surgical and the prosthetic perspectives. Also identify any potential problems and plan in advance on what type, length, and prosthesis would be best suited for the treatment plan.

The surgeon will need a full-mouth series of radiographs and, in general, will use a 3-D image of the patient's jaws to assess the bone contours, and locate anatomical structures, including nerves, blood vessels (i.e., mandibular canal), foramina, and sinuses before implant surgery. Intraoral digital scanning may also be used to digitally capture soft-tissue contours as well and these images can be combined with cone beam computerized tomography (CBCT) bone-level data as well.

In general, in the dental office, the use of cone beam computerized tomography (CBCT) scan technology is the most common diagnostic 3-D radiograph ordered prior to implant placement (see Figure 4.15). A CBCT scan offers a diagnostic 3-D view of an implant site (topography of the osseous structures) with the lowest radiation (87–89). CBCT scan technology is an extremely valuable diagnostic tool with software that allows the surgeon to preplan placement of the implants by length and diameter, and identify the anatomical anatomy to avoid (i.e., mandibular canal, alveolar nerve). The CBCT can also provide the necessary data to fabricate the surgical guide used in surgery for accurate placement of the implants. Surgical guides that are based upon bone and tissue-level digital images can allow for more exact implant placement and guided surgery (refer to Figures 4.15 and 4.16).

The dentist is the quarterback of the implant team and can coordinate care with an implant surgeon, laboratory, and any other specialists who will be involved in the patient's treatment case (i.e., orthodontist, periodontist, or prosthodontist). The implants, abutments, and choice of restorative prosthesis need to be identified by the surgeon/restorative doctor team and agreed upon prior to surgery. All members of the team can work together to develop a plan that allows for optimal restorative results. Having team members with a variety of perspectives is ideal to allow for treatment that is prosthetically driven and biologically executed. The integration of digital planning into the treatment planning armamentarium has allowed for integration of this through review and approval of digital files and can speed the treatment planning process (refer to Figures 4.17 and 4.18).

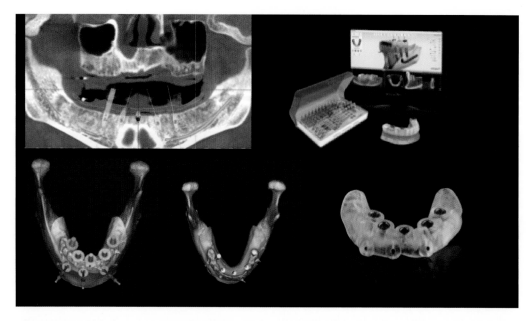

Figure 4.15 Digital treatment lanning, CBCT, and surgical guide fabrication. Courtesy of Dr. M. Geisinger.

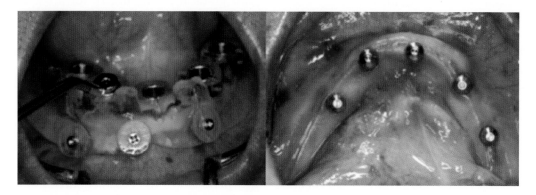

Figure 4.16 Surgical guide and flapless implant placement surgery. Courtesy of Dr. M. Geisinger.

Once the treatment plan is complete, the restoration/prosthesis is chosen, adjunctive procedures planned the treatment conference with the patient can be scheduled. At the treatment conference the treatment plan is discussed, including the restorative/provisional options, and the time sequencing agreed on by dentist and patient. The patient then needs to sign a consent form stating that he or she understands all that has been presented to him or her. *Be sure all the i's are dotted and t's are crossed before the implant surgery is performed*. The patient is given a proposed time schedule and appointment dates, and all the possible variables have been explained.

The laboratory will prepare for the temporary phase of treatment with customized or lab-created prosthesis ahead of surgical date. The surgeon or dentist will do the implant surgery and determine when the implant is ready to be restored. Once the implant is restored and functional, the patient will be scheduled for his or her first implant maintenance appointment.

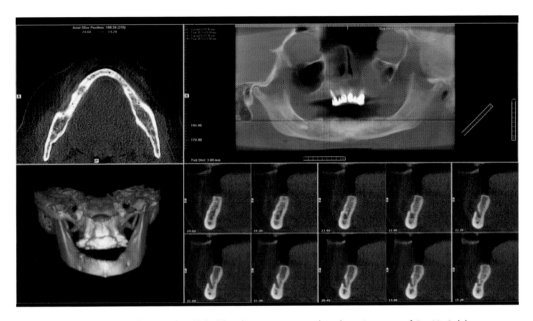

Figure 4.17   CBCT images for digital implant treatment planning. Courtesy of Dr. M. Geisinger.

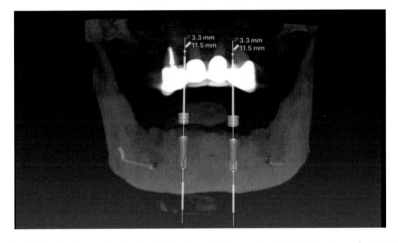

Figure 4.18   Digital software for implant planning with bone level CBCT. Courtesy of Dr. M. Geisinger.

Summary

Hygienists play the key role to clearly define the patient's wants, needs, and expectations. Understand the patient's motivation and time commitments. The hygienist can discuss with the patient all restorative and adjunctive procedure options if they feel comfortable or schedule an implant consultation appointment with office implant coordinator and/or doctor.

Implant dentistry is here to stay and can be a valuable procedure to offer to your patients. It is important the entire team is consistent in the answers given to patients and to learn all the implant terminology associated with implant surgery and adjunctive procedures (see Chapter 1 and Appendix), for implant terminology.

Enjoy sharing this opportunity of implant dentistry with your patients!

References

1. Pietrokovski J, Massler M Alveolar ridge resorption following tooth extraction. J Prosthet Dent. 1967; 17: 21–27.

2. Amler MH, Johnson PL, Salman I Histological and histochemical investigation of human alveolar socket healing in undisturbed extraction wounds. J Am Dent Assoc. 1960; 6: 46–48.

3. Horowitz RA, Mazor D Atraumatic extraction: advantages and implementation. Inside Dent. 2010; 6(7).

4. Schlee M, Steigmann M, Bratu E, Garg A Piezosurgery: basics and possibilities. Implant Dent. 2006; 15(4): 334–340.

5. Fickl S, Zuhr O, Wachtel H, Bolz W, Huerzeler M Tissue alterations after tooth extraction with and without surgical trauma: a volumetric study in the beagle dog. J Clin Periodontol. 2008; 35(4): 356–363.

6. Tal H, Artzi Z Porous bovine bone mineral in healing of human extraction sockets. Part 1: histomorphometric evaluations at 9 months. J Periodontol. 2000; 71(6): 1015–1023.

7. Clokie C, Sennerby L, Urist MR, Becker BE Histologic findings after implantation and evaluation of different grafting materials and titanium micro-screws into extraction sockets: case reports. J Periodontol. 1998; 69(4): 414–421.

8. Stavropoulos F, Dahlin C, Ruskin J, Johansson C A comparative study of barrier membranes as graft protectors in the treatment of localized bone defects: an experimental study in a canine model. Clin Oral Implants Res. 2004; 15(4): 435–442.

9. Becker W, Becker B Guided tissue regeneration for implants placed into extraction sockets and for implant dehiscences: surgical techniques and case reports. Int J Periodontics Restorative Dent. 1990; 10: 377–391.

10. Zitzmann NY, Naef R, Scharer P Resorbable versus nonresorbable membranes in combination with Bio-Oss for guided bone regeneration. Int J Oral Maxillofac Implants. 1997; 12: 844–852.

11. Horowitz RA Extraction environment enhancement: critical evaluation of early socket in long-term barrier-protected extraction sockets. Compend Contin Educ Dent. 2005; 26(10): 703–713.

12. Hoffmann O, Bartee BK, Beaumont C, Kasaj A, Deli G, Zafiropoulos GG Alveolar bone preservation in extraction sockets using non-resorbable dPTFE membranes: a retrospective non-randomized study. J Periodontol. 2008; 79(8): 1355–1369.

13. Carmagnola D, Adriaens P, Berglundh T Healing of human extraction sockets filled with Bio-Oss. Clin Oral Implants Res. 2003; 14(2): 137–143.

14. Becker W, Becker BE, Caffesse R A comparison of demineralized freeze-dried bone and autologous bone formation in human extraction sockets. J Periodontol. 1994; 65: 1128–1133.

15. Sottosanti JS Calcium sulfate: a valuable addition to the implant/bone regeneration complex. Dent Implantol Updat. 1997; 8(4): 25–29.

16. Vance GS, Greenwell H, Miller RL, Hill M, Johnston H, Scheetz JP Comparison of an allograft in an experimental putty carrier and a bovine-derived xenograft used in ridge preservation: a clinical and histologic study in humans. Int J Oral Maxilofac Implants. 2004; 19(4): 491–497.

17. Mazor ZP, Horowitz R, Ricci J, Alexander H, Chesnoiu-Matei I, Mamidwar S The use of a novel nano-crystalling calcium sulfate for bone regeneration in extraction socket. J Implant Adv Clin Dent. 2011; 3(5): 39–49.

18. Horowitz RA, Mazor Z, Miller RJ, Krauser J, Prasad HS, Rohrer MD Clinical evaluation alveolar ridge preservation with a beta-tricalcium phosphate socket graft. Compend Contin Educ Dent. 2009; 30(9): 588–590, 592, and 594.

19. Pikos MA Mandibular block autografts for alveolar ridge augmentation. Atlas Oral Maxillofac Surg Clin North Am. 2005; 13(2): 91–107.

20. Pikos MA Alveolar ridge augmentation with ramus buccal shelf autografts and impacted third molar removal. Dent Implantol Updat. 1999; 10(4): 27–31.

21. Toscano N, Holtzclaw D, Mazor Z, Rosen P, Horowitz R, Toffler M Horizontal ridge augmentation utilizing a composite graft of demineralized freeze-dried allograft, mineralized cortical cancellous chips, and a biologically degradable thermoplastic carrier combined with a resorbable membrane: a retrospective evaluation of 73 consecutively treated cases from private practices. J Oral Implantol. 2010; 36(6): 467–474.

22. Kuperschlag A, Keršytė G, Kurtzman GM, Horowitz RA Autogenous dentin grafting of osseous defects distal to mandibular second molars after extraction of impacted third molars. Compend Contin Educ Dent. 2020; 41(2): 76–82.

23. Mazor Z, Horowitz RA, Prasad H, Kotsakis GA Healing dynamics following alveolar ridge preservation with autologous tooth structure. Int J Periodontics Restorative Dent. 2019; 39: 697–702.

24. Kurtzman GM, Horowitz RA, Hallas MB, El-Bialy T Improving osseous conditions around teeth

and implants utilizing high frequency vibration. J Osseointegration. 2021; 13(1): 35–42.

25. McGuire MK, Scheyer ET, Nevins M, Schupbach P Evaluation of human recession defects treated with coronally advanced flaps and either purified recombinant human platelet-derived growth factor-BB with beta tricalcium phosphate or connective tissue: a histologic and microcomputed tomographic examination. Int J Periodontics Restorative Dent. 2009; 29(1): 7–21.

26. Nevins ML, Said S Minimally invasive esthetic ridge preservation with growth-factor enhanced bone matrix. J Esthet Restor Dent. 2018; 30(3): 180–186.

27. Jivraj S, Chee W Treatment planning of implants in posterior quadrants. Br Dent J. 2006; 201: 13–23.

28. Carlsson GE, Hedegard B, Koivumaa KK Studies in partial denture prostheses: I. A 4-year longitudinal investigation of dentogingivally-supported partial dentures. Acta Odontol Scand. 1965; 23: 443–472.

29. American College of Prosthodontists. Facts & Figures. https://www.gotoapro.org/facts-figures/

30. Curley AW Dental implant jurisprudence avoiding the legal failures. J Calif Dent Assoc. 2001; 29(12): 847–853.

31. Stein RS Pontic-residual ridge relationship: a research report. J Prosthet Dent. 1966; 16: 251–285.

32. Howard WW, Ueno H, Pruitt CO Standards of pontic design. J Prosthet Dent. 1982; 47: 493–495.

33. Becker CM, Kaldahl WB Current theories of crown contour, margin placement, and pontic design. J Prosthet Dent. 2005; 93: 107–115.

34. Liu S Use of a modified ovate pontic in areas of ridge defects: a report of two cases. J Esthet Restor Dent. 2004; 16: 273–283.

35. Geisinger ML, Calvert Grosso K, Kaur M, et al. Clinical decision making for primary peri-implantitis prevention: practical applications. Clin Adv Periodontics. 2021; 11: 43–53.

36. Dixon DR, London RM Restorative design and association risks for peri-implant diseases. Periodontol. 2019; 81: 167–178.

37. Romanos GE, Delgado-Ruiz R, Sculean A Concepts for prevention of complications in implant dentistry. Periodontol. 2019; 81: 7–17.

38. Esposito M, Hirsch JM, Lekholm U, Thomsen P Biological factors contributing to failures of osseointegrated oral implants. (II). Etiopathogenesis. Eur J Oral Sci. 1998; 106: 721–764.

39. Ashey ET, Covington LL, Bishop BG, Breault LG Ailing and failing endosseous dental implants: a literature review. J Contemp Dent Pract. 2003; 4(2): 1–12.

40. Academy Report: AAP, Rosen P, Clem D, Cochran D, et al. Peri-implant mucositis and peri-implantitis: a current understanding of their diagnoses and clinical implications. J Periodontol. 2013; 84: 436–443.

41. Mombelli A, Müller N, Cionca N The epidemiology of peri-implantitis. Clin Oral Implants Res. 2012; 23(Suppl 6): 67–76.

42. Dierks J, Tomasi C Peri-implant health and disease: a systematic review of current epidemiology. J Clin Periodontol. 2015; 42(Suppl 16): S158–S171.

43. Fransson C, Wennström J, Tomasi C, Berglundh T Extent of peri-implantitis associated bone loss. J Clin Periodontol. 2009; 36: 357–363.

44. Atieh MA, Alsabeeha NH, Faggion CM Jr, Duncan WJ The frequency of peri-implant diseases: a systematic review and meta-analysis. J Periodontol. 2013; 84: 1586–1598.

45. Sgolastra F, Petrucci A, Severina M, Gatto R, Monaco A Periodontitis, implant loss and peri-implantitis: a meta-analysis. Clin Oral Implants Res. 2015; 26: e8–e16.

46. Heitz-Mayfield L, Salvi G Peri-implant mucositis. Proceedings from the 2017 World Workshop. J Periodontol. 2018; 89(Suppl 1): S257–S266.

47. Schwarz F, Derks J, Monje A, Wang H-L Peri-implantitis. Proceedings from the 2017 World Workshop. J Periodontol. 2018; 89(Suppl 1): S267–S290.

48. Jepsen S, Berglundh T, Genco R, et al. Primary prevention of peri-implantitis: managing peri-implant mucositis. J Clin Periodontol; 42(Suppl 16): S152–S157.

49. Clementini M, Rossetti PH, Penarrocha D, Micarelli C, Bonachela WC, Canullo L Systemic risk factors for peri-implant bone loss: a systematic review and meta-analysis. Int J Oral Maxillofac Surg. 2014; 43: 323–334.

50. Schwartz F, Beckter K, Sager M Efficacy of professionally administered plaque removal with or without adjunctive measures for the treatment of peri-implant mucositis. A systematic review and meta-analysis. J Clin Periodontol. 2015; 42(Suppl 16): S202–S213.

51. Costa FO, Ferreira SD, Cortelli JR, et al. Microbiological profile associated with peri-implant diseases in individuals with and without preventive maintenance therapy: a 5-year follow-up. Clin Oral Investig. 2019; 23: 3161–3171.

52. Curtis DA, Lin G-H, Fishman A, et al. Patient-centered risk assessment in implant treatment planning. *Int J Oral Maxillofac Implants*. 2019; 34: 506–520.
53. Araujo MG, Lindhe J Peri-implant health. Proceedings from the 2017 World Workshop. *J Periodontol*. 2018; 89(Suppl 1): S249–S256.
54. Renvert S, Roos-Jansaker AM, Lindahl C, et al. Infection at titanium implants with or without a clinical diagnosis of inflammation. *Clin Oral Implants Res*. 2007; 18: 509–516.
55. Mombelli A, Lang NP The diagnosis and treatment of peri-implantitis. *Periodontol*. 1998; 17: 63–76.
56. Ata-Ali J, Candel-Marti M, Flichy-Fernandez A, et al. Peri-implantitis: associated microbiota and treatment. *Med Oral Patol Oral Cir Bucal*. 2011; 16: e937–e943.
57. Quirynen M, Vogels R, Peeters W, et al. Dynamics of subgingival colonization of 'pristine' peri-implant pockets. *Clin Oral Implants Res*. 2006; 17: 25–37.
58. Hammerle CH, Tarnow D The etiology of hard- and soft-tissue deficiencies at dental implants: a narrative review. *J Periodontol*. 2018; 89(Suppl 1): S291–S303.
59. Monje A, Chan HL, Galindo-Moreno P, et al. Alveolar bone architecture: a systematic review and meta-analysis. *J Periodontol*. 2015; 86: 1231–1248.
60. Monje A, Ravida A, Wang H-L, Helms JA, Brunski JB Relationship between primary/mechanical and secondary/biological implant stability. *Int J Oral Maxillofac Implants*. 2019; 34(Suppl 8): s7–s23.
61. Oh S-L, Shiau HJ, Reynolds MA Survival of dental implants at sites after implant failure: a systematic review. *J Prosthet Dent*. 2020; 123(1): 54–60.
62. Sadid-Zadeh R, Kutkut A, Kim H Prosthetic failure in implant dentistry. *Dent Clin N Am*. 2015; 59: 195–214.
63. Heitz-Mayfield LJ, Needleman I, Salvi GE, Pjetursson BE Consensus statements and clinical recommendations for prevention and management of biologic and technical implant complications. *Int J Oral Maxillofac Implants*. 2014; 29(Suppl): 346–350.
64. Iasella JM, Greenwell H, Miller RL, et al. Ridge preservation with freeze-dried bone allograft and a collagen membrane compared to extraction alone for implant site development: a clinical and histological study in humans. *J Periodontol*. 2003; 74(7): 990–999.
65. Nevins M, Camelo M, De Paoli S, et al. A study of the fate of the buccal wall of extraction sockets of teeth with prominent roots. *Int J Periodontics Restorative Dent*. 2006; 26(1): 19–29.
66. Aimetti M, Manavella V, Corano L, Ercoli E, Bignardi C, Romano F Three-dimensional analysis of bone remodeling following ridge augmentation of compromised extraction sockets in periodontitis patients: a randomized controlled study. *Clin Oral Implants Res*. 2018; 29(2): 202–214.
67. Avila-Ortiz G, Chambrone L, Vignoletti F Effect of alveolar ridge preservation interventions following tooth extraction: a systematic review and meta-analysis. J Clin Periodontol. 2019; 46(Suppl 21): 195–223. Erratum in: J Clin Periodontol. 2020; 47(1):129.
68. Avila-Ortiz G, Gubler M, Romero-Bustillos M, Nicholas CL, Zimmerman MB, Barwacz CA Efficacy of alveolar ridge preservation: a randomized controlled trial. *J Dent Res*. 2020; 99(4): 402–409.
69. MacBeth N, Trullenque-Eriksson A, Donos N, Mardas N Hard and soft tissue changes following alveolar ridge preservation: a systematic review. *Clin Oral Implants Res*. 2017; 28(8): 982–1004.
70. Atieh MA, Alsabeeha NH, Payne AG, Duncan W, Faggion CM, Esposito M Interventions for replacing missing teeth: alveolar ridge preservation techniques for dental implant site development. *Cochrane Database Syst Rev*. 2015; 2015(5): CD010176.
71. Juodzbalys G, Stumbras A, Goyushov S, Duruel O, Tözüm TF Morphological classification of extraction sockets and clinical decision tree for socket preservation/augmentation after tooth extraction: a systematic review. J Oral Maxillofac Res. 2019; 10(3): e3.
72. Galindo-Moreno P, Hernández-Cortés P, Mesa F, et al. Slow resorption of anorganic bovine bone by osteoclasts in maxillary sinus augmentation. *Clin Implant Dent Relat Res*. 2013; 15: 858–866.
73. Troeltzsch M, Troeltzsch M, Kauffmann P, et al. Clinical efficacy of grafting materials in alveolar ridge augmentation: a systematic review. *J Craniomaxillofac Surg*. 2016; 44(10): 1618–1629.
74. Brignardello-Petersen R There seems to be an average gain of 4 millimeters of bone after vertical ridge augmentation procedures. *J Am Dent Assoc*. 2019; 150(7): e111.
75. Pal US, Sharma NK, Singh RK, et al. Direct vs. indirect sinus lift procedure: a comparison. *Natl J Maxillofac Surg*. 2012; 3(1): 31–37.

76. Brånemark PI, Hansson BO, Adell R, et al. Osseointegrated implants in the treatment of the edentulous jaw. Experience from a 10-year period. *Scand J Plast Reconstr Surg Suppl.* 1977; 16: 1–132.

77. Souza AB, Tormena M, Matarazzo F, Araujo MG The influence of peri-implant keratinized mucosa on brushing discomfort and peri-implant tissue health. *Clin Oral Implants Res.* 2016; 27: 650–655.

78. Wennstrom JL, Derks J Is there a need for keratinized mucosa around implants to maintain health and tissue stability? *Clin Oral Implants Res.* 2012; 23(Suppl 6): 136–146.

79. Salvi GE, Ramsier CA Efficacy of patient-administered mechanical and/or chemical plaque control protocols in the management of peri-implant mucositis. A systematic review. *J Clin Periodontol.* 2015; 42(Suppl 16): S187–S201.

80. Chackartichi T, Romanos GE, Sculean A Soft tissue-related complications and management around dental implants. *Periodontol.* 2019; 81: 124–138.

81. Lee A, Fu JH, Wang HL Soft tissue biotype affects implant success. Implant Dent. 2011; 20(3): e38–e47.

82. Avila-Ortiz G, Gonzalez-Martin O, Couso-Queiruga E, Wang H-L The peri-implant phenotype. *J Periodontol.* 2020; 91(3): 283–288.

83. Lin G-H, Curtis DA, Kapila Y, et al. The significance of surgically modifying soft tissue phenotype around fixed dental prostheses: an American Academy of Periodontology best evidence review. *J Periodontol.* 2020; 91(3): 339–351.

84. Rosen PS The merit to phenotypic modification treatment for dental implants: two case reports. Clin Adv Periodontics. 2020; 10(4): 164–168.

85. Tischler M, Ganz S "The first implant": protocol for the GP, part 1, treatment planning. Dent Today. 2011; 14: 27.

86. Chung DM, Oh TJ, Shotwell JL, et al. Significance of keratinized mucosa in maintenance of dental implants with different surfaces. J Periodontol. 2006; 77: 1410–1420.

87. Tischler M In-office cone beam computerized tomography: technology review and clinical examples. Dent Today. 2008; 27: 102, 104, 106.

88. Ganz SD CT scan technology: an evolving tool for predictable implant placement and restoration. Int Mag Oral Implantol. 2001; 1: 6–13.

89. Ganz SD Conventional CT and CBCT for improved dental diagnostics and implant planning. Dent Implantol Update. 2005; 16: 89–95.

5 How to Talk to Patients About Implant Dentistry: Risks, Benefits, and Alternatives

Dental implants procedures are expected to increase by 23% from 2020 to 2026. Currently more than 5 million implants are placed in the United States according to the American Dental Association. The American Academy of Implant Dentistry estimate 69% of Americans 35–44 years old have at least one missing tooth, over 45 years old have a few missing teeth, and 24% of older adults over the age of 74 are completely edentulous (1). Implant dentistry is no longer new, it is here to stay and as hygienists we need to know *how to talk implants*.

What are the risks, benefits, and alternatives to replacing missing teeth?

Hygienists, how and when do you talk to patients about implant dentistry? Hygienists, on an average, spend 40–60 minutes of one-on-one time with their patients, more than any other team member in the office. It is very helpful to the dentist if hygienists attain the verbal skills to talk with patients about the risks, benefits, and alternatives (RBAs) to replacing missing teeth with dental implants. An understanding of the RBAs and being able to pass this information on to patients will truly help patients to have a better understanding of their role, responsibility, and treatment options to make informed decisions about their long-term oral health.

Which patients should hygienists talk to about implant dentistry? The best candidates for implants are your existing patients of record. Identify which of your existing patients are missing one or more teeth with no replacement, patients with a fixed bridge, or currently wear a removable partial or denture. Patients with existing fixed bridges who are at risk for decay, bone loss, or poor aesthetics. Periodontal

Peri-Implant Therapy for the Dental Hygienist, Second Edition. Susan S. Wingrove.
© 2022 John Wiley & Sons, Inc. Published 2022 by John Wiley & Sons, Inc.
Companion website: www.wiley.com/go/wingrove/implant

patients that have the potential for future tooth or bone loss. Also, patients with congenitally missing teeth are patients in whom to plant the seed on the technological advancements in implant dentistry. Refer to Table 5.1 for a comparison of treatment options.

Branemark refers to edentulism as "a serious handicap, to be treated with the upmost respect." The Surgeon General's NIDCR Strategic Plan 2010 outlines the psychological issues of the fully edentulous patient as an oral disease that affects the most basic human needs: "the ability to eat and drink, swallow, maintain proper nutrition, smile, and communicate"(2).

Risks

The ultimate consequence or risk of not replacing the missing tooth with an implant is bone loss. More than 44 million people in the United States have at least one quadrant of posterior missing teeth and are potential implant therapy candidates (3). It is the dental professional's responsibility to discuss the options of replacing missing teeth with every patient.

As a hygienist, one of the first questions that a patient might ask you after an extraction is; *"What if nothing is done to replace it?"* The patient can choose to do nothing, it is a viable option; but there will be consequences. Hygienists can talk to patients about the RBAs to tooth replacement. Then offer to set up an implant consultation with the doctor or implant coordinator if they are interested.

Often, when a tooth is removed, the alignment of the teeth next to the missing tooth starts to shift. As the bite shifts, it can become very difficult, time-consuming, and expensive to repair, and over time atrophy or shrinkage of the jawbone can occur. Remember that the primary job of the jawbone is to retain the teeth, and when

teeth are lost and the bone is not stimulated, it melts away.

Traditional dentistry can provide replacements for missing teeth using bridges, removable partials, and/or dentures; however, each of these has risks. If a tooth is lost or needs to be taken out due to infection, fracture, or bone loss from periodontal disease, it can cause ramifications that extend far beyond that one tooth. Bridgework usually involves altering natural adjunctive teeth to provide a stable foundation for support of replacement teeth. Partials and dentures can, at times, be very unstable, leading to denture sores or speech difficulties. All of these options potentially need to be replaced every 6–10 years.

The ideal treatment is to replace the missing teeth at the time of extraction, before the shifting or jaw atrophy occurs. The longer the patient waits, the more involved and expensive the final solution becomes. Bone atrophy not only affects jaw function, but also facial aesthetics. Aesthetics starts with the integrity of the facial bone structures, so if the teeth are lost and not replaced, the bone melts away and the facial structures sag inward, causing a premature aging appearance.

The consequences to facial appearance illustrated (see Figure 5.1) can be a very dramatic visual to show your patients! Make it visual and real to your patients when discussing the risks of not replacing missing teeth. Also give the patient the statistics of the risks of not replacing the missing tooth with an implant. Bone loss of 25% in width of the ridge and an overall 4 mm of bone height during the first year after an extraction (4). These are important statistics that help the patient understand the urgency of replacing missing teeth before bone loss can occur.

The literature reports that only 60% of patients with partial dentures wear them in 4 years, and after 10 years only 35% are still wearing their partials (5). Oral hygiene can

Table 5.1 Comparison treatment options for missing teeth.

Treatment Option	Benefits	Risks
Implants	■ Can be life-long ■ Preserves bone and maintains facial structure ■ Oral hygiene is similar to natural teeth ■ Cost effective in prevention of further expense in future	■ Potentially longer time to complete a phased treatment plan ■ Can be more expensive initially
Permanent bridge	■ Less time to complete treatment ■ Fills in the space to replace the tooth for aesthetic purposes but does not replace the root	■ Requires grinding down of healthy adjacent teeth and loss of bone under pontic ■ Replacement needed about every 5–10 years ■ Root canal and caries complications possible ■ Oral hygiene is more difficult ■ Bone loss under pontics
Partial denture	■ Less time to complete treatment ■ Can be added to; tooth loss does occur in 44% of clasp attachment teeth in 10 years ■ Can be less expensive	■ Can loosen and fall out unexpectedly, causing embarrassing situations, and can be lost; expensive to replace ■ Replacement needed about every 6–10 years ■ Caries and tooth loss with attachment teeth ■ Difficult to keep biofilm-free ■ Difficult to taste and chew ■ Can make talking more difficult (lisping) and possibility of causing a gagging reflex ■ Does not preserve bone and facial structure preservation
Denture	■ Less time to complete treatment ■ Can be less expensive	■ Extensive bone loss and facial structure, premature aging appearance ■ Difficulty to taste and chew ■ Replacement and reline retention complications ■ Can move and/or fall out unexpectedly, causing embarrassing situations ■ Can make talking more difficult (lisping) and possibility of causing a gagging reflex ■ Psychologically difficult to eat in public, which can affect confidence

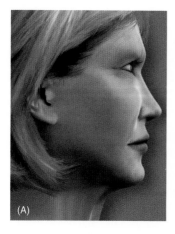 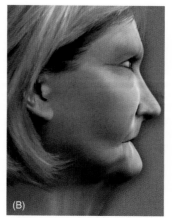 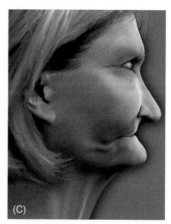

Figure 5.1 Progressive bone loss affects appearance. Courtesy of BioHorizons.

also be affected for patients wearing clasp-retained partials, and this includes an increase in biofilm, bleeding on probing, and inflammation leading to periodontal concerns (6–8). The dental health complications created by increased stress on the attachment teeth leads to mobility, caries, and eventually to loss of the attachment teeth (8–10). The statistics for loss of abutment/attachment teeth range from 23% in 5 years, to 38% in 8 years, to 44% in 10 years (11). Clearly, there are demonstrated risks to not replacing missing teeth and obvious benefits to replacement with dental implants.

Benefits

The Surgeon General's report highlights that *"25% of people without teeth reported that they avoided close relationships because of fear of rejection when their toothlessness was discovered"* (2). To simply be able to chew without pain or laugh without the embarrassment of losing your denture in pubic and have the confidence to start new romantic relationships is priceless to the edentulous patient. Replacing patients' teeth and preserving the bone not only changes patients' smiles, but also improves their quality of life.

Edentulous patients are truly the real winners in the age of implant dentistry. Many edentulous patients have worn dentures since they were 30 years old and now are oral invalids, unable to even wear their dentures except to weddings and funerals. More than 80% of edentulous patients have difficulty with speech and have to continue to spend money on denture adhesives to hold their dentures in place. Without it, these patients could not wear their dentures due to ill fit from serious bone loss that has occurred over time, which can lead to serious quality of life issues (12).

Hygienists, share the benefits of dental implants (Box 5.1) with your patients. Explain how it is possible to restore their smile and function to its most natural state. This will be highly motivational to patients. Aesthetics is the number one reason patients say YES to treatment and improved function in terms of chewing and tasting food ranks a close second. The nutritional

Hygiene Tip:

Hygienists, have a conversation with your patients about the options for tooth replacement. Talk about all the benefits of dental implants compared with the alternatives to bridges and partial and full dentures.

Box 5.1 Benefits of dental implants

■ Improved health through nutrition, digestion, taste, and appetite
■ Implants look, feel, and function like natural teeth
■ Increased bone density and facial structure preservation
■ Improved aesthetic appearance
■ Improved ability to function without pain or gum irritation
■ Improved retention for implant-supported removable denture
■ Improved quality of life and increases life expectancy

---

health benefit of being able to chew more healthy foods, such as raw vegetables, opens up a variety of food options that the edentulous patient has had to give up and could not taste because everything tasted like plastic.

What patient would not want the cosmetic effect of looking younger as an added benefit to function? *Relate the benefits of maintaining and increasing the bone density for an* **internal face lift**, preserving the patient's facial structure. Functionally explain the benefits of better digestion and how ability to chew food enriches the patient's quality of life and can extend the patient's life expectancy (12–14). Other benefits include improved taste, appetite, and that dental implants are not susceptible to decay. This makes implants a very good option for a stable diabetic patients or other immune-compromised patients who are also at risk for dental decay.

The choice of dental implant allows the patient the most conservative option that does not compromise adjacent teeth. Once the adjacent teeth are prepped, tooth structure is removed to sustain a crown, and a bridge is fabricated, the failure rate and the risk of root canal treatment is increased (15, 16).

Bridgework and dentures address the cosmetic problem of missing teeth, but do not prevent bone loss in the long term. Dental implants maintain proper chewing function, stimulating the bone to keep it functional and healthy. The primary benefit is that implants look, feel, and function like natural teeth and help preserve the jaw structure by preventing atrophy from bone loss. Implant therapy is also the number one choice for improved quality of life. Many times, there are several options with implant dentistry and the patient's financial and lifestyle choices can be important factors in the final treatment plan.

Hygienists need to listen and address to the patient's expectations for both aesthetic appearance and choice of removable or nonremovable prosthesis. The dentist and surgeon will also make suggestions that hold a higher success rate and it may be necessary to compromise. Ultimately it is what the patient wants that is important. What are the alternatives and why should patients consider dental implants?

Alternatives

Understanding the alternatives and the options of implant tooth replacement therapy is essential for hygienists to be able to *plant the seed* with patients. There are many considerations in implant tooth replacement therapy. To maintain and increase bone density and preserving facial structure. Implant-supported prostheses also enhance appearance, restore normal eating, and improve removable denture retention.

The patient may not accept implant therapy the first time you have the conversation on the RBAs. It may be months, but one day the patient will be ready to move forward with the recommended treatment.

As a hygienist, familiarize yourself with the restorative options for tooth replacement therapy. Be able to explain the restorative options for implants and explain the alternatives of traditional tooth replacement therapy to bridge, partial or traditional denture. These alternatives do not compare with the longevity, improved function, and most of all patient psychological results that implants can offer.

Bridges

The main advantage of a bridge for the patient is less treatment time to complete. It does fill in the space for aesthetic purposes when it is seated, but over time the bone under the pontic will melt away (see Figure 5.2). When explaining this to a patient, (refer to Box 5.2) on the key points of tooth replacement with implants. The bone width decreases 25% and the height of the ridge decreases 4 mm just in the first year (5, 17). For the patient this will create a higher sense of urgency to have the implant placed as soon as possible after extraction.

Of patients who were asked if they had known about the bone loss with missing teeth, and that implants basically stop the bone loss, most would have had an implant. When talking to patients about implants, refer to the point of having to cut into the healthy adjacent teeth for crowns to support the bridge. The facts show that tooth decay and endodontic failures can occur in the adjacent abutment teeth and cause the bridge to fail (15, 16). It is estimated that 15% of abutment teeth will require

> **Box 5.2** Key points for hygienist to remember and quote to patients when having a conversation on tooth replacement with implants:
>
> - Bone width decreases 25% in the first year after a tooth is lost or extracted (12).
> - Bone height decreases 4 mm in the first year (12).
> - 40–60% of ridge width can be lost in first 2–3 years (12).
> - 0.5–1% bone continues to resorb yearly for the patient's life (25).

endodontic treatment, compared with natural teeth of 3% single crowns. The abutment teeth are also at greater risk for periodontal disease and bone loss complications. These complications have resulted in loss of abutment teeth at 30% in 14 years (12).

One of the key factors to compare a three-unit bridge to an implant for single tooth replacement is *cost over time*. At first the bridge may seem like the better deal to the patient, a faster treatment and on average slightly lower cost than a single restored implant. However, if the patient presents for treatment at age 40, it could cost the patient a much higher *price over time*. A three-unit bridge has an estimated 75% survival rate of a fixed prosthesis over 10 years (18). If the patient lives to be 80 years old, the bridge could need to be replaced four times and there may be possible significant complications on adjacent teeth. Single tooth implants can boost a 90% or higher survival rate and could, with good oral hygiene and implant maintenance, last a lifetime (19). The success rate can vary depending on many factors such as occlusion, health of patient (i.e., whether the patient is a smoker), or poor implant placement, but currently implant therapy boosts the highest success rate of treatments we provide in dentistry today.

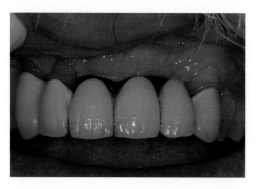

Figure 5.2 Traditional three-unit bridge; note the bone loss. Courtesy of Dr. Kevin Frawley.

Fixed full and partial denture

The main advantage of traditional dentures over implant-supported prosthesis is less time to complete treatment and lower cost. It is interesting that one of the advantages to a partial denture is that prosthetic teeth can be added to the partial if patient loses more teeth. Loss of clasp attachment teeth for partial dentures is reported to be 23% in 5 years, 38% in 8 years, and 44% within 10 years (10). Additionally, the survival rate of a partial denture is less than 6 years (12).

Oral hygiene is also questionable with traditional dentures with a greater risk of oral biofilm and periodontal issues (5, 7). More than 60% of clasp attachment teeth are in need of repair due to caries, mobility (bone loss), bleeding on probing, and endodontic complications (15, 16). Based on these risks, the main focus to compare is cost and complications over time.

For edentulous patients, multiple treatment options are available. Research shows that traditional removable denture patients wear their dentures 80% of the time the first year, 60% in 4 years, 40% in 5 years, and only 20% in 10 years (20–22). Quality of life and life expectancy can be compromised with traditional dentures compared with implant-supported prosthesis mainly due to masticatory function and loss of ability to chew effectively. Patients often may need to take drugs for gastrointestinal disorders that can lead to a decrease in life expectancy due to limited nutritional options and fewer vegetables or healthy food options.

The average patient with natural teeth exerts a bite force of 150–200 psi (22). Patients with stronger buccinators muscles due to grinding or clenching exert a force of 1000 psi. The maximum force of an edentulous patient is reduced to less than 50 psi, and the longer the patient is edentulous the psi can drop as low as 5.6 psi (23).

The top three disadvantages are function, fit, and discomfort, especially with the lower mandibular denture. More than 60% of the patients who complained of mandibular movement had to resort to denture adhesives for retention. The unpleasant taste, need to reapply adhesive, and embarrassing circumstances of dentures falling out lead more patients to strongly consider implant-supported dentures. There is a reason traditional denture patients purchase over 211 million dollars' worth of denture adhesive annually (6, 11, 24).

The goal of partially or completely edentulous patients is to recover normal function, aesthetics, comfort and/or speech, all of which are affected by atrophy of muscle and bone due to traditional dentures (see Figure 5.3).

Summary of risks, benefits, and alternatives

Hygienists, talk to your patients highlighting the serious soft tissue, muscle, and bone consequences that can accelerate the aging process in aesthetic appearance if they do not replace missing teeth. The aesthetic consequences, starting with a decrease in facial height from the collapsed vertical dimension that happens from the resorption of the jaw bones. Also, the atrophy of muscle and bone can cause a loss of facial expressions, thinning of the vermillion border of the lips, deepening of the nasolabial groove, and protrusion of the chin to give the patient a geriatric appearance. Ptosis of buccinators and mentalis muscles leads to jowls and witch's chin, all unfavorable results for any cosmetically driven patient.

Compare the oral hygiene differences for care of an implant-supported crown and a three unit bridge. The patients can care for the implants like they would for their natural teeth, as implants are far easier to care for than threading floss to clean under a three unit natural tooth bridge. Inflammation often occurs, making flossing and caring for the tooth-supported bridge difficult for the patient.

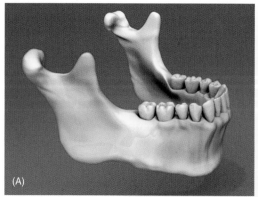
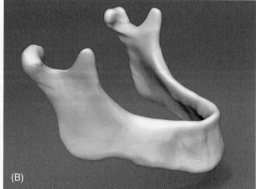
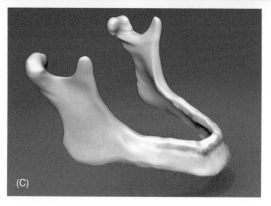

Figure 5.3 Note the progression of bone loss. Courtesy of BioHorizons.

Communication and motivation

The primary job description for a hygienist has been preventive and periodontal care for the patients. Today our job involves good communication as well as exceptional care for our patients (see Figure 5.4). Hygienists are often the patient's first impression of the office. Building a relationship with the patient through good communication skill fosters trust and loyalty for the dental office. The hygienist builds strong, sincere relationships through listening and establishing what the patient wants and needs in regard to his or her dental and overall health. Then the hygienist can convey these wants and needs to the dentist when he or she comes into the operatory to do the comprehensive exam.

Be positive with the tone of your voice and body language or the patient will pick up on it. Keep track of the information on

> **Hygienist Tip:**
>
> Move your patient into an upright position and move your stool to have good eye contact. Now you are in the right position to present treatment options and/or explain oral hygiene recommendations.

the patient's needs, desires, and concerns. Ask the right open-ended questions, questions that cannot be answered with a yes or no answer.

The what is in it for me? (WIFM) motivation expectation of the patient for dental implant therapy: *Edentulous patients often have different concerns; ask the questions and sit back and listen!*

■ What are your expectations? What would you like; removable or nonremovable?

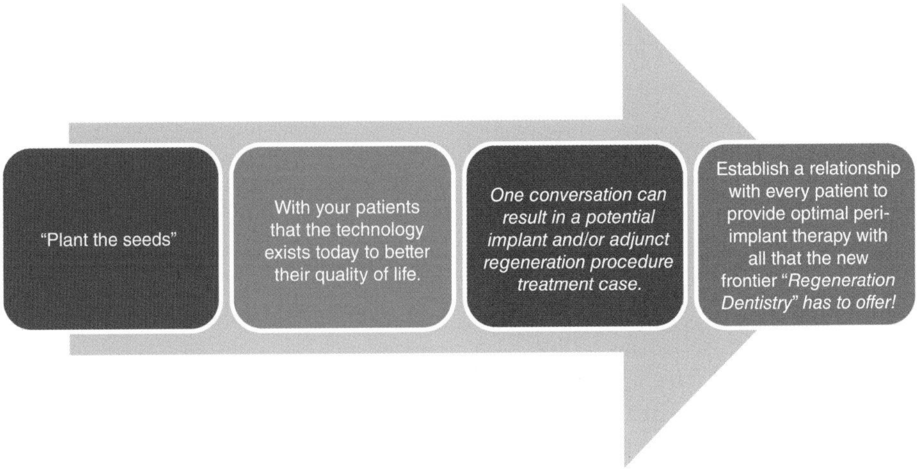

| "Plant the seeds" | With your patients that the technology exists today to better their quality of life. | *One conversation can result in a potential implant and/or adjunct regeneration procedure treatment case.* | Establish a relationship with every patient to provide optimal peri-implant therapy with all that the new frontier *"Regeneration Dentistry"* has to offer! |

Figure 5.4 Communication with patients.

■ What would you change about your smile?

■ What are your long-term dental goals?

■ What do you like to do in terms of activities, lifestyle?

Finally, when the dentist presents for the patient's exam, *bring the dentist into the conversation.* Relate to the dentist a quick explanation of what you and the patient have been discussing. As dental professionals, *be on the same page,* know what treatment options the dentist would like to offer to this patient and which procedures are to be referred to a specialist. Relay the patient's chief concerns, wants, and needs. Represent and convey the overall mission statement of your dental practice.

Review the treatment plan with the patient that day. However, too much information can be overwhelming to the patient. For larger treatment or complex treatment plans, it is often best to have the patient return for a separate treatment conference after the doctor has had time to review all the diagnostic records and determine comprehensive treatment plan options for the patient.

Through a focused conversation with your patients, you will be able to better understand their motivations, define their expectations, and relay this to the dentist to help develop a treatment plan based on those expectations.

How do you introduce value?

Eighty-five percent of our patients will move toward behavior that makes them feel good or positive, shying away from behavior that makes them feel bad or negative. This is why experts tell us that we need to create the *want in the patient's mind.* Patients do not buy what they need; they buy what they want.

As a team, discuss the practice's vision and philosophies and write an office mission statement. Once you have established what the dentist wants for the practice and his/or her philosophy you can present optimal, sincere treatment plans to your patients. The purpose of communicating dental value to a patient is not to sell patients something, but to guide them to the optimal treatment plan that will improve their quality of life and overall health.

As a hygienist, you are one of the front-line educators for ideal treatment in dentistry. You have the time and tools to educate patients, and national statistics show that 40–80% of dental treatment is found in the hygiene maintenance appointment. Inform and document that you have talked to the patient about the RBAs to implant therapy. Build value for the implant consult by summarizing the key benefits of implants and the differences in alternative treatment options, defining the patient's wants and desires.

Talk in terms of replacing the root of the tooth in reference to the implant and relay the benefits of implants versus traditional tooth replacement. Remember to educate the patient on the consequences of missing teeth and the bone resorption that will follow. Relate the treatment to what the patient wants and needs. The patient may not commit to the treatment from your first conversation, *plant the seed*. Patients may need to hear the RBAs until it clicks or their dental health becomes painful, urgent, or a priority for them.

Implants are the future! Not all patients will be able to afford ideal treatment, but all should be educated on the options available today. Traditional dentistry still has its place, but implant dentistry can be *staged*, in phases over time, to offer all patients the best treatment available!

Presenting treatment to patients

After your conversation with the patient on the RBAs of tooth replacement, *what's next?* The patient will ultimately ask you questions about how much implant therapy costs and how much time is needed for him or her to get his or her teeth.

Explain to the patient that the dentist will first need to do an exam, take some diagnostic records, and see if the patient is a good candidate for implant therapy. Hygienists can have the conversation about the implant treatment options. Have educational brochures, short educational

videos (i.e., implant or adjunctive procedure informational sheets), and patient implant models. If there is not time to have this discussion, ask if you can schedule a separate appointment for the patient to talk to the dentist and/or implant/treatment coordinator (designated team member for implant therapy) about the treatment options. At that visit, the dentist or team member will be able to help answer any questions the patient might have on implants, the proposed treatment, and financial obligations.

Patients can be overwhelmed when first

> **Hygienist Tip:**
>
> Having the educational tools such as implant models, flip charts, brochures on tooth replacement options, and videos in your operatory will make it more comfortable to have a conversation or to *plant the seed* with patients on implant therapy.

presented with implant therapy. They may think implants are transplants of a real tooth or cadaver tooth into their mouth. Implant models are extremely helpful to let the patient visually see what implants look like. For an edentulous patient this can be a *wow factor*, to show how and hear the overdenture snap into place. Or for the patient to see that the final prosthesis is smaller than a traditional denture and will have no palate. They will retain their taste and speech will be easier with implant-supported prosthesis. Implant models are available from different companies (i.e., Kilgore International, Salvin Dental Specialties), see Appendix resource section.

Brochures and flip charts are available from most implant companies. Generic brochures are also available from many dental organizations (i.e., American Dental Association, American Academy of Periodontology, American College of Prosthodontists,

> **Box 5.3 Example of information to consider about patients to YES to Treatment**
>
> ■ Are they task-oriented or people-oriented?
> ■ Are they introverted or extroverted?
> ■ What kind of job or profession do they have?
> ■ Do they work with people or alone?
> ■ Where do they vacation?
> ■ What kind of hobbies do they have?

Academy of Osseointegration, or American Association of Oral and Maxillofacial Surgeons). For more information, see the Appendix, resource section.

Value and perception are directly related to our beliefs that drive our choices and our choices define and create our lives. Before you present treatment to patients, know to whom you are speaking (see Box 5.3).

Know your patients, having the information from Box 5.3 and an understanding of your patient's personality type can allow you to present these options in a nonthreatening way. The four main personality types are dominant, cautious thinkers, interacting socializers, and steady relaters. For example, if you do a treatment presentation to dominant personality patients, present it in a powerful and controlled manner. They prefer treatment needs explained quickly and to the point. *Get in, get it done, next!*

If possible, attend continuing education courses to learn about personality styles, how to talk to patients, and increase your knowledge on peri-implant therapy (see Figure 5.5). It will be a skill that will relax your patient, help to build relationships, and allow you to present treatment to the patient in a way he or she would most like to see it presented. It can increase your effectiveness in interacting with patients and give you greater flexibility in your personal style to match and/or mirror to adapt to the patient's personality style.

Another way to approach presenting treatment is to look at the patient's age. It is on the patient's record (i.e., birthdate) to determine which generation the patient is. A traditionalist (1922–1945), baby boomer (1946–1964), Generation Xer (1965–1980), Millennial (1981–1996), or the Z Generation (1997–2012) patient. When presenting to a patient of a certain generation *what are the key traits and points to truly connect* and *help you increase your office's case acceptance?*

Generation overview*: How to speak the way patient wants to hear*

Traditionalists: born 1922–1945

This is the *silent generation*, shaped by the depression and World War II. This generation appreciates and offers respect. Silent generation patients are often savvy travelers, loving grandparents, budding entrepreneurs, affluent retirees, and life-long learners. They value their financial security, teamwork, sacrifice, and delayed gratification, and they believe in the government.

Traditionalists are vital, active people who are redefining the aging process, interested in any cosmetic procedures that you offer. They will have their teeth whitened and hair dyed, undergo plastic surgery, and are interested in staying in shape. As a rule, they do not like to be rushed or pressured; last chance to act.

In dentistry, they will want to interact with the dentist personally and will value his or her opinion as the expert. They tend to be loyal to a fault, and would not be as likely to change dentists or want to go to a specialist they do not know personally. They see technology as a necessary evil, not something they are particularly impressed or excited about.

From the beginning, your initial meeting should show respect. Meet them in the reception area, address them by name,

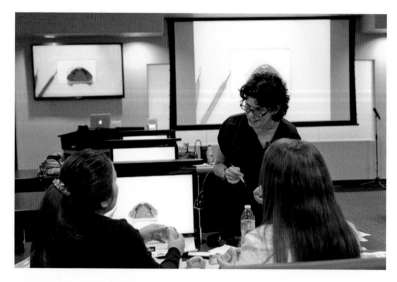

Figure 5.5   Attend continuing education courses, Susan Wingrove presenting. Image courtesy of Glidewell.

shake their hand, and offer your name with your title. Use proper language, refrain from the use of any slang, app, or text-shortened abbreviations that they may not be familiar with the meaning. Listen to their questions, concerns, and stories! Remember they value the dentist as the expert, so they will listen respectfully but will want to hear what you say repeated by the dentist. Once the dentist has diagnosed the treatment they will rarely need any further information and will often schedule for the recommended treatment.

Baby boomers: born 1946–1964

The *me generation*, shaped by the postwar affluence and overindulgent parents who wanted a better life for their children. This generation had a strong awareness of the political and social issues of their time. Baby boomers are disillusioned by the government, big business, traditional religion, and parental hardships, with an increasing divorce rate. The baby boomers launched the sexual revolution and broke down walls for equal rights for women. Idealists, they believe in challenging the status quo and changing the world. Baby boomers,

especially the late baby boomers, are competitive, conscious of their image, and tend to be materialistic, with an *I still matter attitude*.

They value and trust you and your practice, and their loyalty comes from how you make them feel; they value rapport and trust. As far as quality of dentistry, they tend to be more interested in the experience, and the relationship, than the actual quality of treatment. Exceptional customer service is the way to treat this generation. Do not treat them with indifference. They love all the new technology and want to be proud to say their dental office has the latest and greatest!

Patient interaction is key! Get to know them, note any information about them in their patient record to talk to them about it on their next visit. Involve them in their treatment planning, listen to their unique preferences, and make them feel you have their best interest at heart. Baby boomers appreciate knowing you understand their goals, vision, and perception of their dental objectives.

Baby boomers' decision making is completely different from that of traditionalists, who will simply believe what the doctor recommends and it is a done deal. The baby boomer will not do as they are told. They may want second opinions and may even ask different team members in your office, "What do you think?" That is why it is critical to involve them in the treatment planning process, as co-diagnosticians.

As a patient accepting treatment, they will want to be heard through empathetic listening, feel like you have their best interest at heart. They like to be questioned on their goals, vision, and perception of their dental health. Treated like a person, not a disease state. They will want to be shown radiographs and explained the reasons you are recommending the treatment. Boomers, as an example are key candidates for the separate treatment consultation appointment.

They are more likely to say *YES* to treatment if they identify with the treatment as a solution to a problem that they own, not that you found. Baby boomers will be interested in how having implants prevents them from getting sick, looking old, and how it contributes to their overall well-being. Finally, baby boomers will spend money on appearance-enhancing procedures, live on credit, and will say *YES* to the treatment they want!

Generation Xers (Gen Xers): born 1965–1980

Latchkey kids, shaped by growing up in difficult times financially and socially with a struggling economy, sometimes referred to as the *entitlement generation*. Many kids came home from school to an empty home, with both parents working, or in single parent homes, with strong working mothers. More than 60% attended college and believe that there are no absolutes, that one must take care of oneself.

Their loyalty is based on service, believability of the dentist. Once they see the value of the dentistry, and believe in you, they will say *YES* to implant therapy. It will need to be on their terms, what is the most convenient for their time schedule, before the money will be the issue. They want a *cool* office, one recommended by others from social networking (i.e., social media, blogging, tweets, and podcasts). Gen Xers buy what they want. Consumption is a way of life and even having been raised in tough economic times, they have the same desires as the baby boomers.

In decision making, they are skeptical, cynical, pragmatic, and cautious decision makers. Unless they feel a *connection* with you, they probably would not listen to you. Gen Xers also prefer cause marketing and would switch dentists to a provider for one who gives back to the community or another to donate to a cause they believed in. As they begin to take ownership of their health, provide them with enough information to make educated decisions: brochures, interactive video programs, intraoral cameras, or websites.

As a patient accepting treatment they want to be steered through the decision making process, not told what to do. They will want no sugar coating, and they have a high BS meter. They have a take-charge attitude about their appearance and their health combined with a want for it to be easy. Present the implant treatment case in layman's terms and make a connection example with their life that they can relate to. They will spend money and represent a large disposable income. Controlled by today's child who grew up in economic prosperity with a new tool, *the Internet*, for immediate gratification. *Get in, get it done, next!*

Millennial generation (Y Generation): born 1981–1996

The *millennials , Y, or next generation*, sometimes referred to as *trophy children,* growing up being told they were special and receiving multiple trophies for participation. They have strong relationships with their parents, are comfortable with authority, and were shaped by the unraveling era of culture wars, postmodernism, and war on terror. They are being compared to the Greatest Generation from 1901 to 1924 who were optimistic, confident charmers.

Growing up with the Internet, these patients are very open-minded and technology-proficient. Nexters never had negative feedback, so they like being praised for good ideas or thoughts and eased into any negative feedback. They grew up with computers and are very tech savvy and very efficient multitaskers. They celebrate diversity, rewrite the rules, and take technology for granted. For them friends are family and they like a structured and supportive environment. They like extraordinary customer service and technology is important, but do not mention a *cool office*, it would not sound genuine. They want to be treated with dignity and respect.

The *Y generation* wants to be a part of an extraordinary team and will evaluate your office on how you work as a team. They have low tolerance for people who talk a lot, but do not walk the talk. They demand sincerity from their doctors and a sense of purpose. When presenting the treatment plan, be sure to mention your office mission statement and how your office has a purpose. The *meaning is the new money*. Explain how you are making a difference in your community and do not promote and promise any ideals or practices you do not intend to deliver. As a patient, they will want to be treated fairly, define it, and place a high value on it.

Z Generation: born 1997–2012

The *Z generation* is designated for anyone born 1997 and beyond and are now old enough for implants. This generation is characterized as the entrepreneurial generation. They have grown up in the world of global terrorism, social media, and diversity is just the way of the world. They have many of the similar characteristics as the Millennial generation with the exception of being more social like baby boomers.

This generation is on track to be the most educated and diverse generation. Most have parents that were college educated and tend to look to college as a logical step. They do not know a world without internet or smart phones. YouTube, Instagram, and Snapchat are among their favorite online destinations. Traditional dental marketing through a website or Facebook is less popular with this generation.

They are also fiercely independent and would like to be talked to, as an equal. Technology savvy and interested in the *latest and greatest*. When discussing a treatment plan refer to the materials and technology you will be using to create the optimal result. This generation will be financially focused with a value on the environmental impact. Highlight the *green recyclable products* (i.e., Orsing products made from sugar cane and bamboo) that your office uses to lessen the landfills and preserve the planet for their generation and beyond.

Summary

Remember, the best candidates for implant dentistry are your existing patients of record and most hygienists already have a trusting relationship with these patients. Patients come to us for a better smile or to be able to eat a steak, not specifically for dental implants. Use verbal skills to effectively talk with your patients about their treatment options and how choosing implants could be the best long-term treatment choice for tooth replacement.

Hygienists gain an understanding of how the patients want to be talked to and the psychology of partially and fully edentulous patients. This will enhance your ability to discuss and present the patient with their treatment options, which ultimately increases case acceptance and happier, healthier patients!

References

1. Dental Implants Market Size, Share & Trends Analysis Report By Type (Titanium, Zirconium), By Region And Segment Forecasts, 2020-2027. 2020; 3–90.
2. Surgeon General's NIDCR Strategic Plan 2010, www.surgeongeneral.gov
3. Howell AW, Manley RS An electronic strain gauge for measuring oral forces. J Dent Res. 1948; 27: 705.
4. Carr A, Laney WR Maximum occlusal force levels in patients with osseointegrated oral implant prostheses and patients with complete dentures. Int J Oral Maxillofac Implants. 1987; 2: 101–110.
5. Vermeulen A, Keltjens A, Van't Hof M, et al. Ten-year evaluation of removable partial dentures: survival rates based on retreatment, not wearing and replacement. J Prosthet Dent. 1996; 76: 267–272.
6. Carlsson GE, Pearsson G Morphologic changes of the mandible after extraction and wearing of dentures: a longitudinal, clinical, and X-ray cephalometric study covering 5 years. Odontol Revy. 1967; 18: 27–54.
7. Wilding R, Reddy J Periodontal disease in partial denture wearers: a biologic index. J Oral Rehabil. 1987; 14: 111–124.
8. Waerhaug J Periodontology and partial prosthesis. Int Dent J. 1968; 18: 101–107.
9. Agerberg G, Carlsson GE Chewing ability in relation to dental and general health. Acta Odontol Scand. 1981; 39: 147–153.
10. Mattila KJ, Nieminen MS, Valtonen V, et al. Association between dental health and acute myocardial infarction. Br Med J. 1989; 298: 779–782.
11. Aquilino SA, Shugars DA, Bader JD, et al. Ten year survival rates of teeth adjacent to treated and untreated posterior bounded edentulous spaces. J Prosthet Dent. 2001; 85: 455–460.
12. Misch CE. Contemporary Implant Dentistry, 2nd and 3rd ed. St. Louis, MO: Mosby, 1999 and 2008.
13. Sheiham A, Steele JG, Marcenes W, et al. The relationship between oral health status and body mass index among older people: a national survey of older people in Great Britain. Br Dent J. 2002; 192: 703–706.
14. Loeshe WJ Periodontal disease as a risk factor for heart disease. Compend Contin Educ Dent. 1994; 15: 976–992.
15. Carlsson GE Masticatory efficiency: the effects of age the loss of teeth and prosthetic rehabilitation. Int Dent J. 1984; 34: 93–97.
16. Walton JN, Gardner FM, Agar JR A survey of crown and fixed partial denture failures, length of service and reasons for replacement. J Prosthet Dent. 1986; 56: 416–421.
17. Goodacre CJ, Bernal G, Rungcharassaeng K Clincal complications in fixed prosthodontics. J Prosthet Dent. 2003; 90: 31–41.
18. Creugers NH, Kayser HE, Van't Hof MA A meta analysis of durability data on conventional fixed bridges. Community Dent Oral Epidemiol. 1994; 22: 448–452.
19. Binon PP Implants and components: entering the new millennium. Int J Oral Maxillofac Surg. 2000; 15: 76–94.
20. Roberts BA Survey of chrome cobalt partial dentures. N Z Dent J. 1978; 74: 203–209.
21. Koivumaa KK, Hedegard B, Carlsson GE Studies in partial dentures prostheses I: an investigation of dentogingivally-supported partial dentures. Suom Hammaslaak Toim. 1960; 56: 248–306.
22. Carlsson GE, Hedegard B, Koivumaa KK Studies in partial denture prosthesis IV: a 4 year longitudinal investigation of dentogingivally-supported partial dentures. Acta Odontol Scand. 1965; 23: 443–472.
23. Meskin IH, Brown IJ Prevalence and patterns of tooth loss in U.S. employed adult and senior populations, 1985–1986. J Dent Educ. 1988; 52: 686–691.
24. Stafford GD Denture adhesives: a review of their use and compostion. Dent Pract. 1970; 21: 17–19.
25. Sbordone L, Barone A, Ramaglia L, Ciaglia RN, Iacono VJ Antimicrobial susceptibility of periodontopthic bacteria associated with failing implants. J Periodontol. 1995; 66: 69–74.

6 AIM for Implant Success: Assess, Identify, and Monitor

Dental hygienists play a key role as 'first responders' in recognizing potential complications and then referring patients for treatment.
> —Scott Froum, Dept. of Periodontology, SUNY Stony Brook

As the *first responders* (see Figure 6.1), hygienists need to understand and be able to recognize implant complications with protocols for assessment, monitoring, and prevention. Hygienists, by offering a comprehensive assessment/monitoring of implants at every implant maintenance visit, allow the dentists to offer complication treatment procedures early that can save the implant from being lost.

Implants are reported to be over 90% successful in multiple studies and a long-term survival rate of greater than or equal to 10 years, making it one of the most successful treatments that dental professionals can offer patients with absent or lost teeth (1). To achieve implant success, long-term assessment, monitoring, and prevention are critical. The definition of *an ailing implant or peri-implantitis*; inflammation, radiographic evidence of bone loss following healing, and increased probe depths after the allotted 1-year post-restoration. Peri-implant health is defined as the absence of inflammation, soft tissue is pink, keratinized (firm not soft) consistency. No bleeding on probing (BOP), in general probe depth of greater than or equal to 5 mm depending on implant placement, and absence of no progressive bone loss of greater than or equal to 2 mm after healing (i.e., 1-year restoration) (1).

Assess

It is critical to assess, identify, and monitor implants. Implant complications can involve both mechanical (structural), biological (hard and soft tissue), and aesthetic (prosthesis and soft tissue) component considerations (2). Mechanical complications are more structural in nature involving the implant, abutment, or prosthesis. Biological complications affect soft and hard tissue supporting the implant and restoration/prosthesis. Whereas, aesthetic

Peri-Implant Therapy for the Dental Hygienist, Second Edition. Susan S. Wingrove.
© 2022 John Wiley & Sons, Inc. Published 2022 by John Wiley & Sons, Inc.
Companion website: www.wiley.com/go/wingrove/implant

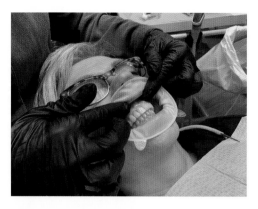

Figure 6.1 Hygienists are first responders, assessment is key! Courtesy of Wingrove Dynamics.

refers to the restoration/prosthesis or the surrounding soft-tissue appearance.

Mechanical, biological, and aesthetic component complications

*Mechanical complicatio*ns are defined as an implant that is affected by stress or occlusal forces resulting in failure and generally becoming mobile. Common mechanical complications associated with single implant restorations and fixed full arch final prostheses are; screw loosening, loss of retention, restoration or prosthesis chipping, or fracturing. As well as, framework fracture, screw fracture, and implant fracture.

Bruxism is a severe, debilitating disease that does not have a known etiology and is a concern for implant therapy. The patient needs to be aware of bruxism and the importance of the need for treatment planning for adjustments and a possible occlusal guard. The bottom line is, implants should still remain a viable treatment option for bruxism patients. If the implant is affected by occlusal forces, a stretch and bending can occur and may result in fracture. Implant fracture is rare, but serious and the treatment is to remove or submerge the implant.

Screw loosen was reported to be a frequent mechanical complication, however, new screw designs and implants with improved internal connection has significantly reduced this occurrence. Dental hygienists can detect mechanical complications by testing for mobility and/or radiographs. If a screw is loose, it needs to be taken care of immediately, by having the dentist retighten and adjust the occlusion for the patient (2). For prevention, it is recommended to consider using new prosthetic screws when implant-borne restorations are removed and replace with new screws according to implant manufacturer (3).

Biological complications are defined as complications in the function of the implant from an infection (i.e., peri-implant disease), fistula, soft-tissue hyperplasia, or loss of the implant including the peri-implant hard and soft tissues that surround the implant (2). Early implant complications can happen during the osseointegration process or even before loading the restoration or prosthesis in place and are generally handled by the surgeon and the dentist. The surgeon will see and treat most early complications, including hemorrhage, damage to adjacent teeth, loss of feeling to the lip or face, and maxillary sinus violations.

Hygienists, on occasion, will see patients on their regular prophylaxis recare visits with implants that are in the cover screw stage. Cover screws can become loose and create an abscess that can be detected visually. It is recommended for the surgeon or the dentist when the cover screw is placed, to take a radiograph and this radiograph can then be compared to future radiographs to evaluate and treat.

Healing abutments, if they are not properly seated, may need to be reseated by the dentist. Any tissue that has migrated into or over the exposed implant platform will need to be removed also by the dentist. Loss of retention, for cement retained restorations can be detected with mobility assessment. The dentist will remove the restoration and recement in place. Hygienists can assist with this, identifying any cement retained implant-borne restoration at approximately the 10-year mark of cement lifespan or if they see flecks of cement in their visual tissue assessment.

Aesthetic component considerations are appearance complications and include missing interdental papillae, mucosal recession, and poor contours of restorations, prosthesis, or pontics (see Chapter 4, Box 4.1 Criteria for pontics). For the most part, this rarely occurs due to proper treatment planning (see Chapter 4). Photographs are sent to the labs for shade matches and augmentation procedures treatment planned prior to final implant-borne restoration or prosthesis placement. When aesthetic complications arise, the dentist can recommend mucogingival tissue grafting procedures or the lab can create a pink, natural looking porcelain to achieve a satisfactory result.

Detecting complications early starts with the hygienist at the implant maintenance visit. Review the American College of Prosthodontists' Clinical Practice Guidelines recommendations for professional in-office maintenance and see implant patients of record at least every 6 months to monitor the implant(s) for any signs of complications (3).

To assess the implant, the hygienist completes a five-step assessment and monitoring protocol at every implant maintenance visit. The hygienist visually inspects the soft tissue that surrounds the implant (i.e., inflammation, keratinized, or nonkeratinized). Probes and palpates for signs of infection and uses floss to assess for calculus and/or residue to determine whether debridement is necessary. The hygienist continues with mobility assessment, pain. if present, and have the dentist check occlusion. Finally, the most critical step is to assess the bone level by taking appropriate radiograph(s) to establish the health of the implant, see five-step assessment and monitoring protocol (Figure 6.2).

Assessment: visual soft tissue

To assess the implant, the hygienist starts with a visual soft-tissue assessment (see Figure 6.1). Record any signs of inflammation or change in tissue color (i.e., red inflammation and pink for healthy), or any signs of swelling in the soft tissue, and consistency (i.e., firm for healthy tissue) (1). Healthy tissue ideally will appear pink, see Figures 6.3A,B for examples of normal and inflamed tissues, respectively.

One of the most used inflammation indexes is the Loe and Silness Gingival Index; mild, moderate, or severe (4). Mild, slight color change and slight edema. Moderate, redness, and edema more pronounced. Severe marked redness, edema, and/ or ulceration (see Figure 6.3B). Note in the patient's record if any inflammation is present with the Gingival Index or any signs of swelling or infection.

If there is presence of a fistulous tract this could be a sign of a serious biologic complication or an implant fracture (5). Evidence

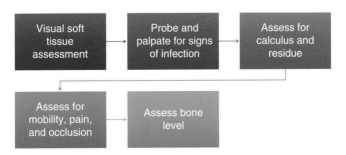

Figure 6.2 Steps for assessment and monitoring implants. Courtesy of Wingrove Dynamics.

(A)   (B)

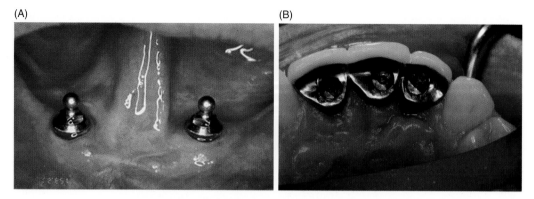

Figure 6.3   (A) Normal, healthy tissue. (B) Inflammation.

also now shows the benefits of 2 mm of keratinized tissue around the implant for biofilm control, patient comfort, and reduced risk of crestal bone loss (6). Maintaining a band of keratinized mucosa greater than or equal to 2 mm can reduce the severity of peri-mucositis in healthy implant patients and previous periodontal disease patients (6–8). If the band of tissue that surrounds the implant is less than 2 mm and inflammation is present, the dentist may recommend a tissue grafting surgical procedure by a periodontist. It is very similar to root coverage for a natural teeth for prevention and long-term success of the implant.

An optional tool to use with a soft-tissue assessment is an intraoral camera or digital camera. A photo of the soft tissue surrounding the implant is helpful as a *baseline to monitor any inflammation* and can also be used to educate the patient about the appearance of healthy tissue or inflammation. An excellent visual tool to reinforce the importance of good at-home care.

Hygienist can help patients to achieve healthy, keratinized tissue around their implants where possible with a rubber tip stimulator to use for at-home care. There are indications that nonkeratinized tissue can lead to peri-implant disease (6–8). Take note if inflammation or infection signs are present, as it can indicate a great deal about what is going on beneath the surface and the health of the implant.

Assessment: probe and palpate for signs of infection

To evaluate any signs of infection around the implants, the hygienist should probe and palpate. An important, but sometimes controversial component of the assessment is probing the dental implant (see Figure 6.4). Probing is not the same for an implant as it is for a natural tooth. Studies have shown that periodontal probe depths (PPD), bleeding points (BOP), and clinical attachment (CAL) as surrogate markers for assessment with implants, however

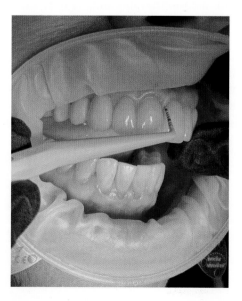

Figure 6.4 Probing the implant, courtesy of Wingrove Dynamics.

more recent information suggests a more conservative approach might be used in the case of implants.

Probe depth, bleeding points, and clinical attachment are not reliable assessments to the overall health of the implant as an endpoint (9). Crestal bone loss measurement with a radiograph or cone beam scan are needed to verify the health of an implant and palpating used to assess an implant for signs of inflammation has been found to be more reliable. It is simply impossible to correlate a specific probe depth or a range of probe depths with the variety of surgical placement of implants. You would first need to know if implant placement was tissue or bone level (with no grafting). All assessments probing or palpating needs to be followed by a radiographic assessment of crestal bone levels to verify if patient is at risk for peri-implant disease.

Research does show, to wait 6 months post load of the restoration or prosthesis to not interfere with regeneration process and it is ideal to wait until 1-year post load, bone remodeling is complete, to probe. Use caution when probing an implant, the perimucosal seal (tissue that surrounds the implant) is fragile and penetration during probing can introduce pathogens and jeopardize the success of the implant (10). It is recommended to obtain a probe depth measurement at *1-year post load as a baseline*, and monitor pocket depth at least once a year (1).

According to Revert et al., in the 2017 World Workshop report on Classification of Peri-Implant Diseases and Conditions, it may be more difficult to interrupt bleeding on probing (BOP) around implants due to the lack of a periodontal ligament (PDL). A suggested scale of *"0" for healthy no bleeding sites noted to a score of "1" for isolated dot of BOP recorded.* Record BOP at least once a year with *light pressure of 0.25 N and pocket depth in general should be less than 5mm pocket depth* (1). BOP alone, is not a

determination of peri-implantitis. Peri-implantitis requires inflammation, infection, and progressive bone loss collaborated with a radiograph to determine the health of the implant (1).

The hygienist should record a *baseline probing measurement at 1-year* after restoration or prosthesis has been loaded and crestal bone remodeling is complete. Every hygienist should take a custom probe reading on each implant patient of record. Then use their probe reading base-line to monitor the patient at each implant maintenance visit thereafter. This gives the hygienist a way to distinguish health from disease or loss of osseointegration. Also, if more than one hygienist is employed in the office, have all the hygienists measure with a compatible probe in millimeters for implant inflammation, exposed threads, or bone loss on radiographs to allow for more accurate monitoring and consistency.

What probe is safe to use around implants? First, determine the complexity of implant-borne restoration, if it is a platform-switching implant, narrow-based implant, or fixed full arch final prosthesis. A plastic or flexible probe, if helpful to access for probe depth measurement. It is safe to use a flexible probe in plastic, titanium or stainless steel (see Figure 6.5). The tip ideally needs to be flexible to follow the anatomy of the implant to get an accurate reading and to reduce trauma to the perimucosal seal.

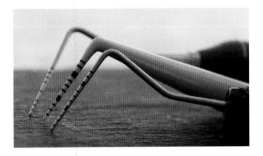

Figure 6.5 Use a flexible probe in plastic (PDT), titanium (Brasseler) or stainless steel (ACE flexible probe PDT). Courtesy of Wingrove Dynamics.

Second, record a probe baseline measurement at a specific location to establish a clinical parameter for the patient's record, ideally 1-year post load and at least once a year thereafter. Place the probe parallel to the long axis of the buccal/lingual surfaces of the implant if possible. Take six measurements (i.e., mesial-buccal [MB]), direct buccal (B), distal buccal (DB), mesial lingual (ML), direct lingual (L), and distal lingual (DL) per implant and identify a location on the restoration as a monitor marker (i.e., MB, DB) (see Box 6.1).

Record this baseline in the patient's record notes and remember to take a custom probe depth the first time the patient presents for implant maintenance at least 1-year post load. Probe depths can be deceiving, deep probe depths can be recorded if the patient's implant was placed at bone level with no bone grafting or an average 0.5 mm for an implant placed at tissue level. The key is to take note if there are *any changes in probe depths after the 1-year baseline* and alert the dentist.

Box 6.1 Protocol for probing dental implants

■ Identify the complexity of the implant-borne restoration, select a flexible tip plastic, stainless steel, or titanium with 1 mm markings probe.
■ Take six measurement sites if possible (i.e., MB, B, DB, LB, L, and DL). Record the baseline measurements at *1-year post load* (restoration/prosthesis in occlusion) and at least once a year thereafter.
■ Use a flexible probe with 1 mm markings to record six measurements
■ Place the probe parallel to the long axis of the implant and identify a location on the restoration as a monitor marker (i.e., MB, DB).
■ Gently probe using light pressure, only 0.25 N, record pocket depth and record any BOP.
■ Report findings to the dentist at time of exam

Bleeding on probing (BOP) should not occur in the sulcus of a healthy implant and is difficult to assess. If redness, inflammation, or bleeding upon probing is present, check for biofilm or the presence of calculus deposits around the implant. Remember to include in the visual tissue assessment using Loe and Silness Gingival Index (mild, moderate, or severe) and any BOP sites if inflammation is present. For new patients, record a baseline probe depth and any BOP at the first new patient visit to use and monitor therafter. Note on the patient's record implant placement date, doctor who restored the implant, type of implant, cemented, or screw retained and any other details that the patient provides.

Exudate may also be present, also referred to as suppuration or pus and consisting of fluids, cells, and cellular debris usually from inflammation. Exudate may not always be apparent upon probing. The hygienist needs to palpate the implant for signs of infection; bleeding or exudate (see Figure 6.6).

To palpate an implant, place a finger on the buccal and lingual of the ridge, just below the implant. If the implant had an apex you would be there. Keep pressure on each side of the ridge and move toward the restoration in a milking type action. Blood and/or exudate will ooze up if present (see Box 6.2). If probe depths have changed or if inflammation (i.e., bleeding or exudate are

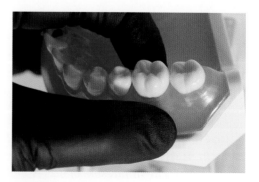

Figure 6.6 Palpate for signs of infection. Courtesy of Wingrove Dynamics.

Box 6.2 Steps to palpate for signs of infection

■ Place a finger on buccal and lingual of the ridge just below the implant.
■ Keep pressure on each side of the alveolar bone ridge and palpate from the apex of the implant, draw upward/downward toward the restoration in a milking action.
■ If the implant is infected, blood and/or exudate will ooze up from the sulcus surrounding the implant.

present), note in the patient's record and bring to the dentist's attention.

Assessment: calculus and/or residue

Is it calculus or residue on the implant? Do you need to debride the implant? Current studies reveal that implants have rough and porous surfaces that can become contaminated with trace elements of plastic, graphite, carbon, or stainless steel from implant scalers and some ultrasonic tips. The use of plastic or graphite instruments and/or ultrasonic tips is not recommended for implant instrumentation. In vitro research shows that calculus, plastic, graphite, and cement can all adhere (i.e., residue) to the implant surfaces. Studies show that implants with residue build-up can develop a foreign body reaction that triggers an inflammation cascade and ultimately can cause the loss of the implant (11).

To assess for calculus and/or residue on implants, use dental tape (not thin or heavy wax floss) and insert the floss in contacts on mesial and distal of the implant. Crisscross the floss in front, switch hands, and move in a shoe-shine motion in the peri-implant crevice. Remove the floss carefully, from the mesial then the distal and ***DO NOT pull through***, (see Chapter 8, Box 8.5, and Figure 8.10) for flossing protocol for implants. Pulling the floss through

may result in floss residue left behind on rough exposed implant surfaces that can trigger the inflammation cascade (12).

As dental professionals, we can use floss (i.e., dental tape) to identify if calculus or residue is left behind on the implant, remove the floss properly and examine. If the floss is *frayed, roughened, or blood* is present on the floss, calculus and/or residue is present. If there is blood on the floss, assess further for the source of the inflammation and plan to debride with a proper scaler or ultrasonic tip. If calculus or residue is detected, often is not easy to discern which is present. Use the appropriate titanium scaler to dislodge calculus and if it is difficult to dislodge, chances are it is cement or instrument residue. If the roughness remains, the doctor may need to assist to remove the excess residue (i.e., cement or instrument residue). *It is critical that all residue be removed or it could cause bone loss, and ultimately lose the implant.*

Assessment; mobility, pain, and occlusion

Assessing for mobility, pain, and occlusion is a very important step. Any sign of mobility could mean loss of implant osseointegration. If there is mobility of the implant itself or a broken screw, it can be a greater cause for concern. Mobility due to failure to osseointegrate generally occurs in the initial postsurgical period. The hygienist will primarily be assessing mobility following osseointegration which could be due to a loose fixed restoration, an infection, a loose or fractured abutment thread, an implant fracture, or trauma.

Natural teeth are held in the jaw with a periodontal ligament that allow for forces to be absorbed and the tooth to move slightly to accommodate these forces. An implant is held in place by being osseointegrated directly to the bone, anchored like a cement post into the ground. If the patient grinds or clenches his or her teeth (bruxism), it is detrimental to the implant and can cause the implant to fail. The dentist or specialist can eliminate this complication by treatment planning for a custom mouth guard for the patient to wear at night or during the day.

Loose retained restorations or fixed restorations may also present as mobility. Dental implant restorations/prostheses are screwed or cemented in place for retention. Screws that connect the abutment to the restoration or prosthesis can become loose. This is remedied by the dentist retightening the loose screw. However, if the internal screw is the problem it can be much more serious because of the micromovement that can occur and threaten to cause loss of osseointegration.

If bubbling of saliva occurs along the gingival margin of the restoration, the internal screw may be loose (see Figure 6.7). If no bubbling occurs, it is likely the external screw or cement is not retaining, therefore the restoration is loose. If the mobility is due to a loose crown, it can be re-cemented or if attached to a screw-retained abutment, the dentist can use the proper screw driver to tighten to the implant. Record if there are any unusual signs of wear (i.e., chipping) to the restoration or prosthesis and alert the dentist with your findings.

As a part of the implant maintenance appointment or if the patient feels the

implant is loose, test for mobility of both the restoration and the implant. Testing for mobility can be conducted using two mirror handles or a mirror handle and end of instrument to gently push on either side of each implant or restoration. Gently rock back and forth with light pressure to assess if any mobility is present (see Figure 6.8). *If mobility is present, take a radiograph, and bring to the dentist's attention.*

If the patient presents with discomfort around the implant, pain may be the first sign of a failing implant even before it is evident on a radiograph. Severe pain lasting more than 3 days immediately after placement is a definite symptom, as well as severe bleeding. If the patient presents with numbness of the lip, gums, or chin after the anesthesia is worn off, along with constant pain, an impingement on the nerve may have occurred and removal of the implant may be necessary to restore the nerve function. In both cases a radiograph and, if possible, a cone beam computed tomography (CBCT) scan would be helpful to diagnose and provide treatment.

What can a hygienist do? As a part of the monitoring and assessment process, ask

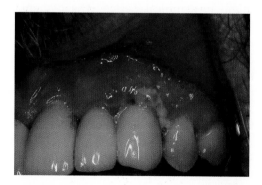

Figure 6.7 Signs of internal loose screw. Notice the bubbling around the crown margin. Courtesy of Dr. John Remien.

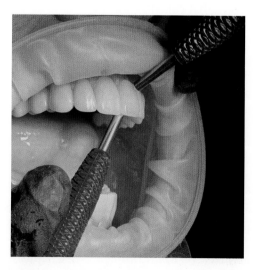

Figure 6.8 Testing for mobility. Courtesy of Wingrove Dynamics.

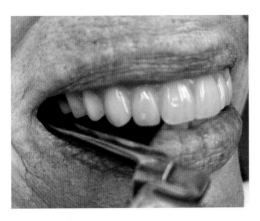

Figure 6.9 Dentist checks the occlusion with blue articulating paper. Courtesy of Dr. Tom Lambert.

the patient "if he or she is experiencing any discomfort with his or her implant(s)." Use the VAS scale (1–10, with 10 being the greatest amount of pain) to determine the pain of the patient. Record this number in the patient chart for future reference, and report findings to the dentist.

If pain is present, the dentist will need to evaluate if the pain is from occlusal trauma, lack of osseointegration, or infection and if the patient needs to be referred to the surgeon or other specialist for an evaluation.

Have the dentist check occlusion at the time of the exam for each and every implant maintenance recare visit. The dentist will have the patient bite on the blue occlusion articulating paper to assess if implant is recording light or heavy pressure (see Figure 6.9). The implant does need to have some occlusion contact to retain the bone in the jaw, just like natural teeth. However, an indication of heavy biting forces, grinding, or clenching could lead to mobility and ultimately could lead to the implant

Hygiene Tip:

Hygienists include blue occlusion articulating paper and holder in your implant maintenance recare set-up to have ready for dentist to assess the occlusion.

failure. If occlusion is heavy on the implant restoration, the dentist can do an occlusal adjustment and/or prescribe fabrication of an occlusal guard.

The American College of Prosthodontists' Guidelines professional maintenance specify; "when clinical signs indicate need for occlusal device, professionals should educate patient and fabricate an occlusal device to protect implant-borne fixed restorations" (3). Monitoring the mobility and occlusion is critical to assure long-term prevention of peri-implantitis.

Assessment; bone level

The final step is the most critical one for assessing and monitoring the health of the peri-implant environment. *It's all about the bone!* A radiographic assessment is the most valuable tool in evaluating the health of an endosseous dental implant (1). The dentist looks for crestal bone remodeling, biological width invasion, and bone loss due to trauma or residue (i.e., cement) left behind. To identify cement residue on a radiograph, look for a saucer-like radiolucent area surrounding the implant (see Figure 6.10). However, due to the lack of radiopacity in many implant-specific cements, the cement may not be evident on a radiograph (13).

Radiographs should be taken at strategic times; during surgical placement, at the cover screw stage/healing cap, during restoration/prosthesis placement, after 6 months, and at 1-year intervals (14). It is critical to verify at each stage that the component parts are seated properly. Important to take a radiograph at the time of impressions for the final restoration and when the abutment is placed to verify the restoration is properly seated.

It is recommended to make a *base-line radiograph at 1-year post load* after the restoration/prosthesis is in occlusion, bone crestal remodeling is complete (1). Retain this radiograph to use to monitor every

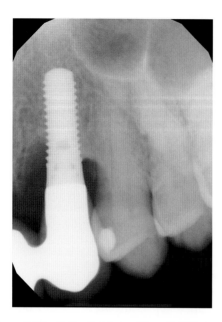

Figure 6.10 Notice the saucer-like radiolucent area. This signifies cement. Courtesy of Dr. John Remien.

year thereafter. At 1-year, bone loss of 0.5–2.0 mm is acceptable, however any changes greater than or equal to 2 mm at any time during or after the first year should be considered pathologic (1).

Vertical bitewings are ideal for implants that fall in the bitewing location or make a periapical (PA) radiograph. A PA radiograph, panoramic film or cone beam computerized tomography (CBCT) is ideal for five or more implants (see Box 6.3). Take the base-line radiograph to assess the bone level at *1-year post load* and retain to monitor any changes for signs of peri-implant

---

Box 6.3   Radiographic guidelines to monitor bone level (14)

■ For one to four implants: Make a vertical bitewing or PA film of each implant
■ For five implants: Take panoramic, CBCT scan, or individual PA radiographs of each implant.
■ Alert dentist of any changes ≥2 mm during or after first year, consider pathologic.
■ Monitor at least once a year.

---

disease. At 1-year, bone loss of 0.5–2.0 mm is acceptable, monitor by taking a radiograph *at least every year* to access any bone level changes and the health of the implant (1).

To take a correct, in-focus implant radiograph, line up the cone–X-ray beam perpendicular to the implant/abutment interface. All radiographs taken of implants must show all indentations in the implant or the threads clearly, *in focus* (see Figure 6.11). If the implant or threads are blurry, the evaluation could be improperly diagnosed. It is critical to retake the radiograph to comprehensively deliver the accurate records to the dentist.

Subsequent radiographs are used to determine if any crestal bone loss has occurred around the implant; if so, it is measured and recorded. A measurement of 0.5–2.0 mm horizontal bone loss and evidence of bone loss to the first thread of the implant is acceptable in the first year (1, 15). It is unacceptable to see a vertical defect or radiolucency along the side of the implant, resembling a periodontal

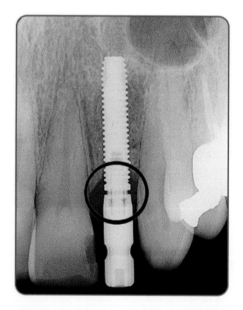

Figure 6.11 Line up the diagnostic radiograph of implant correctly. Threads clearly in focus. Courtesy of Jeff Carlson, CDT.

disease tooth or radiolucency around the apex. If more than 1.0 mm of horizontal or vertical bone loss is detected in the first year, an evaluation by the implant surgeon is recommended. Progressive bone loss around a dental implant of greater than 2 mm is indicative of an ailing or failing implant.

During the radiographic evaluation, no radiolucent areas should be present between the implant and the bone. If bone loss has occurred, it generally indicates an infection, calculus, residue, or a failure to osseointegrate (1). Any signs of peri-mucositis, peri-implantitis, mobility, or bone loss of greater than or equal to 2 mm need to be brought to the attention of the dentist or specialist and treated (1). To accurately monitor the implant, follow the radiographic guidelines (see Box 6.3). If unexplained inflammation and bone loss for two consecutive recare visits, obtain a CBCT scan. This facilitates detection of bone lesions on the facial, lingual, and proximal aspects of the implants, not visible on 2D radiographs. For new implant patients with no previous radiographs, radiographic bone loss of greater than or equal to 3 mm and inflammation, BOP, with probe depths of greater than or equal to 6 mm is suggestive of peri-implantitis (1).

A healthy implant is described as the absence of tissue inflammation, bleeding, suppuration and bone loss of less than two millimeters at one-year evaluation.

Monitoring

Failing implant

A failed implant by definition is *to have lost its osseointegration*. If an implant does fail, it is generally due to bacterial infection (mucositis, peri-implantitis), a poorly designed prosthesis, over-extended occlusal force (occlusal overload), inadequate home-care, and/or change in patient's health (16). Hygienists, record as many assessment factors as possible to assist the dentist to determine the cause of the complication and develop a treatment plan.

An understanding of the signs of a failing implant is necessary for the hygienist to monitor and provide comprehensive implant maintenance therapy (see Box 6.4). The hygienist can assist the dentist by recording a visual soft-tissue assessment, probe/ palpate for signs of infection, assess for calculus/ residue, check the mobility/occlusion (checked by doctor), and take a diagnostic radiograph for bone level. The hygienist can also identify mucositis and recognize any signs of peri-implantitis and outline an at-home care routine for the patient's long-term implant success.

Box 6.4 Signs of a failing implant

■ Bleeding on probing, exudate on palpation
■ Residue (i.e., cement or instrument) present
■ Mobility or pain present
■ Radiographic evidence of unacceptable bone loss >2 mm.

Summary

The hygienist's role is critical in assessment, monitoring, and treatment of implants for their patients. Identify any failing implants, which can be a slow and gradual process, before they become failed implants if not treated in a timely manner. Monitoring for signs of failing implants as a hygienist is a vital part of the implant maintenance appointment (see Box 6.4 and Table 6.1). For more information on treatment planning refer to Chapters 4 and 7 on peri-implant disease.

Table 6.1 Assessment and monitoring summary.

Assessment	Summary
Visual soft tissue	Assess for any signs of inflammation. ■ Record any sign of inflammation, infection, or changes in color, contour, or consistency. Texture; keratinized or nonkeratinized ■ If inflammation is present; note the Gingival Index #1–3 in the patient record; mild, moderate, or severe.
Probe	Assess for any signs of infection. ■ Identify the complexity of the implant-borne restoration, select a flexible tip probe, wait 6 months after implant has been restored. ■ Take six measurement sites if possible (i.e., MB, B, DB, LB, L, and DL). Record the baseline measurements at 1-year post load, restoration/prosthesis in occlusion and at least every year thereafter. ■ Use a *flexible* probe with 1 mm markings to record six measurements. ■ Place the probe parallel to the long axis of the implant and identify a location on the restoration as a monitor marker (i.e., MB, DB). ■ Gently probe using light pressure, only 0.25 N, record pocket depth and BOP (0,1) if present.
Palpate	Assess any signs of infection. ■ Place a finger on buccal and lingual of the ridge just below the implant. ■ Keep pressure on each side of ridge and palpate upward/downward toward the restoration. ■ If the implant is infected, blood, and/or exudate will ooze up from sulcus.
Calculus/residue	Assess the need to debride the implant with a proper scaler or ultrasonic tip by flossing with dental tape. ■ Insert floss in the mesial/distal contacts, crisscross in front, and move in shoe-shine motion. ■ Remove from mesial/distal—DO NOT pull through. ■ Check floss; if frayed, roughened, or blood is present on the floss, calculus and/or residue is present. Assess and debride with a proper scaler/ultrasonic tip.
Mobility/pain/ occlusion	Assess mobility, pain, and occlusion. ■ Use two mirror handles to gently push on either side of the implant or restoration. Gently rock back/forth with light pressure to assess if mobility is present. ■ If patient reports any discomfort around an implant, use the VAS scale (1–10, with 10 being the greatest amount of pain). ■ If mobility or pain is present, take a radiograph, and bring to the attention of the dentist. ■ Doctor check occlusion at time of exam. If occlusion is heavy on implant restoration, the dentist can do an occlusal adjustment and/or prescribe fabrication of an occlusal guard.
Bone level	Take a radiograph to monitor bone level and assess implant health. ■ For one to four implants: vertical bitewing or periapical film of each implant ■ For five or more implants: panoramic, CBCT scan, or individual radiographs of each implant. ■ Alert dentist of any changes ≥2 mm during or after first year, consider pathologic. Note: Take the base-line radiograph to assess the bone level at *1-year post load* and at 1-year, bone loss of 0.5–2.0 mm is acceptable, monitor by taking a radiograph ***at least once a year.***

References

1. Renvert S, Persson GR, Pirih FQ, Camargo PM Peri-implant health, peri-implant mucositis, and peri-implantitis: case definitions and diagnostic considerations. J Clin Periodontol. 2018; 45(Suppl 20): S278–S285.

2. Vere J, Bhakta S, Patel R Prosthodontic complications associated with implant retained crown and bridgework: a review of the literature. Br Dent J. 2012; 212: 267–272.

3. Bidra A, Daubert D, Garcia L, et al. 2016 ACP Clinical Practice Guidelines for Recall and maintenance of patients with tooth-borne and implant-borne dental restorations. J Prosthodont. 2016; 25: S32–S40.

4. Rateitschak KH. Periodontology. In: Rateitschak KH, Rateitschak EM, Wolf HR, *et al.* editors, *Color Atlas of Dental Medicine.* 2nd ed. New York: Thieme, 1989.

5. Silverstein L, Kurtzman GM Oral hygiene and maintenance of dental implants. Dent Today. 2006; 25(3): 70–75.

6. Linkevicius T, Puisys A, Linkeviciene L, Peciulience V, Schlee M Crestal bone stability around implants with horizontal matching connection after soft tissue thickening: a prospective clinical trial. Clin Implant Dent Relat Res. 2015; 17(3): 497–508.

7. Kabir L, Stiesch M, Grischke J The effect of keratinized mucosa on the severity of peri-implant mucositis differs between periodontally healthy subjects and the general population: a cross-sectional study. Clin Oral Investig. 2021; 25(3): 1183–1193.

8. Greenstein G, Cavallaro J The clinical significance of keratinized gingiva around dental implants. Compend Contin Educ Dent. 2011; 32: 24–31.

9. Faggion CM Jr, Listl S, Tu YK Assessment of endpoints in studies on peri-implantitis treatment—A systematic review. J Dent. 2010; 38: 443–450.

10. Bauman GR, Mills M, Rapley J, et al. Clinical parameters of the evaluation during implant maintenance. Int J Oral Maxillofac Implants. 1992; 7: 220–227.

11. Avila-Ortiz G The dental hygienist plays an important role in the prevention, detection, and clinical management of peri-implant diseases. Dimens Dent Hyg. 2013; 11(5): 57–64.

12. Montevecchi M, Blasi V, Checchi L Is implant flossing a risk-free procedure? Int J Oral Maxillofac Implants. 2016; 31: 79–83.

13. Wadwani C, Hess T, Faber T, et al. A descriptive study of the radiographic density of implant restorative cements. J Prosthet Dent. 2010; 103: 295–302.

14. Misch CE. Contemporary Implant Dentistry, 3rd ed. St. Louis, MO: Mosby, 2008: 1061.

15. Cochran DL, Nummikoski PV, Schoolfield JD, Jones AA, Oates TW A prospective multicenter 5-year radiographic evaluation of crestal bone levels over time in 596 dental implants placed in 192 patients. *J Periodontol.* 2009; 80: 725–733.

16. Misch CE Density of bone: effect on treatment plans, surgical approach, healing, and progressive bone loading. Int J Oral Implantol. 1990; 6: 23–31.

7 Implant Complications: Peri-Implant Disease, Biofilm, and Corrosion

With contributions by Dr. Maria L. Geisinger, Dr. Gerrarda O'Beirne, and Dr. Luciana Safioti

What is the hygienist's role in restoratively driven implant complications?

The biocompatibility of titanium has been well researched, ceramic (zirconia) are available, and implants are well established as a valuable tooth replacement modality. In 2015 in the United States, over two million dental implants are placed annually with a survival rate after 10 years of 91.6%. Peri-mucositis rates of 33 and 16% of implants placed developed peri-implantitis (1).

Implants have proven to be an excellent treatment option for our patients. However, there is still some confusion that exists when it comes to the long-term assessment of these sophisticated medical devices. It is important to address this and to understand the role of the team members. The team members include the surgical dentist, restorative dentist, dental assistants, dental laboratory technician, dental hygienist, and the patient.

All members of the team should understand what to look for and how to detect potential complications. *The dental hygienist will have the most important role in long-term maintenance and should be able to recognize what signs and symptoms to look for.* He or she should also understand when surgical intervention is required. The other team members will depend on the dental hygienist for any information that may be pertinent to the long-term success of the implant.

The high survival rate of osseointegrated implants is well documented, but if an implant does fail it is generally due to bacterial infection, a poorly designed prosthesis, or overextended occlusal force (occlusal overload) (2). Studies are now showing that

Peri-Implant Therapy for the Dental Hygienist, Second Edition. Susan S. Wingrove.
© 2022 John Wiley & Sons, Inc. Published 2022 by John Wiley & Sons, Inc.
Companion website: www.wiley.com/go/wingrove/implant

only a small percentage of implant failures are due to occlusal overload (3), and the majority of the late failures of already integrated implants can be attributed to biofilm, peri-implant infections, residue (i.e., cement, instrument), and corrosion.

In Peri-Implant Therapy for the Dental Hygienist First Edition, cement residue implantitis was highlighted. Studies have reported a correlation between excess cement and the prevalence of peri-implant disease (4). Staubli et al., completed a systematic review that concluded that the rough surface structure of cement remnants may facilitate retention and biofilm formation and excess cement is a potential risk factor for peri-implantitis (5) (see Chapter 9 Assessment and treatment for implants with cement residue).

This chapter will focus on the complications that can lead to peri-implant disease (mucositis and implantitis) and includes special contributions from by Dr. Maria L. Geisinger (implant complications and peri-implant disease), Dr. Gerrarda O'Beirne (biofilm), and Dr. Luciana Safioti (corrosion) (see Figure 7.1A–C). It is important as hygienists to understand these complications and their role in peri-implant disease detection, diagnosis, and treatment.

Implant complications: prevention, identification, and treatment

Contribution by Dr. Maria L. Geisinger DDS, MS

We have established that dental implant complications are common and may be due to a variety of etiologies and may be classified as prosthetic or biologic. While dental implants enjoy a high level of success, all members of the dental team need to be aware of common dental implant complications and be prepared to identify and intervene in these cases. As dental hygienists are on the front lines in examining and treating intraoral inflammation, they have a critical role in the prevention of peri-implant diseases and in the long-term maintenance of dental implants. As such, a thorough understanding of the signs and symptoms of peri-implant health, peri-implant mucositis, peri-implantitis, and other implant complications and the potential effective therapies for these implant complications is critical.

In our discussion of treatment planning, we focused on best practices to *set the stage* to establish long-term health and discussed both biologic and prosthetic complications (see Chapter 4 treatment planning). We will review risk factors for both biologic and prosthetic complications. What are common implant complications?

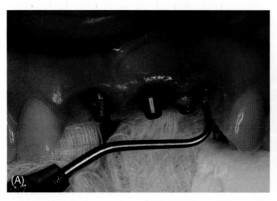
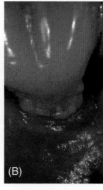
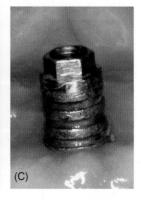

Figure 7.1 (A) Peri-implantitis. Courtesy of Dr. John Remien. (B) Biofilm present on implant. Courtesy of Dr. Pam Maragliano-Muniz. (C) Corrosion implant. Courtesy of Dr. Georgios Kotsakis.

Peri-implant disease; mucositis and peri-implantitis

Peri-implant mucositis has been defined as an inflammatory lesion of the mucosa surrounding an implant without loss of supporting peri-implant bone (6,7). Peri-implant mucositis has been shown to develop when biofilm deposits accumulate within the mucosal sulci at osseointegrated dental implants (6–8). While these lesions have been characterized as analogous to gingivitis lesions around teeth, it has been noted that the histologic inflammatory lesions associated with peri-implant mucositis are larger and require a longer time of pristine oral hygiene to reverse than gingivitis lesions (9, 10). The overall incidence of peri-implant mucositis has been reported to be observed in up to 65% of subjects with dental implants (11). Clinical signs associated with peri-implant mucositis include bleeding upon gentle probing, erythema, edema, and suppuration (6–9). Additionally, while peri-implant mucositis is reversible and may be present for long periods of time without progression to peri-implantitis, it is considered a precursor to peri-implantitis and may progress if left untreated (8, 9, 12).

Peri-implantitis is a pathological condition occurring in tissues around dental implants, characterized by inflammation of the peri-implant mucosa and loss of supporting peri-implant bone (7, 13) (see Figure 7.2). Clinically, these lesions are characterized by swelling, erythema, pain, bleeding upon probing, increasing probing depths, and radiographic bone loss (7). Peri-implantitis lesions have been demonstrated to commence early in the post-restorative period and to progress more rapidly than is seen with periodontitis lesions (14, 15).

Risk factors that have been associated with peri-implantitis include a history of periodontitis, smoking, hyperglycemia, retained cement, restorative design, implant-abutment interface, and previous implant failure at the implant site (13, 16–20). Overall incidence of peri-implantitis varies in different reports and have been reported to range from 10 to 47% (11, 21, 22). Given the highly prevalent nature of peri-implantitis and the relative difficulty in treating peri-implant lesions, identification of high-risk patients is critical in clinical practice. *What predisposing factors are associated with biologic and prosthetic complications?*

Biologic and prosthetic complications

Factors associated with biologic complications

Systemic Disease

Many common systemic diseases may also directly affect the rates of implant survival. In particular, we will discuss diabetes mellitus, osteoporosis/osteopenia, and autoimmune disorders, but emerging evidence suggest that many other systemic conditions may influence implant health.

Dental implants placed in patients with diabetes have been shown to have higher failure rates than those placed in nondiabetic patients (23, 24). In humans, hyperglycemia is known to impair wound healing, impair host defense against pathogens, prolong the inflammatory response to injury, and impair new bone formation and bone repair (24). Future studies are needed to identify distinct cut-off points and quantify the risks, if any, associated with diabetes and development of peri-implantitis.

Osteoporosis/osteopenia have common risk factors with periodontal and peri-implant diseases, including cigarette smoking, dietary factors, and medications, but periodontal disease has also been independently associated with bone density and osteoporosis diagnosis (25, 26). It is important to note that individuals with osteoporosis have decreased alveolar bone

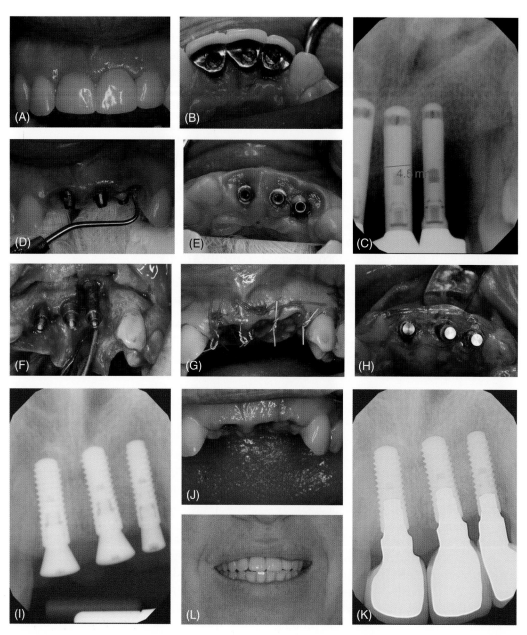

Figure 7.2 Peri-implantitis case. Courtesy of Dr. John Remien. (A) Peri-implantitis (facial view). (B) Peri-implantitis (lingual view). (C) Periapical X-ray. (D) Notice the exudate. (E) Occlusal view. (F) Full thickness flap elevation/removal of implants and granulomatous tissue. (G) GBR with xenograft (bovine), mineralized bone, and resorbable collagen membrane. (H) Implant placement after 6 months healing utilizing a surgical stent. (I) Periapical X-ray placed implants. (J) Tissue facial view pre-restorative. (K) Restored at 3 months post-implant placement. (L) Final photo. Courtesy of Dr. John Remien.

Table 7.1 Case definitions for peri-implant health, peri-implant mucositis, and peri-implantitis (7).

	Peri-implant health	**Peri-implant mucositis**	**Peri-implantitis**
Definition	Implant without signs and symptoms of disease at either the soft- or hard-tissue attachment and without noted pathology	Reversible inflammation of the soft-tissue mucosal attachment around dental implants without concomitant bone loss	An inflammatory lesion around dental implants that affects the soft- and hard-tissue attachment and characterized by bone loss.
Visual inspection	No noted erythema No noted edema Firm mucosal consistency	Erythema may be present Edema may be present Soft mucosal consistency	Erythema may be present Edema may be present Soft mucosal consistency
Patient-reported signs/symptoms	No pain No paresthesia No loss of function	Patients may report pain	Patients may report pain
Bleeding upon probing	Lack of profuse bleeding on probing.	Presence of profuse bleeding and/or suppuration on probing	Presence of profuse bleeding and/or suppuration on probing
Probing pocket depths	Probing pocket depths may vary based upon soft-tissue height, but should not increase over time	Probing depths are increased from baseline levels	Probing depths are increased from baseline levels
Radiographic bone loss	Absence of bone loss after initial remodeling	Absence of bone loss after initial remodeling	Progressive bone loss after initial remodeling

Renvert et al. (7).

density and mass and thinner cortical bone than healthy counterparts, which have the potential to affect primary implant stability (26). While current studies have not shown a definitive association of peri-implantitis with osteoporosis, dental implant placement and the subsequent application of forces to the alveolar bone and the use of bisphosphonate medications in osteoporotic patients may mitigate progressive alveolar bone loss (25–27).

Autoimmune disorders, particularly scleroderma, rheumatoid arthritis, and Sjögren's syndrome have been associated with an increase in bleeding index and marginal bone loss after placement of dental implants, but this does not seem to affect cumulative success rates, which remain high in these patients (28). In patients with systemic diseases that may increase risks of biologic implant complications, more frequent assessments and maintenance may be warranted.

Systemic medications

Some systemic medications have been associated with a decrease in implant success through a decrease in osseointegration. Both selective serotonin reuptake inhibitors (SSRIs) and proton pump inhibitors (PPIs) have been associated with increased implant failure rates (29–32). Patients taking SSRIs saw rates of implant failures that were three times higher than for individuals who were not taking SSRIs (29, 30). Furthermore, individuals taking PPIs also demonstrated a 2–3 increase in failure rates (31, 32).

Smoking status and /or tobacco cessation

Smoking is a known risk factor for periodontal disease and this effect is mediated by a variety of mechanisms including reduction in neutrophil chemotactic response, local vasoconstriction, alterations in immune response, a shift to a more dysbiotic biofilm, and a decrease in fibroblast number and collagen production (13, 33, 34). These effects of smoking can lead to chronic inflammation at periodontal and peri-implant tissues. Smoking is an established predisposing factor for peri-implantitis and patients who smoke have up to two times the failure rate of implants compared to non-smokers (13, 33). In patients who use tobacco, maintenance is increasingly critical as supportive implant therapy for smokers shows a greater benefit in reducing rates of peri-implantitis than in non-smokers (35).

Periodontal health

It is well-established that a history of periodontitis is a risk factor for peri-implant diseases (6, 13, 14). Findings suggest that bacteria associated with periodontal disease and peri-implant diseases are similar (36). Colonization with these bacterial species occurs within the first 28 days after implant exposure to the oral environment and bacteria can be transferred from distant reservoirs, such as periodontal pockets at teeth elsewhere within a patient's mouth (37). Since periodontitis is the most common reason for tooth loss in adult patients, treatment of active periodontal disease and continued maintenance therapy for patients with dental implants is critical in maintenance of both teeth and implants (36–39).

Plaque/Oral biofilm control

Plaque control delivered by patients and professionals can result in a reduction in clinical signs of peri-implant inflammation, which is important in controlling peri-implant mucositis and preventing the shift from peri-implant mucositis to peri-implantitis (40). Furthermore, a lack of adherence to supportive peri-implant therapy results in more sites with mucosal inflammation, increased levels of pathogenic bacteria, and peri-implant bone loss (10). High levels of oral bacteria have also been associated with disruptions to implant surface characteristics and titanium corrosion, which can alter the biocompatibility and potential osseointegration of some dental implant surfaces (20). Personalized oral hygiene instructions, regular implant examination and imaging, and professional implant cleaning must be an ongoing component of all implant treatment plans (10, 20, 40, 41).

Peri-implant soft tissue quality/quantity

It has been proposed that the establishment of a circumferential seal of tightly packed collagen around the implant-oral cavity interface may improve long-term implant success and that this is better facilitated in the presence of keratinized mucosa (42). Given the anatomical differences between soft-tissue attachments around teeth and implants, it should be noted that higher levels of gingival inflammation are associated with a lack of keratinized mucosa (42, 43). Particularly in patients with other biologic risk factors, including increased plaque accumulation and previous history of periodontitis, increased keratinized mucosa may be protective to allow for personal and professional plaque removal (42–45).

Prosthetic complications

While prosthetic complications do not have an underlying microbiological etiology and do not, in most cases jeopardize the osseointegration of the dental implant, they are, nevertheless, a clinical problem during the practice of treating implant patients. A recent review has identified six categories of technical or mechanical failures: loosening of screws, screw fracture, fracture of framework, fracture of abutment, chipping/fracture of veneering material, and decementation (46). As reported in this retrospective analysis, the overall incidence of technical or mechanical complications for all implants in partially edentulous patients was 10.8% for single implant restorations and 16.1% for partial fixed implant-supported prostheses over approximately a 5-year period (46). The most common form of mechanical complication for single implant restorations was screw loosening and was veneering material fracture in partial fixed implant-supported prostheses (46).

Prosthetic design and occlusal load

Overall, prosthetic/occlusal risk factors in the absence of inflammation are not thought to increase the risk of peri-implantitis, but these factors may modify disease progression if inflammation is present.

Occlusal load is influenced by prosthetic design, but hard to study due to lack of quantification of overload. For instance, implants demonstrating off-axis forces demonstrate more peri-implant bone loss after loading, when not engineered in a cross-arch stabilized prosthesis but threshold values are unclear and may vary based upon other implant and patient-specific factors (47). A recent systematic review concluded that occlusal overloading was associated with peri-implant marginal bone loss caused by microtrauma concentrated at the marginal bone (47). The mechanisms for this marginal bone loss may be similar to that seen in natural dentition wherein occlusal trauma may serve to potentiate attachment loss in the presence of inflammation.

Retained cement

Retained cement has been indicated in a large number of peri-implant disease cases (6, 13, 14, 35, 48). This association may be due to residual cement presenting a rough, plaque-retentive surface and therefore lead to peri-implant inflammation (5). Peri-implant disease prevalence is significantly higher at fixtures with cement-retained versus screw-retained restorations (49) and when implants with peri-implantitis were examined subgingivally, 81% had excess cement present whereas no retained cement was found at healthy implants (50).

To reduce the risk of retention of excess cement, practitioners are cautioned to practice techniques to avoid excess cement, including: use of screw-retained restorations, allowing for adequate soft-tissue healing prior to seating of a permanent restoration, and early follow up after initial cementation to detect any early signs of cement retention, see Peri-Implant Therapy for the Dental Hygienist, Clinical Guide to Maintenance and Disease Complication, Chapter 7 Cement residue complication (4).

Parafunctional habits/occlusal dysfunction

Patients with parafunctional habits have been shown to have higher risks of implant failure, over time (51). Implant failure rates in patients with bruxism have been estimated to be up to 3–4 times higher than in nonbruxers (52). Given these increased failure rates, assessment of parafunctional habits and adequate treatment planning to ensure adequate implant number and placement to reduce individual occlusal load and off-axis forces are critical, particularly for patients who may also have other biologic risk factors. In these patients, reinforcement of the importance of the use of an occlusal appliance to manage excessive forces and considerations of a history parafunction should be considered during initial treatment planning.

Examination, diagnosis, and treatment of peri-implant disease

Proper examination, diagnosis, and treatment planning are critical to maintaining health at dental implants. In order to assess the health of a dental implant, a careful clinical assessment and adequate radiographs are necessary to identify signs of both health and disease. Importantly, baseline radiographs with a clear delineation of the crestal bone levels taken at the time of implant placement and prosthetic restoration are important references that will allow clinicians to evaluate any changes to crestal bone height that may occur. Radiographs taken at regular intervals can allow for longitudinal assessment of crestal bone height over time. Patient interview to determine if there are signs of either biologic or prosthetic complications, including pain, occlusal dysfunction, or prosthesis mobility is a critical component to the implant examination.

During the clinical examination, it is important to note that it has been proposed that the soft-tissue mucosal seal exhibits less resistance to probing and gentle probing pressure (<25 N) is required (53). In addition, clinical evaluation including assessment of implant mobility, soft-tissue color and contour, probing depth measurements, quantification of dental plaque accumulation, and assessment of bleeding or suppuration on probing are all required (7). Dental implants should be visually evaluated and probed routinely and periodically as part of comprehensive oral examinations, much like natural teeth. Utilizing a systematic approach to diagnosis is critical to properly identify disease and formulate a proper treatment plan.

Many treatment options are available to address implant complications. Initial assessment of the clinical signs of inflammation is the critical first step and most often provided by dental hygienists in practice (see Figure 7.3). This decision matrix, reviews the potential for initial

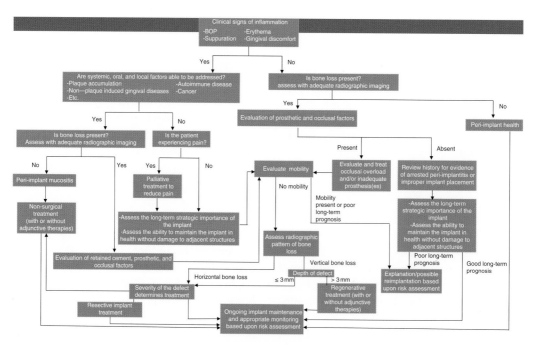

Figure 7.3 A decision matrix to determine treatment for peri-implant diseases. Courtesy of Dr. Maria L. Geisinger.

evaluation and treatment of dental implant complications. Refer to Chapter 9 for protocols for peri-implant disease treatment, mucositis and early peri-implantitis. If the dental hygienist understands what signs and symptoms to look for, early detection and treatment may commence. This will ultimately benefit the implant team and most importantly, the patient. Be ready and be prepared to take on this next, very important challenge in our profession!

The role of *biofilm* in peri-implant disease

Contribution by Dr. Gerrarda O'Beirne BDS, MSD

Dental implants have presented the dental community with an amazing way to restore functionality in the edentulous or partially dentate patient. The replacement of a functioning dentition benefits the individual on many fronts, nutritionally, psychologically, and socially. Initially when implants were introduced, the presumption was that the transmucosal seal around the implant should not be disturbed. Removal of plaque, oral biofilm, from around implants and below the gumline was not a focus. As with everything, our knowledge base has evolved.

We now know that biological complications can arise over time and that routine oral biofilm removal is essential for the long-term stability of the dental fixture. Indeed, there is strong evidence that poor oral biofilm control around dental implants is one of the main risk factors for the development of peri-implant disease (6, 13, 54, 55). *Where do we start?*

We need to educate our patients about the nature of oral biofilms in health and disease and around both natural teeth and implants. They should know that health represents a state of homeostasis between the host and the resident flora, symbiosis (the state of co-existence between the human host and the wide variety of flora,

bacteria, viruses, eukaryotes, and archaea, that live together in a beneficial relationship, contributing to health). Disease represents a loss of equilibrium or dysbiosis (a loss of microbial diversity with an imbalance that means a decrease in beneficial bacteria, an increase in pathogenic species and the onset of disease) (56, 57).

It is also important to consider the fact that dental implants differ with respect to surface composition and texture and the introduction of the varying contours on the implant-supported restorations all bring about unique ecological changes that offer a modified habitat for the flora to grow and a challenge for the patient to manage (58, 59). Finally, the potential for the seeding of a biofilm can occur at many stages of treatment and is not just limited to post treatment plaque accumulation. It is a complex plethora of evolving science that we have to try to share with our patients, so as to empower them in their role as co-therapists in the management of the health of their dentition.

Understanding biofilms

According to the Human Microbiome Project (HMP), 26% of the total microbiome is located in the mouth (60). The mouth is an open ecosystem and host to a wide variety of bacteria at all times. For bacteria to persist they have to become attached to a non-shedding surface (tooth, root, or implant). Sheltering from physical forces of the tongue or cheek, that could potentially dislodge them, the protective niche allows the polymicrobial species to integrate themselves into highly organized communities (see Figure 7.4).

Colonization follows a structured pattern with adhesion of primary colonizers to receptors in the enamel pellicle within hours of first contact followed by growth through interbacterial adhesion of the secondary and tertiary colonizers and finally

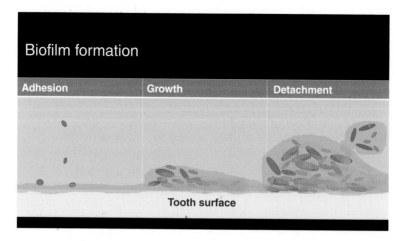

Figure 7.4 Depiction of biofilm formation. Courtesy of Dr. Gerrarda O'Beirne.

detachment to perpetuate the spread of the oral biofilm (61, 62). As the oral biofilm grows, an extracellular matrix is formed to envelope, nourish, and protect the growing mass. There is evidence that a sophisticated community develops with a primitive circulatory system, exhibiting metabolic co-operation and a communication system that works via the release of small diffusible molecules (quorum sensing) (63). This highly evolved ecosystem allows for group co-ordination of the pathogenic potential of the oral biofilm, so that, the compositional flora adjusts favorably to the new conditions and survives (64). In addition, the layering of the microflora within the extracellular matrix affords considerable protection to the embedded bacteria, so that, they are less susceptible to antimicrobials compared to free floating bacteria (65, 66). The oral biofilm that evolves can contain a wide variety of micro-organisms including, predominantly, bacteria but also fungi, viruses, and/or other species (67–69). The exact composition is dictated by microenvironmental conditions of the habitat and that meets the survival requirements of the various species present (56, 63, 67). In the oral cavity alone, studies have shown that several site-specific habitats support unique microbial communities (60, 70).

Biofilm composition and host response in health and disease

As mentioned, the properties of the habitat, both physical and chemical, select out and dictate the colonization profile of the oral biofilm community. Just like teeth, implants have distinctive physical and chemical properties that result in different ecological microenvironments for biofilm formation. Factors such as surface energy, surface roughness, and component implant material influence the make-up and virulence potency of the biofilm (58, 71–73). Oxygen availability for example, differs whether above or below the gingival margin and this affects growth outcomes. Much research has gone into qualitative and quantitative evaluation of the microbiome around teeth and implants in both health and disease. Newer methods of discovery, that are culture independent, have opened up the opportunity to study a wider variety of bacterial species and provide a more complete picture (13, 71).

It was once thought that the oral biofilms around teeth and implants, in both health and disease were similar. Now we believe that, although certain species may be common to both ecosystems, the majority of microflora, particularly those in greater abundance, are distinct when comparing the microbial populations around teeth and implants (74–76). The peri-implant microbiome tends to be less diverse than the periodontal microbiome, and the difference is even more pronounced in health versus in disease (74, 76, 77).

Based on the literature, our current assessment suggests that peri-implantitis lesions are mixed anaerobic infections with periodontal microflora, novel, and even opportunistic species (74, 78–80). The exact characterization of the microbiome of peri-implantitis has not been clarified and continues to be a focus of investigation (13).

In health, the various micro-niches within the oral cavity provide a stable habitat that supports a relatively consistent interdependent community of microflora, *the core microbiome* (the genetic material of all the flora that are shared by all or most humans). These flora are very important to normal biological functioning of the host such as in the generation and uptake of vitamins and in the support of our immune response (60). The stability is due to a dynamic balance or homeostasis between the host and the microbiome (56, 63). The characteristic resident microbiome, also known as the *commensals*, offers benefits to the host through various methods including competitive regulation of potential pathogens *colonization resistance* (56). In short, commensals use up the available resources, outcompeting more virulent species.

The polymicrobial commensal profile tends to feature high levels of Gram +ve cocci bacteria and bacterial loads in the region of 10^2 or 10^3 (61, 81). The community contributes to the host's innate defense mechanism by keeping a surveillance level of inflammatory cells and inflammatory mediators in circulation. The infiltrate released into the sulcus consists of cells and proteins that are involved in killing and/or removal of bacteria (56). This aspect of biofilm containment is particularly important, subgingivally or submu-

cosally, in the case of the implant. The biofilm is protected from contact with saliva and the physical forces that would disrupt the supra-gingival biofilm.

Sites with periodontal disease exhibit a proliferation of Gram −ve flora with bacterial loads in the region of 10^5–10^8 (61, 81), which causes a disproportionate inflammatory response. These observations lead to the idea that the destruction seen in periodontal disease is due to the combined response of bacteria and host (56, 82, 83). The innate host response becomes dysfunctional and the once ordered inflammatory mediator expression that was protective in health becomes destructive in disease. Periodontitis represents a *dysbiotic state*. The inflammatory response perpetuates the dysbiotic cycle with an increase in protein and glycoprotein (GCF) that provides nutritional support for the anaerobic polymicrobial community.

Peri-implant health is also believed to be dependent on a symbiotic state of existence between the microbiome and the host. The introduction of a fixture into the mouth brings into play a number of unique factors that leads to the creation of a selective ecosystem potentially supporting a different microbial composition (74, 76). Again, in health a surveillance level of inflammatory cells circulates in the barrier tissues adjacent to implant-gingival margin in response to the resident microbiome (84). This equilibrium between the implant microbiome and the host's immune response system helps maintains stability of the tissues at the implant site. However, if there is a shift in the local environment with an accumulation of oral biofilm (6) or the introduction of bacterial contamination following installation of the implant-restoration unit (85). We may see the development of the inflammatory cascade leading to peri-mucositis and potentially peri-implantitis.

This is characterized by accumulation of the inflammatory infiltrate, proliferation of the sulcular epithelium and degeneration of the connective tissue matrix that could finally end in the loss of the all-important transmucosal seal (86, 87). The inflammatory infiltrate in peri-implant disease features a predominance of plasma cells and neutrophils (88). The biofilm is not separated from the connective tissue by epithelium as in periodontal disease and only has the barrier membrane for separation (89). The inflammatory lesion is larger in peri-implantitis when compared with periodontitis and spreads out in the adjacent tissues, in close proximity to the bone (87, 89).

It is anticipated that an increase in peri-implant crevicular fluid, with the release of proteins and glycoproteins into the peri-implant space, will alter the nutritional ecosystem of flora by accommodating diverse species, just like in periodontitis (59). The mixed predominantly gram-negative biofilm of peri-implant disease, although likely to be less complex than seen in periodontal disease (74, 76) serves the same function. It alters the biocompatibility of the implant and incites an inflammatory response that perpetuates the dysbiotic state.

The host response to the microbiome may be modified by *acquired factors*, factors that are not inherited and are acquired after birth. Medications, for example, can directly alter the peri-implant biofilm, as in the case of antibiotics, steroids, or drugs that have hyposalivation as a side effect. Obviously, there are a myriad of systemic conditions that can modify the host-microbiome dynamic such as diabetes (90), or other immune-compromised states.

The microbial profile of smokers is also different, supporting less diversity, and greater pathogenicity (67, 91). Lastly, we have to acknowledge that not all at-risk individuals lose implants and indeed patients with no history of periodontal disease can get peri-implant disease (92). The inter-relationships are complex and many factors both host and site specific may come into play (59).

Management of biofilms around implants

We know that biofilm formation starts within 30 minutes of an implant fixture being placed in the mouth (93, 94). Introduction of the implant-supported restoration transforms the ecosystem, altering the microbial profile (95). There are hints that uniqueness of the implant and the restorative abutment connection needs to be considered as this niche has been shown to support some of the known peri-pathogens such as *Porphyromonas gingivalis* and *Tannerella forsythia* (85). It also seems that biofilms can develop on all implant surfaces that have been developed including titanium and ceramic (zirconia) implants (72, 96). Care needs to be taken with the selection of antimicrobial agents so as to favor biocompatibility on the implant surface (97). In addition, investigation of the interaction between the oral biofilm and the implant surface suggests the potential for development of corrosion with concerns that this could have immunologic consequences that alter the biocompatibility of the fixture (77, 98), see "Corrosion Complication" section of this chapter.

Abstention studies indicate that greater oral biofilm accumulation seems to occur around teeth versus implants (10, 99) but this does not correlate to a protective effect for implants. Oral biofilms, by nature, are tenacious and especially challenging to remove if they have accessed and colonized the implant surface. In an ideal situation, the implant is completely encased in bone and the connective tissue and epithelial components are in intimate contact with the abutment surface, creating the peri-implant mucosal protective seal.

What is our best approach to achieving long-term stability?

As mentioned, the patient with a history of periodontal disease is more at risk for developing peri-implant disease (55, 100).

It is unclear whether the perio-pathogens provide a reservoir or that the increased risk reflects the host response of a vulnerable patient (74, 76). In any case, long-term management of periodontal disease is very important (101, 102). The implant-supported prosthesis should be carefully designed to facilitate effective oral biofilm removal, otherwise, there is the likelihood of an increase in the incidence of peri-implant disease over the long term (59, 103). The research tells us that where possible, a supra-gingival restorative margin is more favorable for access (104). We also know that a dysbiotic shift is correlated with increased probing depth; risking development of peri-implant disease (59, 80), hence deep subgingival placement of restorations should be avoided (59).

Once the implant surface becomes exposed it will become colonized with oral biofilm. In addition to the problematic quality of this being a highly textured surface, we also have to deal with the hydrophobic and layered nature of extracellular matrix of the oral biofilm which has the effect of shielding the biofilm community from anti-microbials (66, 105). These challenges have given rise to a body of research focusing on ways to interfere with adhesion of the bacteria and the extracellular matrix. Since interference with the implant surface runs the risk of amplifying the inflammatory response through the possibility of corrosion, researchers have focused on the development of agents that can effectively remove the oral biofilm in the least invasive way, restoring some level of biocompatibility (106).

Research also suggests that peri-mucositis precedes peri-implantitis (107) and that peri-mucositis sites with oral biofilm accumulation over extensive periods of time, are more at risk of transitioning to peri-implantitis (12). Again, prevention is key since we have evidence that institution of effective oral biofilm control reverses the course of peri-implant mucositis, arresting

the arc of deterioration in health at the implant site.

Patients should be clear about their role in the prevention of development of that destructive inflammatory lesion that can lead to loss of integrity of the transmucosal seal. We can explain to them that oral biofilm is not just composed of unicellular micro-organisms living independently, but coordinated, functional colonies attached to the surface as oral biofilms. Hence, a concerted effort needs to be made to access and remove this hydrophobic film. It is important that they understand that it is easy to remove in the early stages of accumulation, when the level of maturation does not pose a serious threat to the health of the implant. Mechanical plaque removal is considered the standard of care for management of peri-implant disease (41, 108). The patient should be coached on the effective use of oral hygiene tools that access and manage the peri-implant oral biofilm.

The transition from peri-implant health to disease is correlated with a decrease in quantity or loss of the health-associated species and an increase in the quantity of disease-associated species. The degree of dysbiosis encountered at peri-implant disease sites has correlations with the individual's risk profile in addition to an interplay of site-specific factors. An exact profile of the peri-implant disease microbiome has not been fully outlined; however, it appears to be less diverse when compared with periodontal disease.

There is a strong evidence that poor plaque control and lack of regular maintenance therapy are risk factors for the development of peri-implant disease. Curtailment of oral biofilm accumulation at all stages of treatment is necessary, including delivery of sterile/decontaminated restorative components and with the regular disruption of the peri-implant oral biofilm as part of a home-care regimen. Our focus should be on maintenance of the protective transmucosal seal and underlying boney support by careful consideration of the host and site factors in favor of a symbiotic ecological micro-environment and peri-implant health.

The role of *corrosion* in peri-implant disease

Contribution by Dr. Luciana Safioti DDS, MSD

Oral bacterial biofilm is the primary etiologic agent for peri-implantitis, and patients with a history of periodontal disease, poor oral hygiene, and no regular periodontal and peri-implant maintenance care have an increased risk of developing peri-implantitis. Despite the lack of a strong evidence, other factors have been linked to or proposed to have a role in the pathogenesis.

Titanium shows excellent biocompatibility and high resistance to corrosion due to the formation of a titanium dioxide (TiO_2) layer on the implant surface (109, 110). However, despite the high resistance to corrosion and the biocompatibility properties that allow cell attachment and osseointegration, corrosion can still happen in the oral environment, with permanent degradation of the implant surface (111). Rodrigues et al. (111), examined implants removed from patients with peri-implantitis for corrosion with magnification digital microscopy. Delamination, deformities, cracking of the bulk of the implant, pitting, discoloration, and scratches are found (see Figure 7.5). The breakdown or dissolution of the biocompatible interface represented by the titanium dioxide layer of the implant surface and the peri-implant bone leads to loss of osseointegration of the implant, which characterizes peri-implantitis.

An association between titanium dissolution and peri-implantitis was found by Safioti et al. (98), in an in vivo study comparing healthy and diseased implants. The

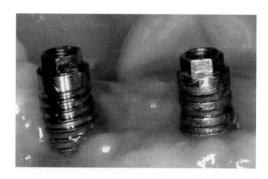

Figure 7.5 Healthy implant and corroded implant example. Courtesy of Dr. Georgios Kotsakis

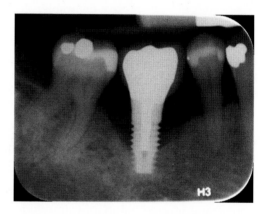

Figure 7.6 Radiograph showing bone loss around an implant. Courtesy of Dr. Luciana Safioti.

authors showed statistically significant increased quantities of titanium dissolution products, measured in the form of titanium particles, in submucosal biofilm collected around implants with peri-implantitis when compared to biofilm collected around healthy implants (see Figures 7.6 and 7.7). In addition, this finding implied the role of the peri-implant oral biofilm as an intermediary pool of titanium particles that can eventually be incorporated into host tissue (98). Titanium particles or elements have also been found in epithelial cells collected from peri-implant mucosal tissues (112), in foreign bodies comprised of titanium and cement in soft tissues of implants with peri-implantitis (113), and in bone and soft-tissue biopsies from sites with peri-implantitis (114).

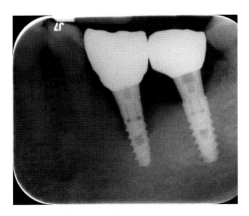

Figure 7.7 Radiographic images of an implant with bone loss adjacent to a healthy implant without bone loss. Courtesy of Dr. Luciana Safioti.

Dissolution of titanium may be triggered by mechanical and biological factors. The corroded surface of the implant may release titanium particles or ions in response to wear from the implant-abutment interface (114), mechanical attempts to debride the implant surface (113), promotion of an acidic oral environment by biofilm (115), and oral solutions such as fluoride (116), among others. The use of ultrasonic metal tips for scaling on titanium implants releases particles and elicits inflammation, which may cause bone loss and aggravate peri-implantitis (117). In addition, the use of titanium brushes has been found to leave marks and cause increased dissolution of the titanium, when the brushes were used on the surface of titanium discs mimicking commercial titanium dental implants (118).

The presence of lipopolysaccharides (LPS) from the walls of gram-negative bacteria combined with local acidification of the peri-implant tissues because of inflammation may decrease the corrosion resistance of titanium promoting dissolution of the titanium surface layer (115). The presence of *Streptococcus mutans*, responsible for the release of oral acid, also renders an acidic environment that reduces the corrosion resistance of titanium (119). The corroded titanium surfaces may become niches for LPS of gram-negative bacteria (115) and colonization of *P. gingivalis* (120), propagating a cycle of interaction between titanium and biofilm, ensuing biocorrosion.

Of special interest in in-office maintenance by a hygienist, is the use of fluoride, present in several oral hygiene products. Solutions that turn the oral environment acidic such as fluoride may cause dissolution of the titanium layer (116). Toniollo et al. (121), evaluated the effect of different concentrations of sodium fluoride (NaF) on the surface of titanium. The study suggested that the use of 0.05% NaF solution was safe, whereas a concentration of 0.2% caused corrosion (121).

In another study, the protective titanium dioxide layer was destroyed by fluoride ions when concentrations were higher than 0.1%, leading to corrosion (122). There seems to be no consensus on the recommendation of fluoride and its impact on the corrosion behavior of titanium implants, although these in vitro studies suggest that both stannous and sodium fluorides are safe to use in patients having titanium implants; however, the higher concentrations above 0.1% should have a neutral pH formulation, (see Chapter 8 for more information on pH and fluoride).

Titanium particles released to the peri-implant tissues as a result of degradation of a dental implant can trigger the immune system and act as inflammatory agents, causing increased release of pro-inflammatory cytokines and factors associated with stimulation of bone resorption, all associated with peri-implantitis (123–126). Moreover, titanium particles were found to be modifiers of the peri-implant microbiome that may result in dysbiosis (77). By eliciting pro-inflammatory immune responses, corrosion can work as a potential etiologic factor in the pathogenesis of peri-implantitis and enhancement of bone loss, especially when combined with peri-implant biofilm.

Kotsakis and Olmedo (127) suggested a new model of infection in peri-implantitis, distinct from the one in periodontitis (see Figure 7.8). This theoretical model includes local and environmental factors including peri-implant biofilm, use of antibiotics, and titanium particles that lead to alterations in microbiome diversity and dysbiosis in peri-implant diseases.

Surgical and non-surgical decontamination of the implant threads that became exposed, because of bone resorption and loss of osseointegration, is a crucial goal during peri-implantitis treatment. However, using the incorrect method to remove the oral biofilm may lead to damage to the implant surfaces with further breakdown of the oxide layer and corrosion, compromising the biocompatibility of titanium surfaces. The evident association between peri-implantitis and dissolved titanium brings up the importance of developing protocols for the treatment of peri-implantitis that aim to control the biofilm while also respecting the properties of the titanium material surface (98).

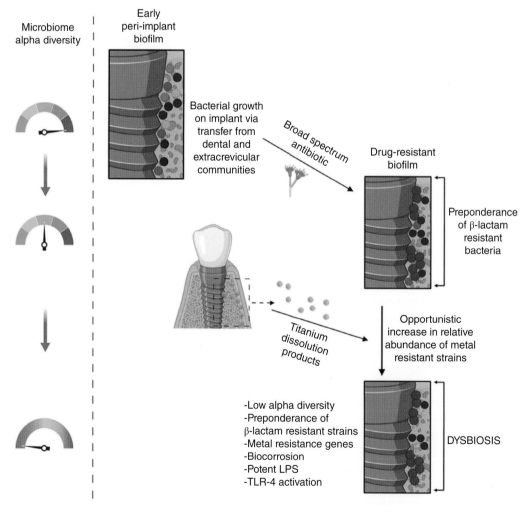

Figure 7.8 Theoretical model of infection in peri-implantitis. Courtesy of Dr. Georgios Kotsakis and Dr. Daniel Olmedo (127).

Using a peri-implantitis model in vitro to simulate implant decontamination and cellular response with different chemotherapeutic agents, *the use of chlorhexidine* demonstrated to have cytotoxic effects on osteoblasts and is not recommended for the treatment of titanium surfaces (97). Kotsakis et al., proposed that saline solution, 20% citric acid, and a mix of 1.5% sodium hypochlorite (NaOCl) with 24% ethylenediaminetetraacetic acid (EDTA) were effective in decontaminating the implant surfaces and restoring biocompatibility in the treatment of peri-implantitis (97).

Non-surgical and surgical modalities have been proposed for the treatment of peri-implant diseases. In general, treatment has limited predictability making peri-implantitis an emerging challenge faced by the dental community. Non-surgical treatment including mechanical debridement with hand instruments and the use of glycine powder air-abrasive devices may result in improvement of the peri-implant inflammation; however, it has limited effect on the definitive reduction of peri-implant probing depth and decontamination of the implant surfaces (128). Surgical treatment may be considered when complete resolution of the disease is not achieved with non-surgical modalities. Surgical treatment may include resective procedures with bone recontouring and decontamination of the implant surface (129), and regenerative procedures with addition of bone grafts to the decontaminated bony defects and implant surfaces (130).

For any treatment modality, it is important to limit the dissolution or breakdown of the titanium surface that can be caused by instruments or brushes used for debridement, and at the same time provide a clean surface to arrest progression of the peri-implant disease and to promote regeneration of the lost osseointegration. Titanium dissolution during decontamination of the implant surface and its effects to the host should become an essential consideration for clinical use and fabrication of instruments for implant non-surgical and surgical debridement. For protocols and proper instruments (see Chapter 9).

Summary

Long-term prevention of peri-implant disease, now more important than ever, starts with using safe, research-based products for in-office and for our patients to use at home. Corrosion is being widely studied as a contributing factor in the etiology and progression of bone loss around dental implants. Bacterial oral biofilm is considered the main etiologic factor in the development of peri-implantitis however, the presence of titanium particles around implants indicating corrosion of the implant surface and the interaction of the oral biofilm with the implant surface cannot be underestimated as factors in the progression of peri-implant disease.

Over the next decade, expect an explosion of dental implants. This will be followed by a tidal wave of ailing and failing implants that will change the way we practice dental hygiene. For long-term implant success, it is necessary to *detect* early signs of any implant complications, *diagnose* these complications to provide early intervention, and perform in-office implant maintenance *treatment* on patients at least once every 6 months, including effective biofilm removal and home-care recommendations (131).

References

1. Daubert DM, Weinstein BF, Bordin S, Leroux BG, Flemming TF Prevalence and predictive factors for peri-implant disease and implant failure: a cross-sectional analysis. J Periodontol. 2015; 86: 337–347.
2. Paquette DW, Brodala N, Williams RC Risk factors for endosseous dental implant failure. Dent Clin N Am. 2006; 50: 351–374.

3. Heitz-Mayfield LJA Diagnosis and management of peri-implant disease. Aust Dent J. 2008; 53(1 Suppl): S43–S48.

4. Wingrove S. Peri-Implant Therapy for the Dental Hygienist: A Clinical Guide to Implant Maintenance and Disease Complications. Oxford: Wiley Blackwell, 2013.

5. Staubli N, Walter C, Schmidt JC, Weiger R, Zitzmann NU Excess cement and the risk of peri-implant disease - a systematic review. Clin Oral Implants Res. 2017; 28: 1278–1290.

6. Heitz-Mayfield LJA, Salvi GE Peri-implant mucositis. 2017 World Workshop for Classification of Periodontal and Peri-implant Diseases and Conditions. J Periodontol. 2018; 89(Suppl 1): S257–S266.

7. Renvert S, Persson GR, Pirih FQ, Camargo PM Peri-implant health, peri-implant mucositis, and peri-implantitis: case definitions and diagnostic considerations. Proceedings from the 2017 World Workshop for Classification of Periodontal and Peri-Implant Diseases and Conditions. J Periodontol. 2018; 89(Suppl 1): S304–S312.

8. Pontoriero R, Tonelli MP, Carnevale G, Mombelli A, Nyman SR, Lang NP Experimentally induced peri-implant mucositis: a clinical study in humans. Clin Oral Implants Res. 1994; 5: 254–259.

9. Zitzmann NU, Berglundh T, Marinello CP, Lindhe J Experimental peri-implant mucositis in man. J Clin Periodontol. 2001; 28: 517–523.

10. Salvi GE, Aglietta M, Eick S, Sculean A, Lang NP, Ramseier CA Reversibility of experimental peri-implant mucositis compared with experimental gingivitis in humans. Clin Oral Implants Res. 2012; 23: 182–190.

11. Dierks J, Tomasi C Peri-implant health and disease: a systematic review of current epidemiology. J Clin Periodontol. 2015; 42(Suppl 16): S158–S171.

12. Costa FO, Takenaka-Martinez S, Cota LOO, Ferreira SD, Silva GL, Costa JEE Peri-implant disease in subjects with and without preventative maintenance: a 5-year follow-up. J Clin Periodontol. 2012; 39: 173–181.

13. Schwarz F, Derks J, Monje A, Wang H-L Peri-implantitis 2017 World Workshop. J Periodontol. 2018; 89(Suppl 1): S267–S290.

14. Derks J, Schaller D, Hakansson J, Wennstrom JL, Tomasi C, Berglundh T Peri-implantitis – onset and pattern of progression. J Clin Periodontol. 2016; 43: 383–388.

15. Fransson C, Tomasi C, Pikner SS, et al. Severity and pattern of peri-implantitis associated bone loss. J Clin Periodontol. 2010; 37: 442–448.

16. Oh S-L, Shiau HJ, Reynolds MA Survival of dental implants at sites after implant failure: a systematic review. J Prosthet Dent. 2020; 123(1): 54–60.

17. Javed F, Romanos GE Chronic hyperglycemia as a risk factors in implant therapy. Periodontol. 2019; 81: 57–63.

18. Koutouzis T Implant-abutment connection as a contributing factor to peri-implant disease. J Periodontol. 2019; 81: 152–166.

19. Dixon DR, London RM Restorative design and associated risks for peri-implant diseases. J Periodontol. 2019; 81: 167–178.

20. Daubert DM, Weinstein BF Biofilm as a risk factor in implant treatment. Periodontol. 2019; 81: 29–40.

21. Mombelli A, Müller N, Cionca N The epidemiology of peri-implantitis. Clin Oral Implants Res. 2012; 23(Suppl 6): 67–76.

22. Fransson C, Wennström J, Tomasi C, Berglundh T Extent of peri-implantitis associated bone loss. J Clin Periodontol. 2009; 36: 357–363.

23. Morris HF Implant survival in patients with type 2 diabetes: placement to 36 months. Ann Periodontol. 2000; 5: 157–177.

24. Iacopino AM Periodontitis and diabetes interrelationships: role of inflammation. Ann Periodontol. 2001; 6: 125–137.

25. Geurs NC Osteoporosis and periodontal disease. Periodontol. 2007; 44: 29–43.

26. Geurs NC, Lewis CE, Jeffcoat MK Osteoporosis and periodontal disease progression. Periodontol. 2003; 32: 105–110.

27. Kribbs PJ, Smith DE, Chesnut CH Jr Oral findings in osteoporosis. Part I: measurement of mandibular bone density. J Prosthet Dent. 1983; 50: 576–579.

28. Weinlander M, Krenmair G, Piehslinger E Implant prosthodontic rehabilitation of patients with rheumatic disorders: a case series report. Int J Prosthodont. 2010; 23: 22–28.

29. Altay MA, Sindel A, Özalp Ö, et al. Does the intake of selective serotonin reuptake inhibitors negatively affect dental implant osseointegration? A retrospective study. J Oral Implantol. 2018; 44: 260–265.

30. Wu X, Al-Abedalla K, Abi-Nader S, Daniel NG, Nicolau B, Tamimi F Proton pump inhibitors and the risk of osseointegrated dental implant failure. A cohort study. Clin Implant Dent Relat Res. 2017; 19: 222–232.

31. Chrcanovic BR, Kisch J, Albrektsson T, Wennerberg A Intake of proton pump inhibitors is associated with an increased risk of dental implant failure. Int J Oral Maxillofac Implants. 2017; 32: 1097–1102.

32. Battaglino R, Fu J, Späte U, et al. Serotonin regulates osteoclast differentiation through its transporter. J Bone Miner Res. 2004; 19: 1420–1431.

33. Curtis DA, Lin G-H, Fishman A, et al. Patient-centered risk assessment in implant treatment planning. Int J Oral Maxillofac Implants. 2019; 34: 506–520.

34. ALHarthi SSY, Natto ZS, Gyurko R, O'Neill R, Steffensen B Association between time since quitting smoking and periodontitis in former smokers in the National Health and Nutrition Examination Surveys (NHANES) 2009 to 2012. J Periodontol. 2019; 90: 16–25.

35. Araujo MG, Lindhe J Peri-implant health. Proceedings from the 2017 World Workshop. J Periodontol. 2018; 89(Suppl 1): S249–S256.

36. Ata-Ali J, Candel-Marti M, Flichy-Fernandez A, et al. Peri-implantitis: associated microbiota and treatment. Med Oral Patol Oral Cir Bucal. 2011; 16: e937–e943.

37. Quirynen M, Vogels R, Peeters W, et al. Dynamics of subgingival colonization of 'pristine' peri-implant pockets. Clin Oral Implants Res. 2006; 17: 25–37.

38. Renvert S, Roos-Jansaker AM, Lindahl C, et al. Infection at titanium implants with or without a clinical diagnosis of inflammation. Clin Oral Implants Res. 2007; 18: 509–516.

39. Mombelli A, Lang NP The diagnosis and treatment of peri-implantitis. Periodontol. 1998; 17: 63–76.

40. Ramanauskaite A, Tervonen T The efficacy of supportive peri-implant therapies in preventing peri-implantitis and implant loss: a systematic review of the literature. J Oral Maxillofac Res. 2016; 7: e12.

41. Salvi GE, Ramsier CA Efficacy of patient-administered mechanical and/or chemical plaque control protocols in the management of peri-implant mucositis. A systematic review. J Clin Periodontol. 2015; 42(Suppl 16): S187–S201.

42. Souza AB, Tormena M, Matarazzo F, Araujo MG The influence of peri-implant keratinized mucosa on brushing discomfort and peri-implant tissue health. Clin Oral Implants Res. 2016; 27: 650–655.

43. Wennstrom JL, Derks J Is there a need for keratinized mucosa around implants to maintain health and tissue stability? Clin Oral Implants Res. 2012; 23(Suppl 6): 136–146.

44. Chackartichi T, Romanos GE, Sculean A Soft tissue-related complications and management around dental implants. Periodontol. 2019; 81: 124–138.

45. Hammerle CH, Tarnow D The etiology of hard- and soft-tissue deficiencies at dental implants: a narrative review. J Periodontol. 2018; 89(Suppl 1): S291–S303.

46. Sadid-Zadeh R, Kutkut A, Kim H Prosthetic failure in implant dentistry. Dent Clin N Am. 2015; 59: 195–214.

47. Fu JH, Hsy YT, Wang HL Identifying occlusal overload and how to deal with it to avoid marginal bone loss around implants. Eur J Oral Implantol. 2012; 5(Suppl): S91–S103.

48. Linkevicius T, Puisys A, Vindasiute E, Linkeviciene L, Apse P Does residual cement around implant-supported restorations cause peri-implant disease? A retrospective case analysis. Clin Oral Implants Res. 2013; 24: 1179–1184.

49. Kotsakis GA, Zhang L, Gaillard P, Raedel M, Walter MH, Konstantinidis IK Investigation of the association between cement retention and prevalent peri-implant diseases: a cross-sectional study. J Periodontol. 2016; 87: 212–220.

50. Wilson T The positive relationship between excess cement and peri-implant dis- ease: a prospective clinical endoscopic study. J Periodontol. 2009; 80: 1388–1392.

51. Chrcanovic BR, Kisch J, Albretsson T, Wennerberg A Bruxism and dental implant failures: a multilevel mixed effects parametric survival analysis approach. J Oral Rehabil. 2016; 43: 813–823.

52. Zhou Y, Gao J, Luo L, Wang Y Does bruxism contribute to dental implant failure? A systematic review and meta-analysis. Clin Implant Dent Relat Res. 2016; 18: 410–420.

53. Lang NP, Wetzel AC, Stich H, Caffesse RG Histologic probe penetration in health and inflamed peri-implant tissues. Clin Oral Implants Res. 1994; 5: 191–201.

54. Berglundh T, Armitage G, Araujo MG, et al. Peri-implant diseases and conditions: consensus report of workgroup 4 of the 2017 World Workshop on the Classification of Periodontal and Peri-Implant Diseases and Conditions. J Periodontol. 2018; 89(Suppl 1): S313–S318.

55. Lindhe J, Meyle J Group D of European Workshop on Periodontology. Peri-implant diseases: consensus report of the sixth European workshop

on periodontology. J Clin Periodontol. 2008; 35: 282–285.

56. Darveau RP The oral microbial consortium's interaction with the periodontal innate defense system. DNA Cell Biol. 2009; 28(8): 389–395.

57. Roberts FA, Darveau RP Microbial protection and virulence in periodontal tissue as a function of polymicrobial communities: symbiosis and dysbiosis. Periodontol. 2015, 2015; 69: 18–27.

58. Teughels W, Van Assche N, Sliepen I, Quirynen M Effect of material characteristics and/or surface topography on biofilm development. Clin Oral Implants Res. 2006; 17(Suppl 2): 68–81.

59. Kumar PS, Dabdoub SM, Hegde R, Ranganathan N, Mariotti A Site-level risk predictors of peri-implantitis: a retrospective analysis. J Clin Periodontol. 2018; 45(5): 597–604.

60. NIH HMP Working Group, Peterson J, Garges S, Giovanni M, et al. The NIH Human Microbiome Project. Genome Res. 2009; 19(12): 2317–2323.

61. Darveau RP, Tanner A, Page RC The microbial challenge in periodontitis. Periodontol. 1997; 14: 12–32.

62. Costerton JW, Lewandowski Z, DeBeer D, Caldwell D, Korber D, James G Biofilms, the customized microniche. J Bacteriol. 1994; 176(8): 2137–2142.

63. Marsh PD, Moter A, Devine DA Dental plaque biofilms: communities, conflict and control. Periodontol. 2011; 55: 16–35.

64. Kolenbrander PE, Andersen RN, Blehert DS, Egland PG, Foster JS, Palmer RJ Communication among oral bacteria. Microbiol Mol Biol Rev. 2002; 66: 486–450.

65. Costerton JW, Montanaro L, Arciola CR Biofilm in implant infections: its production and regulation. Int J Artif Organs. 2005; 28: 1062–1068.

66. Costerton JW Biofilm theory can guide the treatment of device-related orthopaedic infections. Clin Orthop Relat Res. 2005; 437: 7–11.

67. Kumar PS, Matthews CR, Joshi V, de Jager M, Aspiras M Tobacco smoking affects bacterial acquisition and colonization in oral biofilms. Infect Immun. 2011; 79(11): 4730–4738.

68. Schwarz F, Becker K, Rahn S, Hegewald A, Pfeffer K, Henrich B Real-time PCR analysis of fungal organisms and bacterial species at peri-implantitis sites. Int J Implant Dent. 2015; 1: 1–9.

69. Jankovic S, Aleksic Z, Dimitrijevic B, Lekovic V, Camargo P, Kenney B Prevalence of human cytomegalovirus and Epstein-Barr virus in subgingival plaque at peri-implantitis, mucositis and healthy sites. A pilot study. Int J Oral Maxillofac Surg. 2011; 40: 271–276.

70. Socransky S, Haffajee AD, Cugini MA, Smith C, Kent RL Jr Microbial complexes in subgingival plaque. J Clin Periodontol. 1998; 25: 134–144.

71. Han AF, Tsoi JKH, Rodrigues FP, Leprince JG, Palin WM Bacterial adhesion mechanisms on dental implant surfaces and the influencing factors. Int J Adhes Adhes. 2016; 69: 58–71.

72. Egawa M, Miura T, Kato T, Saito A, Yoshinari M in vitro adherence of periodontopathic bacteria to zirconia and titanium surfaces. Dent Mater J. 2013; 32(1): 101–106.

73. Grössner-Schreiber B, Teichmann J, Hannig M, Dörfer C, Wenderoth DF, Ott SJ Modified implant surfaces show different biofilm compositions under in vivo conditions. Clin Oral Implants Res. 2009; 20(8): 817–826.

74. Kumar PS, Mason MR, Brooker MR, O'Brien K Pyrosequencing reveals unique microbial signatures associated with healthy and failing dental implants. J Clin Periodontol. 2012; 39: 425–433.

75. Kumar PS, Leys EJ, Bryk JM, Martinez FJ, Moeschberger ML, Griffen AL Changes in periodontal health status are associated with bacterial community shifts as assessed by quantitative 16S cloning and sequencing. J Clin Microbiol. 2006; 44: 3665–3673.

76. Dabdoub SM, Tsigarida AA, Kumar PS Patient-specific analysis of periodontal and peri-implant microbiomes. J Dent Res. 2013; 92(12 Suppl): 168S–175S.

77. Daubert D, Pozhitkov A, McLean J, Kotsakis G Titanium as a modifier of the peri-implant microbiome structure. Clin Implant Dent Relat Res. 2018; 20: 945–953.

78. Mombelli A, Decaillet F The characteristics of biofilms in peri-implant disease. J Clin Periodontol. 2011; 38(11): 203–213.

79. Kormas I, Pedercini C, Pedercini A, Raptopoulos M, Alassy H, Wolff LF Peri-implant diseases: diagnosis, clinical, histological, microbiological characteristics and treatment strategies. A narrative review. Antibiotics (Basel). 2020; 9(11): 835.

80. Kröger A, Hülsmann C, Fickl S, et al. The severity of human peri-implantitis lesions correlates with the level of submucosal microbial dysbiosis. J Clin Periodontol. 2018; 45(12): 1498–1509.

81. Tanner A, Kent R, Maiden MFI, Taubman MA Clinical, microbiological and immunological profile of health, gingivitis and putative active periodontal subjects. J Periodontal Res. 1996; 31: 195–204.

82. Darveau RP, Hajishengallis G, Curtis MA *Porphyromonas gingivalis* as a potential community activist for disease. J Dent Res. 2012; 91: 816–820.

83. Lang NP, Bartold PM Periodontal health. J Clin Periodontol. 2018; 45(Suppl 20): S9–S16.

84. Araujo MG, Lindhe J Peri-implant health. J Periodontol. 2018; 89(Suppl 1): S249–S256.

85. Canullo L, Peñarrocha-Oltra D, Covani U, Rossetti PH Microbiologic and clinical findings of implants in healthy condition and with peri-implantitis. Int J Oral Maxillofac Implants. 2015; 30(4): 834–842.

86. Tonetti MS, Imboden M, Gerber L, Lang NP Compartmentalization of inflammatory cell phenotypes in normal gingiva and peri-implant keratinized mucosa. J Clin Periodontol. 1995; 22: 735.

87. Berglundh T, Gislason Ö, Lekholm U, Sennerby L, Lindhe J Histopathological observations of human periimplantitis lesions. J Clin Periodontol. 2004; 31: 341–347.

88. Carcuac O, Albouy J-P, Abrahamsson I, Linder E, Larsson L, Berglundh T Experimental periodontitis and peri-implantitis in dogs. Clin Oral Implants Res. 2013; 24: 363–371.

89. Carcuac O, Berglundh T Composition of human peri-implantitis and periodontitis lesions. J Dent Res. 2014; 93: 1083–1088.

90. Ferreira SD, Silva GL, Cortelli JR, Costa JE, Costa FO Prevalence and risk variables for peri-implant disease in Brazilian subjects. J Clin Periodontol. 2006; 33: 929–935.

91. Tsigarida AA, Dabdoub SM, Nagaraja HN, Kumar PS The influence of smoking on the peri-implant microbiome. J Dent Res. 2015; 94: 1202–1217.

92. Da Silva ES, Feres M, Figueiredo LC, Shibli JA, Ramiro FS, Faveri M Microbiological diversity of peri-implantitis biofilm by Sanger sequencing. Clin Oral Implants Res. 2014; 25(10): 1192–1199.

93. Quirynen M, Vogels R, Peeters W, van Steenberghe D, Naert I, Haffajee A Dynamics of initial subgingival colonization of 'pristine'peri-implant pockets. Clin Oral Implants Res. 2006; 17(1): 25–37.

94. Fürst MM, Salvi GE, Lang NP, Persson GR Bacterial colonization immediately after installation on oral titanium implants. Clin Oral Implants Res. 2007; 18(4): 501–508.

95. Danser MM, van Winkelhoff AJ, van der Velden U Periodontal bacteria colonizing oral mucous membranes in edentulous patients wearing dental implants. J Periodontol. 1997; 68(3): 209–216.

96. Al-Ahmad A, Wiedmann-Al-Ahmad M, Faust J, et al. Biofilm formation and composition on different implant materials in vivo. J Biomed Mater Res B Appl Biomater. 2010; 95B(1): 101–109.

97. Kotsakis GA, Lan C, Barbosa J, et al. Antimicrobial agents used in the treatment of peri-implantitis alter the physiochemistry and cytocompatibility of titanium surfaces. J Periodontol. 2016; 87(7): 809–819.

98. Safioti LM, Kotsakis GA, Pozhitkov AE, Chung WO, Daubert DM Increased levels of dissolved titanium are associated with peri-implantitis - a cross-sectional study. J Periodontol. 2017; 88: 436–442.

99. Schincaglia GP, Hong BY, Rosania A, et al. Clinical, immune, and microbiome traits of gingivitis and peri-implant mucositis. J Dent Res. 2017; 96: 47–55.

100. Lang NP, Berglundh T Working Group 4 of Seventh European Workshop on Periodontology. Periimplant diseases: where are we now? -Consensus of the Seventh European Workshop on Periodontology. J Clin Periodontol. 2011; 38(11): 178–181.

101. Matarasso S, Rasperini G, Siciliano VI, Salvi GE, Lang NP, Aglietta M A 10-year retrospective analysis of radiographic bone-level changes of implants supporting single-unit crowns in periodontally compromised vs. periodontally healthy patients. Clin Oral Implants Res. 2010; 21(9): 898–903.

102. Martinez-Hernandez M, Olivares-Navarrete R, Almaguer-Flores A Influence of the periodontal status on the initial-biofilm formation on titanium surfaces. Clin Implant Dent Relat Res. 2016; 18(1): 174–181.

103. Serino G, Strom C Peri-implantitis in partially edentulous patients: association with inadequate plaque control. Clin Oral Implants Res. 2009; 20: 169–174.

104. Heitz-Mayfield LJ, Salvi GE, Botticelli D, Mombelli A, Faddy M, Lang NP Anti-infective treatment of peri-implant mucositis: a randomized controlled clinical trial. Clin Oral Implants Res. 2011; 22: 237–241.

105. Costa RC, Souza JGS, Bertolini M, Retamal-Valdes B, Feres M, Barão VAR Extracellular biofilm matrix leads to microbial dysbiosis and reduces biofilm susceptibility to antimicrobials on titanium biomaterial: an in vitro and in situ study. Clin Oral Implants Res. 2020; 31(12): 1173–1186.

106. Lupi SM, Granati M, Butera A, Collesano V, Rodriguez Y, Baena R Air-abrasive debridement

with glycine powder versus manual debridement and chlorhexidine administration for the maintenance of peri-implant health status: a six-month randomized clinical trial. Int J Dent Hyg. 2017; 15(4): 287–294.

107. Jepsen S, Berglundh T, Genco R, et al. Primary prevention of periimplantitis: managing peri-implant mucositis. J Clin Periodontol. 2015; 42(Suppl. 16): S152–S157.

108. Schwarz F, Becker K, Sager M Efficacy of professionally administered plaque removal with or without adjunctive measures for the treatment of peri-implant mucositis. A systematic review and meta-analysis. J Clin Periodontol. 2015; 42(Suppl. 16): 13.

109. Kasemo B Biocompatibility of titanium implants: surface science aspects. J Prosthet Dent. 1983; 49: 832–837.

110. Niinomi M Recent research and development in titanium alloys for biomedical applications and healthcare goods. Sci Technol Adv Mater. 2003; 4: 445–454.

111. Rodrigues D, Valderrama P, Wilson T, et al. Titanium corrosion mechanisms in the oral environment: a retrieval study. Materials. 2013; 6: 5258–5274.

112. Olmedo DG, Nalli G, Verdú S, Paparella ML, Cabrini RL Exfoliative cytology and titanium dental implants: a Pilot Study. J Periodontol. 2013; 84: 78–83.

113. Wilson TG Jr, Valderrama P, Burbano M, et al. Foreign bodies associated with peri-implantitis human biopsies. J Periodontol. 2015; 86(1): 9–15.

114. Fretwurst T, Buzanich G, Nahles S, Woelber JP, Riesemeier H, Nelson K Metal elements in tissue with dental peri-implantitis: a pilot study. Clin Oral Implants Res. 2016; 27(9): 1178–1186.

115. Yu F, Addison O, Baker SJ, Davenport AJ Lipopolysaccharide inhibits or accelerates biomedical titanium corrosion depending on environmental acidity. Int J Oral Sci. 2015; 7: 179–186.

116. Mabilleau G, Bourdon S, Joly-Guillou ML, Filmon R, Basle MF, Chappard D Influence of fluoride, hydrogen peroxide and lactic acid on the corrosion resistance of commercially pure titanium. Acta Biomater. 2006; 2: 121–129.

117. Eger M, Sterer N, Liron T, Kohavi D, Gabet Y Scaling of titanium implants entrains inflammation-induced osteolysis. Sci Rep. 2017; 7: 39612.

118. Kotsakis GA, Black R, Kum J, et al. Effect of implant cleaning on titanium particle dissolution and cytocompatibility. J Periodontol. 2020; 92: 1–12.

119. Souza JC, Ponthiaux P, Henriques M, et al. Corrosion behavior of titanium in the presence of Streptococcus mutans. J Dent. 2013; 41: 528–534.

120. Barao VA, Yoon CJ, Mathew MT, Yuan JC, Wu CD, Sukotjo C Attachment of Porphyromonas gingivalis to corroded commercially pure titanium and titanium-aluminum-vanadium alloy. J Periodontol. 2014; 85: 1275–1282.

121. Toniollo MB, Galo R, Macedo AP, Rodrigues RCS, Ribeiro RF, Mattos MGC Effect of fluoride sodium mouthwash solutions on cpTi: evaluation of physicochemical properties. Braz Dent J. 2012; 23: 496–501.

122. Huang HH Effects of fluoride concentration and elastic tensile strain on the corrosion resistance of commercially pure titanium. Biomaterials. 2002; 23: 59–63.

123. Nishimura K, Kato T, Ito T, et al. Influence of titanium ions on cytokine levels of murine splenocytes stimulated with periodontopathic bacterial lipopolysaccharide. Int J Oral Maxillofac Implants. 2014; 29: 472–477.

124. Liu FX, Wu CL, Zhu ZA, et al. Calcineurin/NFAT pathway mediates wear particle-induced TNF-a release and osteoclastogenesis from mice bone marrow macrophages in vitro. Acta Pharmacol Sin. 2013; 34: 1457–1466.

125. Pettersson M, Kelk P, Belibasakis GN, Bylund D, Molin Thorén M, Johansson A Titanium ions form particles that activate and execute interleukin-1b release from lipopolysaccharide-primed macrophages. J Periodontal Res. 2016; 52: 21–32.

126. Wachi T, Shuto T, Shinohara Y, Matono Y, Makihira S Release of titanium ions from an implant surface and their effect on cytokine production related to alveolar bone resorption. Toxicology. 2015; 327: 1–9.

127. Kotsakis GA, Olmedo DG Periimplantitis is not periodontitis: scientific discoveries shed light on microbiome-biomaterial interactions that may determine disease phenotype. Periodontol. 2000; 86: 1–10.

128. Wang C, Renvert S, Wang H Nonsurgical treatment of periimplantitis. Implant Dent. 2019; 28(2): 155–160.

129. Carcuac O, Derks J, Abrahamsson I, Wennström JL, Petzold M, Berglundh T Surgical treatment of peri-implantitis: 3-year results from a

randomized controlled clinical trial. J Clin Periodontol. 2017; 44(12): 1294–1303.

130. Roccuzzo M, Pittoni D, Roccuzzo A, Charrier L, Dalmasso P Surgical treatment of peri-implantitis intrabony lesions by means of deproteinized bovine bone mineral with 10% collagen: 7-year-results. Clin Oral Implants Res. 2017; 28(12): 1577–1583.

131. Wingrove, S. Long-term prevention of peri-implant complications: assessment, mainte-nance, and home-care protocols. Straumann.com/490.600-en_low.pdf

8 Biofilm-Focused Implant Home Care

Home care, like implant maintenance, has shifted to a biofilm focus. The research shows that the elimination of over 80–85% of biofilm on a daily basis is critical to oral health and overall health of the patient (1). When does biofilm-focused home care begin for the implant patient? Once the implant is exposed to the environment and restored, a pellicle is formed followed by bacteria with the formation of plaque/oral biofilm (2).

There are biological differences to understand between a natural tooth and an implant. Dental implants are a medical device which make implants more susceptible to inflammation and bone loss from bacterial plaque/oral biofilm (3). Oral biofilm acts as a *trigger* for pro-inflammatory responses that can induce a systemic *toxic effect*. This amplifies biofilm and makes it a major risk factor for peri-implant disease infection and an oral systemic issue for the patient's overall health (4).

As hygienists, we can help our patients to understand the importance of implant biofilm-focused home care for long-term success of their implants. As well as, an awareness of the importance of healthy keratinized tissue surrounding the implant. It has been well documented that the absence of keratinized tissue can make the implant more susceptible to pathogenic bacteria/oral biofilm, thus leaving the implant vulnerable to peri-implant disease (5). What home care products should patients use, what not to use? Examples of home care products and hygiene tools are listed in this chapter to give you a place to start on what to recommend. Many more products are available or will be emerging, do your own research to help your patient sort through the multiple options (Figure 8.1). Keep it simple!

Peri-Implant Therapy for the Dental Hygienist, Second Edition. Susan S. Wingrove.
© 2022 John Wiley & Sons, Inc. Published 2022 by John Wiley & Sons, Inc.
Companion website: www.wiley.com/go/wingrove/implant

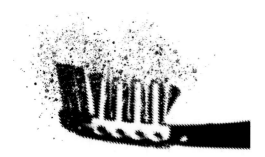

Figure 8.1 Image by Marc Swanson Photography/ Design.

Patients are concerned about their oral hygiene for their new implant(s) and implant-borne restoration/prosthesis. *Do they brush and floss their implants like regular teeth? Does food get underneath the fixed implant prosthesis?* All of these oral hygiene questions need to be addressed and an individualized, easy-to-follow home care protocol needs to be recommended by the hygienist. "Patients with implant-borne restorations should be advised to use these oral hygiene aids; dental floss, water flosser, air flossers, interdental cleaners, and electric toothbrushes," to disrupt biofilm according to American College of Prosthodontists' Clinical Practice Guidelines (6).

Good oral hygiene must take place before, during, and after placement of dental implants to ensure the success of the implant, but also the systemic health of the patient. Peri-implant disease prevention starts with a successful implant home care protocol, along with regular assessment, monitoring, and proper implant maintenance. Follow the protocols listed in this chapter to develop new and innovative ways to help your patients achieve their goal of good dental implant oral hygiene home care!

Postsurgical home care

The patient's oral hygiene starts with a good postsurgical protocol for adjunctive regenerative procedures and after implant placement during the healing phase. Home care begins immediately after regenerative and/or implant placement surgical procedure with postsurgical guidelines to maintain a healthy field and to initiate healing. Hygienists can prepare their patients by providing a biofilm-focused regimen based on their individual treatment case.

Post-regenerative surgical home care

A soft- or hard-tissue adjunctive procedure is often needed prior to implant placement, or bone particulate may be added at the time of implant placement. If bone loss has occurred, a bone graft or sinus lift may be needed to prepare the edentulous area for an implant. After any of these regenerative surgical procedures, the patient generally needs a healing period prior to implant placement. The following protocol listed in Box 8.1 will help the patient with home care recommendations for post-regenerative

---

Box 8.1 Post-regenerative surgical procedures home care protocol

■ Use ice packs *twice daily* externally, 15–20 minutes on/off for first 48–72 hours.
■ Drink only clear liquids, soft diet for the first few days, avoid chewing in surgical site
■ Take all antibiotics, if prescribed, to prevent infection
■ Take pain medication, if prescribed, as needed for pain
■ Brush *twice daily*, avoiding surgical incision area. Use an extra soft toothbrush and wait to use electric brush on surgeon's recommendation.
■ Wait to use water flosser or floss on surgeon's recommendations
■ Rinse *twice daily* with antimicrobial or prescribed mouthrinse by surgeon.
■ Avoid any undue pressure over a grafted extraction site while healing or wearing removable prosthesis as directed by surgeon.
■ Return for postoperative evaluation as directed by surgeon.

surgical procedures, prior to implant placement during the surgical healing period.

As a hygienist, encourage your patients to follow the surgeon's recommendation. Use ice packs externally, approximately 15–20 minutes on and 15–20 minutes off for the first 48–72 hours. Ensure good nutrition, but eat softer, cooler foods, and avoid chewing in the surgical site. Avoid any undue pressure over the graft extraction site while healing, including avoiding wearing removable prosthesis as directed by surgeon. The surgeon may even recommend *not to brush or floss the area for a specific time* and/or prescribe a prescription mouthrinse.

Following the post-regenerative procedure surgery, the surgeon will instruct the patient on the care of the surgical site following adjunctive procedures and/or implant placement surgery. It is important to follow all the surgeons instructions. New epithelial attachment seals are generally formed in 6–7 days following surgical procedure. In the case of a nonresorbable barrier, used in some guided tissue/bone regeneration procedures,

hygienist can prepare their patients to continue with post-regenerative home-care protocol until it has been removed (7) (see Box 8.1).

During the healing phase of the surgical phase of treatment (i.e., regenerative and/or implant placement), antimicrobial mouthrinses/chemotherapeutic agents (ChAs) can be very beneficial. ChAs (i.e., antimicrobial mouthrinses, gels, and sprays), to prevent biofilm formation and reduce inflammation (see Figure 8.2 for examples). Other ChAs, previously thought to be the standard of care are not currently recommended, chlorhexidine gluconate (CHXG) in 0.12% formulation.

Safioti et al. and Kotsakis et al. demonstrate research that shows that CHXG mouth rinse can alter the physiochemistry and cytocompatibility of the titanium dental implant surface, and can remove the titanium oxide layer which can make the titanium implant more susceptible to corrosion (8, 9). This compromises the biocompatibility of the body and one factor in *WHY* it is not recommended to detoxify titanium implants.

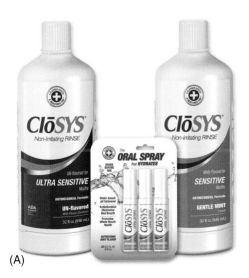

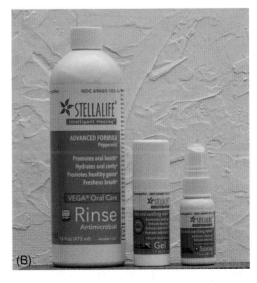

Figure 8.2 Examples of pre- and postsurgical implant safe products. (A) CloSYS mouthrinse and spray. Courtesy of Rowpar Pharmaceuticals. (B) StellaLife® VEGA® Oral Care Recovery Kit; mouthrinse, sublingual spray, and gel. Courtesy of StellaLife®.

In new studies, CHXG mouthrinse has shown to lower pH and alter microbiome after only seven days (9). These studies show the relationship of CHXG adversely affecting the osteoblastic response for bone formation, and negatively impacting cellular inflammatory response of gingival fibroblasts that has shown to be directly related to patient pain (7, 9, 10). Dental professionals and patients are seeking non-Opioid alternatives for pain and ways to promote healing (11). Research on pre- and postsurgical products (i.e., CloSYS and StellaLife® VEGA®) that can be used safely before/after surgical procedures and safe to use with implants. They promote healing, and help to alleviate inflammation, thus reduce pain for the patient (see Figure 8.2).

Chlorine dioxide, uniquely qualified as a pre- and postsurgical mouthrinse, does not interfere with prescription drugs and more importantly does not interfere with osteoblasts and fibroblastic activity, which initiate healing (7). Once activated, the antimicrobial strength of chlorine dioxide will kill most oral pathogens and more importantly inhibit their regrowth. Multiple chlorine dioxide products are on the market. One example: CloSYS, alcohol free, near neutral, antimicrobial mouthrinse is a stabilized chlorine dioxide with Cloralstan® which is an effective oxidant, naturally activated by the amino acids in patient's saliva (Figure 8.2A). Research studies show CloSYS, available in mouthrinse and spray, used *twice daily pre- and postsurgery*; "kills oral bacteria up to 99% in 10 seconds and is less toxic than chlorhexidine to human gingival cells in vitro" (12).

Another, excellent option, StellaLife® VEGA® Oral Care Recovery Kit, well researched for pre-and postsurgical healing and Opioid free pain relief (10, 11), (Figure 8.2B). This kit consists of three products; antimicrobial mouthrinse, sublingual spray, and a gel. The spray and gel decrease inflammation thus deliver pain relief postsurgical. The spray is used sublingually or can be sprayed directly on the surgical site if the surgeon does not want the graft or surgical site disturbed. Apply gel with Q-tip or lightly with patient fingertip and the rinse has good efficacy against pathogens as well as fungus (10). It is recommended to use StellaLife products, *three times daily, 3 days prior to procedure and 7–10 days following surgery* for optimal results.

It is important to remind the patient to follow all the surgeon's postsurgical recommendations. Connect with the surgeon and agree on a postsurgical home-care protocol. If possible provide the patient with an extra soft toothbrush (can be hard to find), pre/postsurgical mouthrinse, and a post-regenerative or postsurgical implant placement home-care instruction sheet (see Boxes 8.1 and 8.2), for the patient's healing phase.

Box 8.2 Postsurgical implant placement home-care protocol

- Use ice packs *twice daily* externally, 15–20 minutes on/off for first 48–72 hours.
- Drink only clear liquids, soft diet for the first few days, avoid chewing in surgical site
- Take all antibiotics, if prescribed to prevent infection
- Take pain medication, if prescribed as needed for pain
- Brush, *twice daily* avoiding surgical incision area. Use an extra soft toothbrush and wait to use electric brush on surgeon recommendation.
- Wait to use water flosser or floss on surgeon recommendations
- Rinse *twice daily* with antimicrobial or prescribed mouthrinse by surgeon.
- Avoid wearing temporary prosthesis (except fixed full-arch hybrid) at night to let tissue heal.
- Return for postoperative evaluation as directed by surgeon.

Postsurgical implant placement home care

After the implant is surgically placed, the healing phase begins which is generally 3–6 months, unless the implant has been immediately loaded with a restoration. The healing phase allows the implant to integrate with the patient's own bone, to osseointegrate. Instruct patients to follow *postsurgical implant placement home-care protocol* (Box 8.2), all subject to the surgeon's specific recommendations, until the surgeon's postop evaluation is complete. Use ice packs externally, approximately 15–20 minutes on and 15–20 minutes off for the first 48–72 hours. Ensure good nutrition, but eat softer, cooler foods, and avoid chewing in the implant placement site. It is imperative that the patient keep the implant placement area biofilm-free, biofilms can affect healing. The patient will return for postoperative evaluation as directed by surgeon. Once the surgeon has assessed that the patient's initial healing is complete, have the patients follow the protocol for *pre-restorative implant home care* until the implant is loaded (restoration/final prosthesis placed) (see Box 8.3).

Single implant home care

Oral care for single, implant-borne restorations needs to be customized for the patient based on dexterity and type of implant. Healthy single implant home care includes; *single implants, mini implants, ball or Locator implants, and bar-supported implants.* Home care for single implants does not differ significantly from home care for a natural tooth, but there are some differences. What to use, what not to use, and keep in mind that implants are a medical device (see Box 8.4).

The single implant patient should be instructed on some specific points, brushing twice daily with an electric toothbrush and if possible to use a water flosser. Use a water flosser or floss twice daily in the peri-implant crevice circumferentially to remove any oral biofilm present. Stimulating the tissue once daily is also extremely important, especially for the bar-retained implant patients. For the bar-supported implants, the tissue can migrate into the space between the bar and the ridge due to inflammation, making cleaning more difficult, and increase the chance of peri-implant disease. Rinse twice daily with antimicrobial mouthrinse or add to water flosser unit 1:10 dilution or dental professional's recommendation.

Box 8.3 Pre-restorative implant home-care protocol

- Brush *twice daily* with soft manual, electric toothbrush on sensitive mode, interdental, sulcabrush, or end-tuft toothbrush.
- Use a water flosser *twice daily* on low to medium setting or as directed by the surgeon. Avoid directing water flow perpendicular to the gingiva.
- Use a stimulator *once daily* to massage soft tissue that surrounds implant, if accessible.
- Rinse *twice daily* with antimicrobial mouthrinse or add to water flosser unit in 1:10 dilution or dental professional recommendation.

Box 8.4 Single implant home-care protocol; single, mini, ball or Locator, and bar-supported

- Brush *twice daily* with soft manual, electric, or interdental toothbrush.
- Use a water flosser or floss *twice daily*.
- Use a stimulator *once daily* to massage (stimulate) soft tissue that surrounds the implant.
- Rinse *twice daily* with antimicrobial mouthrinse or add to water flosser unit 1:10 dilution or dental professional recommendation.

To ensure optimal peri-implant health, the patient must maintain *daily biofilm removal, every 8–12 hours and it is critical to maintain regular professional in-office maintenance recare at least every 6 months* (6). The negation of early microbial accumulation on the dental implant surfaces and the elimination of at least 85% of oral biofilm by the patient with meticulous home care is essential for long-term implant success (2).

Brushing implants

Due to the focus on biofilm disruption, prevention of regrowth/ attachment of biofilm, and implants as a medical device, it is important to review brushing and which dentifrice to recommend to your patient. The patient should brush the implant(s) twice daily with a low-abrasive neutral pH dentifrice to remove bacterial plaque/oral biofilm. Brushing an implant is similar to brushing a natural tooth with a crown; however, note that the patient needs to be aware of the type of dentifrice they chose to use on their implant. With single tooth implants, patients may not think they need to be that cautious about their choice of dentifrice, but using a low-abrasive dentifrice ensures that it will not scratch the restoration or irritate the tissue cuff surrounding the implant (13).

This is important for the practitioner to determine which oral care products should be used in combination with titanium-alloy implants in light of the new corrosion risk factor for titanium implants (see Chapter 7, Corrosion). Titanium-alloy, is the most frequently used biomaterial for dental implants because of its titanium oxide layer that prevents corrosion. Although highly resistant to stress and corrosion, titanium–alloy implants do have the potential to corrode under certain environmental conditions. One condition to be keenly aware of is high fluoride, low pH products use around titanium-alloy implants. The titanium oxide layer can become mottled, roughened and can leave the implant prone to corrosion (8, 14) (see Figure 8.3). *Ceramic (zirconia) implants do not have this oxide layer and therefor are not affected the same way.*

What are the ins and outs of fluoride use around titanium-alloy dental implants? A 30-day study on the chemical effects of stannous and sodium fluoride (NaF) dentifrice used on titanium-alloy implant surfaces revealed that both stannous fluoride (SnF_2) containing dentifrices and gel products are safe to use, but *must be near-neutral pH* (14) (see Figures 8.3 and 8.4). This study also evaluated the chemical effects of NaF and acidulated phosphate fluoride gels (APF) on titanium-alloy surfaces. NaF dentifrices are safe to use with titanium-alloy implants but when NaF concentration is *higher than 0.1% and the product in not a neutral pH*, the protectiveness of titanium oxide layer can be destroyed by fluoride ions, leading to severe corrosion of titanium (14).

The overall conclusion, both sodium (NaF) and stannous fluoride (SnF_2) dentifrices are safe to use with titanium-alloy implants in a neutral pH. Caution needs to be used with high fluoride, low pH products around titanium-alloy implants. Acidified NaF or SnF_2 gels in low pH should not be used in trays or office treatments, shown to cause surface deposits and changes in the oxide layer making it prone to corrosion (see Figure 8.4 study

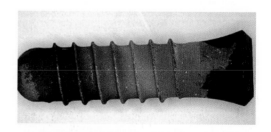

Figure 8.3 Titanium implant in 30 day study, high fluoride low pH, note results.

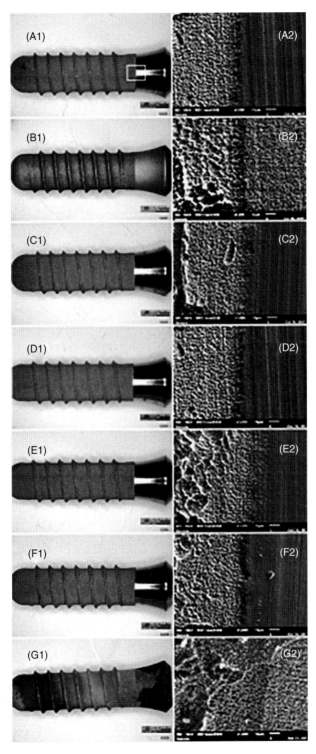

Figure 8.4   Light microscopy and SEM assessment of the 30-day exposure study show: controls. (A) Deionized water pH 5.20, negative control, *no changes in implant*. (B) Acidified 0.1 M NaF pH 2.21, positive control. *Testing show the surface effects, corrosion*. (C) APF gel, low pH 3.84, *shows surface deposits, changes in the oxide layer*. (D) Tin, no fluoride SnCl$_2$-Sol pH 5.8, *shows no surface effects*. (E) NaF-TP pH 6.97 pH, *neutral pH, shows no surface effects*. (F) SnF$_2$-TP 5.67 pH, *neutral pH, shows no surface effects*. (G) SnF$_2$-Gel 3.32 pH, *low pH, surface changes in oxide layer (14)*.

results). The bottom line, titanium oxide layer on the outside of titanium-alloy implants can be removed by continual use of high fluoride, low pH concentrations with patients with titanium-alloy implants (14–17).

What about higher concentrated fluoride dentifrice? Recent studies have shown that 1100 ppm NaF is comparable in effectiveness to 5000 ppm fluorides dentifrices (18). This is good news because many of the 5000 ppm dentifrice do not pass the near neutral pH testing. Manufacturers are now developing more 1100 ppm dentifrices that contain neutral PH values (i.e., MI Paste® ONE by GC America). An excellent choice for any implant patient and orthodontic patients with TAD implants (see Chapter 1).

Stannous fluoride dentifrice, safe for implants in neutral pH value and has shown to be 36.5% greater protection against plaque/oral biofilm than other fluorides. It is uniquely qualified for biofilm elimination with the stannous fluoride molecule bioavailability for 8–12 hours when incorporated in dentifrice, gel, or mouth rinses (19). Multiple companies have included stannous fluoride that follows the biofilm elimination body of research (i.e., examples Crest® + Oral-B GUM Detoxify™, and Colgate® Total SF). Bioavailability varies for stannous fluoride products by manufacturer; 8, 10, or 12 hours. When the product is used in mouth, it is activated to achieve the desired therapeutic result. The key to bioavailability is largely in the stabilizer to achieve the perfect balance that allows the stannous fluoride to be stable in the tube or mouth rinse bottle, but once in the oral cavity it is released and bioavailable (20).

For implants, keep in mind when customizing a patient's home care protocol that many implants have deep sulcus like pocket that surrounds the implant and an increased oral biofilm virulence that exists around implants (21). Adding a dental neutral pH dentifrice and/or a mouth rinse to patient's home care regimen can make a significant difference in prevention of oral biofilm for the recommended 8–12 hours, used twice daily.

What type of brush is the best to use for dental implants? Options for brushes include electric (i.e., iO micro-vibration or sonic), manual or specialty soft-bristled toothbrush, sulcus, end-tuft, or interdental brushes (see Table 8.1 and Figure 8.5 for examples).

Electric toothbrush

The use of an *electric toothbrush* cannot be over emphasized for patients with dental implants due to the fact that implants are ruff and porous thus collect more biofilm than natural teeth. The peri-implant crevice around implants (where the implant/abutment connects) is highly susceptible to

Table 8.1 Examples of brushes to use with implants.

Brushes	Examples	Manufacturer
Manual	Soft-compact size, end-tuft, sulcabrush Implant Orthodontic™	Multiple manufacturers TePe Oral Health Care, Inc.
Electric	Oral-B® Genius™, Oral-B® iO™ Philips Sonicare® Sonic-fusion® 2.0	Crest + Oral-B Philips, N. America Corp. Water Pik, Inc.
Interdental	GUM® Go-Between® Proxabrush Tapered or thinline TePe original and angled	Sunstar Americas, Inc. Multiple manufacturers TePe Oral Health Care, Inc.

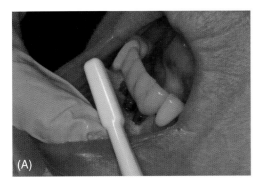
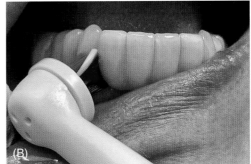
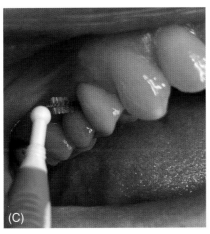

Figure 8.5 (A) Manual specialty toothbrush, TePe Implant Orthodontic™. Courtesy of Dr. Peter Fritz. (B) Electric, Oral-B® iO™, Targeted Clean™ brush head. Courtesy of Dr. Tom Lambert. (C) Interdental, Go-Between® Proxabrush® by Sunstar Americas, Inc. Courtesy of Dr. Tom Lambert.

inflammation, biofilm can accumulate, and can lead to peri-implant disease (21). Biofilm-focused care research demonstrates patients compliance of twice daily and the significance of effective biofilm control with removal of 80–85% biofilm twice daily (2). Therefore, now with the focus on biofilm elimination, the electric toothbrush should be recommended over the manual toothbrush especially for patient with risk factors to systemic diseases (see Figure 8.6).

If an electric toothbrush is used, choose the smallest head, set it on a setting to disrupt the plaque/biofilm around the tissue cuff surrounding the implant (see Figures 8.6 and 8.7). Select an electric toothbrush with a soft tissue setting (i.e., GUM care mode) to massage/stimulate the soft

tissue around restorations and implants. Stimulating the soft tissue around implants can prevent the biofilm from getting into the permucosal seal, which can lead to inflammation.

The oscillating-rotating electric toothbrushes (i.e., Oral-B®Genius and iO™) are different from other toothbrushes. Studies show a 50% greater reduction in bleeding sites over manual brushes and 28% greater reduction in bleeding sites versus sonic brushes (22). The iO brush is different from sonic electric toothbrushes as it has a linear magnetic drive, oscillation-rotations with micro-vibrations. This creates concentrated energy at the bristles, a more effective, smoother, and quieter brushing experience. The iO brush also includes a smart sensor to confirm for the patient that they

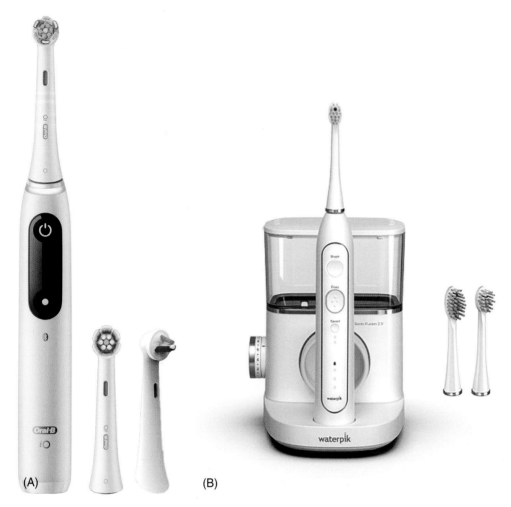

(A)   (B)

Figure 8.6 Examples of electric toothbrush. (A) Oral-B® iO™ with Ultimate Clean, Gentle Care, and Targeted Clean™ brush heads. Courtesy of Crest + Oral-B. (B) Waterpik® Sonic-fusion® 2.0, Full size and compact brush heads. Courtesy of Water Pik, Inc.

are effectively disrupting the biofilm with the right amount of pressure; green light if they are brushing with right amount to disrupt the biofilm and a red light if brushing too hard (23).

Another option is an electric toothbrush and water flosser all in one (i.e., Sonic-fusion® 2.0 by Waterpik, Inc.), enables sonic electric toothbrushing and water flossing to be accomplished with one tool (24) (see Figure 8.6). To use the Sonic-fusion 2.0, fill the water reservoir, replace in the unit. Place brush in mouth, press brush button. Use light pressure and clean all the tooth/

implant surfaces. Next press the floss button, and pointing the head into the sink, set the water setting. Keep lips partially closed to allow the water to flow into the sink. Water floss interproximal of all the teeth and implant-borne restorations.

Instructing patients on how to use an electric toothbrush is also important. Most electric toothbrushes will have a sensitive mode, a good place to start especially if the patient has never used an electric toothbrush. As soon as the patient feels comfortable, move up to the daily clean mode and brush each quadrant for 30 seconds, a total

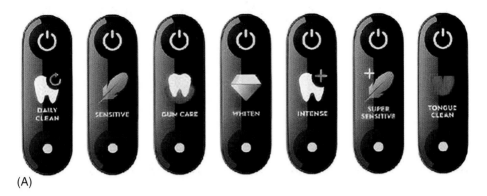

(A)

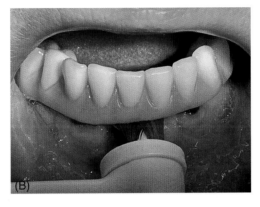

(B)

Figure 8.7 (A) Example of brushing modes on electric toothbrushes. (Note Oral-B® iO™ daily clean, sensitive, and GUM care modes.) Courtesy of Crest + Oral-B. (B) Example of specialized brush head for implants; Oral-B® iO™ electric toothbrush with Targeted Clean™ brush head, in use to brush around implants and under fixed final prosthesis. Courtesy of Dr. Tom Lambert.

of 2 minutes is ideal. If available, move to the soft tissue setting (i.e., GUM care mode), to stimulate (massage) the soft tissue that surrounds the implant.

To stimulate the soft tissue, start in the mandibular and trace the bristles along the gingival tissue gumline in a *SMILE face*, outlining the gingiva with the brush head. Repeat on the lingual. Move to the upper, outline the facial soft tissue along the gingival gumline with a *FROWN face* and repeating on the lingual for a total of one minute is ideal.

Many electric toothbrush models have different brushing modes (i.e., daily clean or sensitive, low or high mode) (see Figure 8.7). If possible select an electric toothbrush with a soft tissue setting to stimulate blood circulation and massage

the soft tissue around implants. This is especially helpful to keep the soft tissue under the bar for bar-retained implants healthy. Also, look for electric toothbrushes with specialized brush heads to specifically reach around and target the peri-implant crevice (i.e., Oral-B® Targeted Clean™) (see Figure 8.7).

Interdental brushes

Interdental brushes, nylon-coated wire proxabrushes, are also helpful for tight or hard-to-access areas around implants/prostheses and will not scratch the implant or prosthesis (see Figure 8.8). Interdental brushes can be used to clean around single implant-borne restorations, under a Hader/

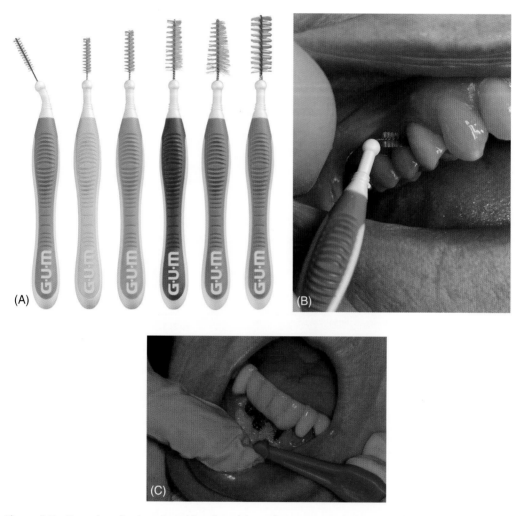

Figure 8.8 Examples of a interdental brushes. (A) GUM® Go-Betweens® Proxabrush®, note all the different sizes. Courtesy of Sunstar Americas, Inc. (B) Using GUM go-between proxabrush. Courtesy of Dr. Tom Lambert. (C) Example of TePe Angle™ interdental brush. Courtesy of Dr. Peter Fritz.

Miller bar, and around ball and Locator implants.

Help your patients to select the correct size and shape of an interdental brush. Pick an interdental brush that is tight, but not too difficult for the patient to use. If inflammation is present, also give the patient the next size larger brush to use after the inflammation is gone. *To use an interdental brush,* insert between or around implants, implant-borne restorations/prostheses and scrub to disrupt the biofilm twice daily.

Ultimately, the restoration/prosthesis (adaptation), oral anatomy, and patient dexterity will dictate which brush will be most effective for you to recommend and for the patient to use (i.e., manual, electric, or interdental) (see Table 8.1). Educate your patients on the transmission of microorganisms and advise them to change manual toothbrush or electric brush head at least every 3 months (see Table 8.1). Interdental brushes should be changed at least once a month. The main objective for you, as a hygienist, is to assist your patients in finding a toothbrush that the patient feels comfortable using, can adapt to remove the plaque/biofilm effectively, and will use twice daily. Remember, *80–85% removal of all plaque/oral biofilm daily every 8–12 hours* is critical to the long-term success of implants (2).

Flossing an implant

Flossing has been used as a method of interdental cleaning for a very long time. However, with implants it has been used with marginal success and some studies have shown it to be detrimental. The studies showed that tufted floss can be retained as a filamentous foreign body. Once removed, proper home care reverted back to a healthy environment (25) (see Figure 8.9).

Dr. Marco Montevecchi DDS, PhD, Periodontal Professor from Bologna University, Italy, completed a 6-year scanning electron microscope (SEM) study of a patient with recurrent swelling, perimucositis, and after 10 days had complete remission. Following this patient for 6 years showed that the microflora reverted back to a healthy environment and stable condition (26) (see Figure 8.9).

Dr. Montevecchi has continued his research with a study to evaluate implant flossing leaving residue in three different implant-prosthetic conditions. A healthy connection control group, group two with 220–230 μm between implant platform and abutment with no threads exposed, and group three with partial exposure of implant threads. Twenty-one implant micro-structured, tapered, threaded implants divided into the three groups were flossed in a strict controlled movement and a standardized magnification of 10× was used to examine any floss residue left behind in the three groups. Results

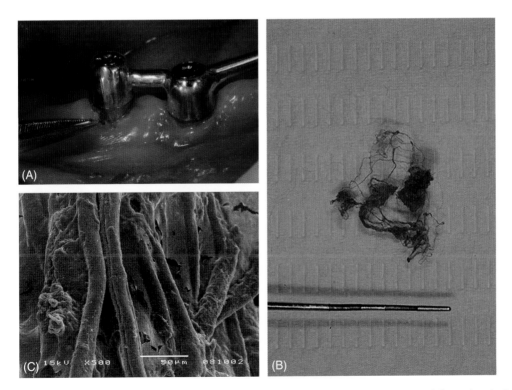

Figure 8.9 (A) Removing floss from around single implant. (B) Floss remnants removed from the single implant. (C) SEM shows the bacterial biofilm present on the floss remnants. Courtesy of Dr. Marco Montevecchi, University of Bologna, Italy.

showed no floss residue in the healthy implant group, but floss residue was detected in the form of microfilaments and amorphous particles in group two and three (26). Therefore, flossing may not be the ideal option but no clear evidence exists that a healthy well-fit implant/abutment titanium implant patient should not floss an implant. However, this recent study showed; "exposed threads and misfit can induce the release of floss residue," (27).

For ceramic implants, flossing is not recommended due to the possibility that it will interfere with tissue attachment/adherence. More studies on flossing ceramic implants are needed, but caution should be used if flossing a ceramic implant and water flossing should be recommended. Flossing is also not recommended for implant-supported fixed or removable final prosthesis patients, due to multiple clinical observations of retained filamentous foreign body (floss) left behind to cause inflammation (see Figures 8.9).

If the patient prefers to floss rather than use a water flosser for their single, healthy titanium implant with no thread exposure, hygienists should demonstrate the proper technique to prevent retained floss (see

Box 8.5, Figure 8.10). Note in the patient's record that they are flossing and monitor for inflammation and/or floss remnants left behind at all future implant maintenance recare visits.

There are many types of floss on the market and currently it is recommended to use tape, not tufted or thin waxed floss, to protect the tissue surrounding the implant and not leave residue behind on any rough or exposed implant threads. The objective is to remove the biofilm in the peri-implant crevice, flossing the entire circumference of the implant, not just the contact points.

Box 8.5   Protocol for flossing implants

1. Insert tape floss through contact on mesial and distal, without removing the floss.
2. Criss-cross in front (buccal), switch hands.
3. Move in shoe-shining motion to remove plaque/biofilm from peri-implant crevice.
4. Important to remove the floss from the contact points (mesial, distal), DO NOT PULL THROUGH
5. Check floss: if frayed or blood present, alert dental professional.

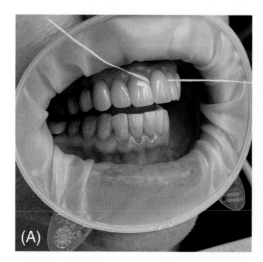 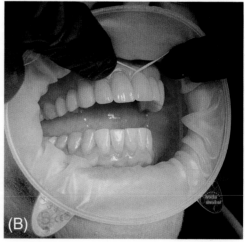

Figure 8.10   Flossing an implant. (A) Insert on the mesial and distal, (B) crisscross the floss and move in shoe-shine motion in the peri-implant crevice. Remove from the mesial and distal, DO NOT pull through. Courtesy of Wingrove Dynamics.

To floss a titanium implant, use dental tape or specialized floss (see Box 8.5 and Figure 8.10). Insert in the contact points (mesial, distal), then crisscross the floss in front. Move the floss in a shoe-shine motion in the peri-implant crevice to remove the oral biofilm and remove floss from contact points (mesial, distal) DO not pull through. This will help prevent remanent floss from retaining on the ruff or exposed implant threads (Figure 8.9). Have the patient check the floss, if fraying or blood is present on the floss, alert the dental professional.

Water flossers/water irrigation units

One of the key challenges for hygienists is what to recommend that will cleanse the entire circumference around implants other than flossing. The peri-implant crevice around implant is highly susceptible to inflammation and oral biofilm can accumulate that can lead to peri-implant disease (21). Water flosser lends itself perfectly to this task, directing the water pressure specifically to flush out the oral biofilm around the peri-implant cervices in a circular motion up to *6 mm probe depth*, not just interproximal.

At the University of Southern California Center for biofilms, Dr. Amita Gorur, conducted a 2009 study to evaluate the ability of water flossers to remove biofilm (28). The scanning electron microscope (SEM) results demonstrated that the hydraulic water forces of a water flosser on medium pressure setting (1200 pulsations per minute, approximately 70 psi), can significantly remove biofilm. Using a Classic Jet tip by Waterpik, Inc., *removed 99.99% oral biofilm ex vivo and in vivo in 3 seconds* (28) (see Figure 8.11). Other studies have compared the use of electric sonic toothbrushes in conjunction with a water flosser verses traditional manual toothbrushing and flossing for biofilm removal. Results showed a *significant difference in biofilm removal* using an electric toothbrush and a water flosser in comparison to traditional manual toothbrushing and flossing (29).

Removal of oral biofilm from the circumference around dental implants with a water flosser or flossing with string floss is *essential twice daily*. To use a water flosser or string floss as a method to remove oral biofilm has been well studied and the results are conclusive that a patient does not need to do both. Magnuson et al., completed a study of water flossing with a Plaque Seeker® Waterpik tip at medium setting to using string floss. Water flossing was *two times as effective* at reducing bleeding around implants (30). Making water flossing a significant improvement over flossing in the care of dental implants.

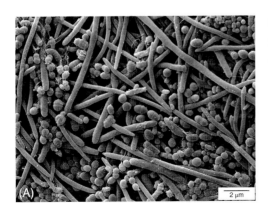 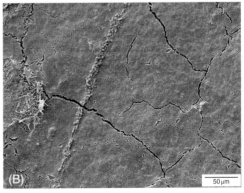

Figure 8.11 SEM results hydraulic water forces on biofilm. (A) Oral biofilm prior to cleansing. (B) Results after using a water flosser for 3 seconds at 70 psi. Courtesy of Dr. Amita Gorur and Water Pik, Inc.

Follow the proper instructions for use by each water flosser manufacturer and instruct implant-borne restoration patients on the importance of directional flow. Using a nonmetal tip, instruct the patient to direct the water flow ¼ inch from a flat surface or at 90° horizontally. Start a new water flosser patient on low power with their eyes facing into the sink not looking in the mirror. Recommend that they move up to medium or higher setting (all settings are safe to use with implants), as soon as they feel comfortable. Most studies have the participants using medium or higher settings to properly disrupt the biofilm. The water flosser can be used with an antimicrobial mouthrinses/ChAs in the reservoir, to precisely deliver the antimicrobial benefits. Dilute the ChAs in 1 part to 10 parts water or as directed by the dental professional to deliver the antimicrobial benefits specifically where it is needed (see Box 8.6).

To keep reservoir of the ultrasonic unit clean, fill the reservoir with white vinegar at full strength and run the vinegar through the lines, pointing the tip into the sink. Refill the reservoir with only water and run the unit again to flush out the vinegar to complete the cleaning process of the water flosser unit.

Box 8.6 How to use a water flosser/water irrigation unit

1. Read and follow manufacture directions for use
2. Fill reservoir with lukewarm water and add antimicrobial rinse if recommended.
3. Select tip, attach, and insert tip into mouth, close lips slightly to prevent splashing.
4. Lean over a sink, eyes into the sink not looking in the mirror and turn ON unit. Dial setting to medium to high.
5. Direct the water flow ¼ inch from the teeth/implant at 90° horizontally, and follow the gumline.
6. When complete pause to shut unit off, then remove the tip from your mouth.

Water flosser units have been a true advantage to access difficult-to-clean areas surrounding implants to disrupt and remove the biofilm present. This is extremely helpful in controlling the oral biofilm accumulation, and in preventing inflammation. There are many water flosser units on the market by multiple manufacturers, (i.e., Crest+Oral-B and Waterpik, Inc.).

Waterpik® has multiple unit models; Aquarius®, Whitening with glycine tablets, Cordless, Kids, and traveler size units. The tips that are currently available; Classic Jet, Plaque Seeker®, Pik Pocket™, Orthodontic, and Implant Denture tip (see Figure 8.12). It is recommended to replace water flosser tips every 6 months.

Specialized tips like Waterpik Pik Pocket and Implant Denture tips are especially needed for hard to access single implants and implant-supported fixed final prothesis. The Pik Pocket tip has a small aperture to direct the water flow in hard to access areas, it can only be used on a low setting (i.e., 2 power setting). The Implant Denture tip is designed for the implant-supported fixed full-arch final prosthesis patients and can be used on all power settings. The hypodynamic shear forces of pulsating water removes oral biofilm and food debris between the final prosthesis and around the supporting implants of the fixed final prosthesis patient. It is best to instruct the patient to start at one end of the prosthesis, place the Implant Denture tip under the lingual of the fixed final prothesis, and slowly follow around to the other side of the prosthesis, use twice daily.

Another water flosser unit example is the handheld cordless water flosser, Oral-B® Water Flosser Advanced with new *Oxyjet technology*. The Oxyjet™ technology enriches the water with microbubbles of air (see Figure 8.13). The microbubble air, which is composed of 78% nitrogen, 21% oxygen, 0.93% argon, and 0.04% carbon dioxide, exposes the anaerobic bacteria to

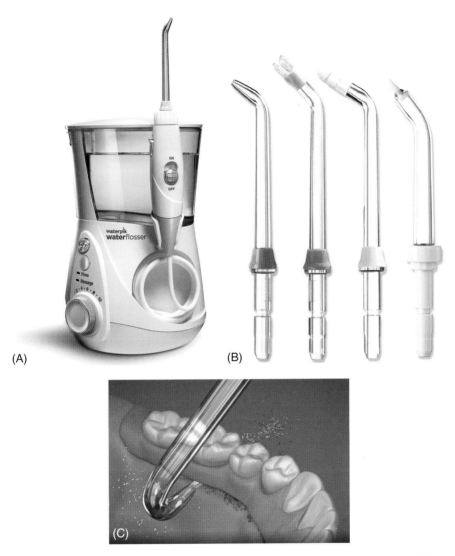

Figure 8.12 Examples of Waterpik water flosser unit and tips. (A) Aquarius® Water Flosser. (B) Waterpik tip options; Classic Jet, Plaque Seeker®, Pik Pocket™, and Orthodontic tips. (C) Implant denture tip, insert on the lingual of the prosthesis. Courtesy of Water Pik, Inc.

oxygen. The oxygen is toxic to the anaerobic bacteria, and as a result, attacks the anaerobic bacteria that contributes to several conditions including inflammation and mucositis (31). It comes with two tip options, the Aquafloss and the Precision Jet nozzle with two setting modes on both for target cleaning and soft-tissue stimulation (Figure 8.13).

The *Aquafloss nozzle* has a focused stream for targeted cleaning and a rotational stream for *gum care (tissue stimulation)*. In addition, the *Precision Jet nozzle* offers a precision stream for targeted cleaning (at a higher intensity than the Aquafloss-focused stream) and a multi-jet stream mode for *gum care (tissue stimulation)*. The gum care mode on both tips makes it uniquely beneficial for implant home care *to stimulate* the soft tissue around implants to keep the tissue firm and healthy around the implant(s).

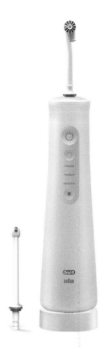

Figure 8.13 Example of a cordless water flosser. Oral-B® Water Flosser Advanced Oxyjet™ technology with Aquafloss and Precision Jet Tips. Courtesy of Crest + Oral-B.

In terms of at-home care for implants, water flossers are becoming one of the most valuable tools for implant home care. Mechanical oral biofilm control is the foundation for prevention of peri-implant disease and water flossing has shown to be *twice as effective to traditional brushing and flossing* (30). Access and the ability to direct an antimicrobial mouthrinses/ChAs directly to cleanse the implant makes a water flosser a brilliant choice for patients with implants.

Stimulators

A critical step, use a stimulator once daily to massage and stimulate the soft-tissue surrounding implants. The tissue surrounding the implants *does not get stimulated like natural teeth*. The goal for a healthy implant is to prevent biofilm from attaching in the peri-implant crevice by promoting tight, keratinized tissue surrounding the implants. Patients need to stimulate the tissue once daily or inflammation can occur, starting the inflammation cascade. If the soft tissue is less than 2 mm with inflammation, it can lead to bone loss and ultimately to peri-implantitis (32). Linkevicius et al., noted in studies that "tissue *greater than 2 mm thick* will have less chance of bone loss around implants; 0.17 mm after 2 months and 0.21 after one year." "If the tissue is *less than 2 mm thick,* there is more of a chance of bone loss around the implant; 0.79 mm after 2 months and 1.17 mm after 1 year (32).

What is our role as dentists and hygienists? Motivate patients to use a stimulator after implant placement to stimulate soft tissue around the healing cap or around the temporary crown on a one-piece implant to promote blood circulation and healing. After the restoration or prosthesis is loaded (restoration/prosthesis is placed), use a stimulator or patients can use a soft tissue setting on an electric toothbrush to stimulate the soft tissue that surrounds the implant once daily and keep the tissue healthy.

The most frequently used soft tissue stimulators are rubber-tip stimulators made by multiple manufacturers and for single implants dental picks can be used (i.e., Precision Clean Picks by Crest + Oral-B, Soft-Picks® by Sunstar Americas, Inc. or TePe Picks). Stimulators have been found to keep the tissue around implants or implant-borne restorations, tighter and healthy, less likely to allow biofilm to get into the peri-implant crevice (see Figures 8.14 and 8.15).

To use a rubber-tip stimulator, instruct the patient to place the side of the tip of the rubber-tip stimulator so it lays flat against the soft tissue, *not poking into the tissue,* and with light pressure rolls in a circular motion to massage and stimulate the tissue (see Figure 8.14). If done with correct pressure, the tissue blanches or changes to a lighter

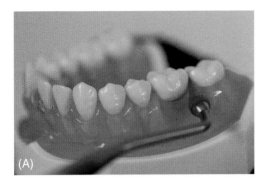
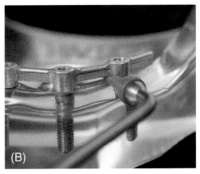

Figure 8.14 Example GUM® rubber tip stimulator, use the flat side of the tip not the point. (A) Single implants. (B) Around and under bar on bar-supported implants. Courtesy of Wingrove Dynamics.

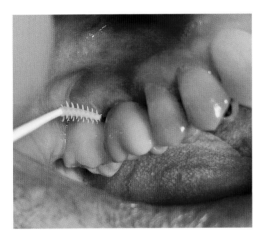

Figure 8.15 Example of a dental pick to stimulate soft tissue on single implants, use the side of the pick, GUM Soft-Picks®. Courtesy of Dr. Tom Lambert.

color. Repeat this 5–10 times on the mesial and distal of each implant or implant-borne restoration crown once daily to stimulate the soft tissue to remain healthy. This is extremely helpful for the soft tissue under the bar of bar-supported implants where the tissue tends to grow up and become inflamed. Walk the rubber tip under the bar, pressing the flat side against the tissue as you go. When you reach an implant, press up against the implant on both sides, and then continue for the full arch (see Figure 8.14).

For single implants patients, use a rubber tip stimulator or dental picks (Figures 8.14A and 8.15). *To use dental picks*

for stimulation, instruct patients to insert the dental pick next to the implants and press the soft tissue with firm pressure, using the side only of the dental pick to stimulate the tissue. The soft tissue will blanch in color when the correct pressure is used and repeat on both sides of the implant/ implant-borne restoration crown. Use stimulators (i.e., rubber tip or dental pick for single implants) to keep the soft tissue firm and healthy. Note that patients will still need to brush, floss or use a water flosser to remove the oral biofilm twice daily.

Antimicrobial mouthrinses/chemotherapeutic agents

The American Dental Association (ADA) and the Robert Koch institute both recommend the use of antimicrobial mouthrinses/ chemotherapeutic agent (ChA) (33). Antimicrobial mouthrinses are particularly beneficial before and after dental surgeries for reduction of bacterial bioburden and as a critical part of a home care daily routine (see Figure 8.16). There has been a paradigm shift in the components for selecting a long-term mouthrinse to recommend to implant patients. The antimicrobial mouthrinse should kill bacteria, prevent biofilm from attachment to the implant, and eliminate volatile sulfur compounds (VSCs) for 8–12 hours.

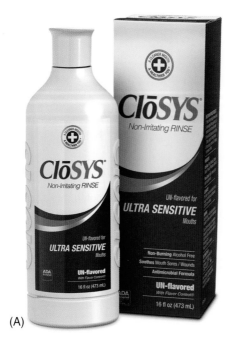

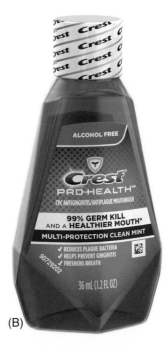

(A)   (B)

Figure 8.16 Antimicrobial nonalcohol mouthrinses (A) CloSYS mouth rinse, effective for 8 hours. Courtesy of Rowpar Pharmaceuticals. (B) Multi-protection clean mint, effective for 12 hours. Courtesy of Crest + Oral-B®.

Chlorhexidine gluconate (CHXG) 0.12%, thought to be the standard antimicrobial mouthrinse is NOT recommended for long-term use or with the latest science for biofilm-focused care. General directions for use are only for supragingival gum infections for 3–6 weeks. Staining of natural teeth and restorations, an alteration in taste perception, and calculus build-up have been reported as side effects for CHXG and can be severe after 6 weeks (34). The latest research shows that CHXG mouthrinse can alter the physiochemistry and cytocompatibility of the titanium-alloy dental implant surfaces (8, 9). It can make the titanium implant more susceptible to corrosion by removing the titanium oxide layer (layer on the titanium implant to protect against corrosion) (see Chapter 7).

New research has also emerged that shows CHXG can also alter microbiome after just 7 days (9). Therefore, CHXG is not recommended for long-term use or prior to implant-borne restoration placement. It can leave residue on the implant surfaces

that can alter the titanium physical chemistry and adversely affect the osteoblastic (bone cells) response (7). Therefore, clinicians should not dip floss into CHXG or painted with cotton applicator on to an implant to detoxify implants (8).

Antimicrobial nonalcoholic mouthrinses (Figure 8.16) with chlorine dioxide or cetylpyridinium chloride (CPC) are highly recommended for all implant-borne restoration/prosthesis patients to kill germs, prevent biofilm attachment, and to eliminate the volatile sulfur compounds (VSCs) every 8–12 hours. Antimicrobial mouthrinses are the primary product to provide elimination of the VSCs, the missing link in biofilm elimination and inflammation in periodontal/peri-implant disease.

Chlorine dioxide and CPC mouthrinses are good examples of over-the-counter mouthrinses that are safe to use long-term with ceramic and titanium dental implants. They also meet the biofilm science standards to kill germs that cause peri-implant disease for 8–12 hours.

Single bacteria is not that hard to kill, antimicrobial mouthrinses need to inhibit the biofilm from attaching to the implant surface and causing inflammation. Alcohol and CHXG mouthrinses only kill single bacteria, they do not breakup biofilm or eliminate VSCs (7). Therefore, antimicrobial mouthrinses are also beneficial in prevention of infection until surgical healing has been achieved (34) (see Boxes 8.1 and 8.2). Instruct patients to use antimicrobial nonalcohol mouthrinses twice daily or add to a water flosser unit in 1:10 dilution or as directed by dental professional.

Specialized home care

Patients with an implant-supported full-arch fixed and removable final prosthesis can find oral hygiene difficult and home care for patients with peri-implant disease (i.e., mucositis, early peri-implantitis). Hygienists can recommend and educate their patients using the following recommended protocols (see Boxes 8.6–8.8).

Implant-supported full-arch fixed final prosthesis

For the *implant-supported fixed full-arch final prosthesis* patients, brush the supporting implants and under the final prosthesis,

---

Box 8.6 Implant-supported full-arch *fixed* final prosthesis home care protocol

- Brush implants/prosthesis *twice daily* with soft manual, electric, or interdental toothbrush.
- Use water flosser *twice daily*, around implants and under prosthesis.
- Rinse *twice daily* with antimicrobial rinse or add to water flosser unit 1:10 dilution or dental professional recommendation.

Box 8.7 Implant-supported full-arch *removable* final prosthesis (overdenture) home care protocol

- Remove the overdenture and do a visual check of attachments.
  - If O-rings, caps or clips are worn or missing alert dental professional
- Brush implants and underside of overdenture *twice daily*.
  - Use soft manual, electric, or interdental toothbrush. Do not use denture brush on overdenture.
  - Soak overdenture, specific time and solution *once a week*, remove and rinse.
- Use water flosser *twice daily* around implants and bar of bar-supported implants.
- Use a stimulator *once daily* to massage (stimulate) soft tissue, around implants and under the bar of bar-supported implants.
- Rinse *twice daily* with antimicrobial rinse prior to reinserting the overdenture.
- Reinsert overdenture into place, leave out overnight if possible.

Box 8.8 Peri-implant mucositis/early peri-implantitis home care protocol

- Brush *twice daily* with soft manual, electric, or interdental toothbrush.
- Use water flosser *twice daily*
- Use a stimulator *once daily* to massage (stimulate) soft tissue that surrounds implant, if accessible.
- Rinse *twice daily* with antimicrobial rinse or add to water flosser unit in 1:10 dilution or dental professional recommendation.
- Optional, apply antimicrobial gel, if directed by dental professional to infected area *twice daily* (morning/bedtime).

---

twice daily to remove all biofilm present (see Box 8.6). If the patient has an electric toothbrush with a soft-tissue care mode, set to the GUM mode to stimulate the gum tissue under the prosthesis and around the implants (see Figure 8.7B).

Next, use a water flosser twice daily on medium to high power. Flossing is not recommended for the fixed full-arch final prosthesis patient. More research is needed, but currently studies show that floss could be retained and not visual to the patient, and cause inflammation or infection (25–27). Rinse with an antimicrobial mouthrinse twice daily or add to a water flosser in a 1:10 dilution or as directed by a dental professional.

Access under a fixed final prosthesis can be difficult. Specialty tips for the water flosser and electric toothbrush have been designed to make this easier for the fixed final prosthesis patients (i.e., Implant Denture Tip by Waterpik® for use with Aquarius® water flosser unit [Figure 8.12C], Precision Jet tip for use with Oral-B® Water Flosser Advanced unit [Figure 8.13], and Oral-B® Targeted Clean™ brush head [Figure 8.7B] for use with the Oral-B® iO™ electric toothbrush).

Implant-supported full-arch removable prosthesis (overdenture)

For *implant-supported full-arch removable overdenture patient*, follow the home care protocol (Box 8.7). Home care for removable full-arch prosthesis patient starts with removing the overdenture. Educate the patient on proper way to remove the overdenture, removing improperly can cause unnecessary wear on the attachments.

Oral biofilm can accumulate on the overdenture inside and out, causing wear to the attachments and can be an oral–systemic health concern. Educate the patient to do a visual check on the attachments that are located in the overdenture and attach to the implants and/or bar (Figure 8.17). The attachments (i.e., O-rings, Locator caps, and/or clip system), assist with retention, allowing the patient to talk or laugh without the fear of the denture coming out of their mouth and the ability to chew more effectively. Have the patient check for wear and tear, or if the attachments are missing.

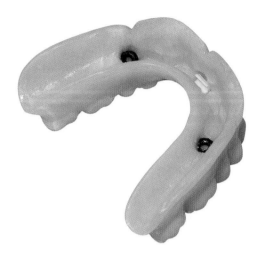

Figure 8.17 Example of attachments in overdenture. Courtesy of Salvin Dental Specialties.

Direct the patient to alert dental office, if attachments are worn or missing, and make an appointment to replace.

Instruct the patient to use a soft manual toothbrush or an electric toothbrush twice daily, on the implants and the outside/underside of the removable overdenture to eliminate the oral biofilm, do not use a denture brush on the overdenture it can remove the attachments. Instruct the patient to soak the overdenture according to manufacturer's directions for a specific time and solution safe to use on overdentures, once a week. A dilution of one-part household vinegar to one-part water can also be used. It is not recommended to soak the implant overdenture overnight; it can deteriorate the attachments.

A water flosser can be used twice daily around the implants and bar of bar-supported implants. Flossing is not recommended for the fixed full-arch removable final prosthesis patient. More research is needed, but currently the studies show that floss could be retained and not visual to the patient, and cause inflammation or infection (25–27) (see Figure 8.9).

Use a stimulator once daily to massage (stimulate) soft tissue, around implants and under the bar of bar-supported implants (see Figure 8.14). If the patient has an electric toothbrush with a soft tissue care mode, use to stimulate the gum tissue around the implants and under the bar of bar-supported implants. Remove the overdenture if soaking in solution and rinse thoroughly to remove the cleaner or vinegar.

Have the patient *rinse orally twice daily with an antimicrobial mouthrinse* for 30 seconds and reinsert the overdenture. If possible instruct the patient to leave the overdenture out at night to let the tissues under the overdenture breath. The patients will be less likely to develop inflammation or candidiasis under the overdenture.

Hygienists, help the patients understand how to reinsert the overdenture properly. Emphasize the patient not to bite the overdenture into place which can damage the attachments. Remind the patient to do a visual attachment check. If the patient notices anything different with the attachments, he or she should notify the dental office and set up an appointment for replacement.

Peri-implant mucositis/early peri-implantitis

For implants with peri-implant disease (mucositis, early implantitis), the patient needs to follow the home care protocol for the type of implant or prosthesis, plus add antimicrobial therapy (see Box 8.8). Home care is a critical component for peri-implant mucositis, inflammation that affects the soft tissue with no signs of supporting bone loss, and early peri-implantitis with less than 25% bone loss.

Instruct the patient to brush twice daily with soft manual, electric, or interdental toothbrush. Educate and motivate your patient to use an electric toothbrush and/or water flosser unit to achieve 80–85% of biofilm elimination. If an electric toothbrush is used, brush all the implants or complete dentition for 2 minutes and 1 minute on the

soft-tissue care mode to stimulate the gum tissue for a total of 3 minutes. Use a water flosser twice daily and direct patient to add an antimicrobial mouthrinse to the water flosser unit in a 1:10 dilution or as directed by dental professional. Use a stimulator once daily to stimulate the soft tissue if accessible and rinse twice daily with an antimicrobial mouthrinse if patient has not already used in the water flosser unit. Optionally, apply an antimicrobial gel, if directed by dental professional on the infected area of inflammation twice daily (i.e., morning and before bed). Continue with this home care protocol until reevaluation appointment (see Chapter 9, peri-implant disease treatment).

Educate and motivate

Dental hygienists are educators as well as dental care providers. Providing the implant maintenance is only one part to a well-rounded maintenance appointment. As dental hygienists, we need to *be the educator* and *motivate the patient to commit to a biofilm-focused home care routine* for long-term prevention of peri-implant disease. The patient must be motivated to learn before education can begin. Education and motivation can occur together if you have established a rapport with the patient first. Supply patients with written home care recommendations on your office letterhead (see Table 8.2 list of home care protocols). Patients can feel anxious at the dental office and do not always retain information presented at the time of the appointment. It is easy to forget how many times per day, amounts to use, or the order in which to do specific recommendations. There are some basic motivational teaching points to consider (see Box 8.9).

Your office can offer your patients an implant care kit, with home care instructions on your letterhead. Home care and products specifically for implants can be

Table 8.2 Oral hygiene home care protocol summary.

Implant Type	Oral Home Care Protocol Summary
Post-regenerative surgical procedures	■ Use ice packs *twice daily* externally, 15–20 minutes on/off for first 48–72 hours ■ Drink only clear liquids, soft diet for the first few days, avoid chewing in surgical site ■ Take all antibiotics, if prescribed to prevent infection ■ Take pain medication, if prescribed as needed for pain ■ Brush, *twice daily* avoiding surgical incision area. Use an extra soft toothbrush and wait to use electric brush on surgeon recommendation ■ Wait to use water flosser or floss on surgeon recommendations ■ Rinse *twice daily*, antimicrobial or prescribed rinse by surgeon ■ Avoid any undue pressure over a grafted extraction site while healing or wearing removable prosthesis as directed by surgeon ■ Return for postoperative evaluation as directed by surgeon
Post-surgical implant placement	■ Use ice packs *twice daily* externally, 15–20 minutes on/off for first 48–72 hours ■ Drink only clear liquids, soft diet for the first few days, avoid chewing in surgical site ■ Take all antibiotics, if prescribed to prevent infection ■ Take pain medication, if prescribed as needed for pain ■ Brush *twice daily* avoiding the surgical incision area, with an extra soft toothbrush and wait to use electric on surgeon recommendations ■ Wait to use water flosser or floss on surgeon recommendations ■ Rinse *twice daily*, antimicrobial or prescribed rinse by surgeon ■ Avoid wearing temporary prosthesis (except fixed full-arch hybrid) at night to let tissue heal ■ Return for postoperative evaluation as directed by surgeon
Pre-restorative implant	■ Brush *twice daily* with soft manual, electric toothbrush on sensitive mode, interdental, sulcabrush, or end-tuft toothbrush ■ Use a water flosser *twice daily* on low to medium setting or as directed by surgeon. Avoid directing water flow perpendicular to the gingiva ■ Use a stimulator *once daily* to massage soft tissue that surrounds implant, if accessible ■ Rinse *twice daily*, antimicrobial rinse or add to water flosser unit in 1:10 dilution or dental professional recommendation
Single implants: *Single, mini, ball or Locator, and bar-supported implants*	■ Brush *twice daily* with soft manual, electric, or interdental toothbrush ■ Use a water flosser or floss *twice daily* ■ Use a stimulator *once daily* to massage (stimulate) soft tissue that surrounds the implant ■ Rinse *twice daily*, antimicrobial rinse or add to water flosser unit 1:10 dilution or dental professional recommendation
Implant-supported full-arch *fixed* final prosthesis	■ Brush implants/prosthesis *twice daily* with soft manual, electric or **interdental toothbrush** ■ Use water flosser *twice daily*, around implants and under prosthesis ■ Rinse *twice daily*, antimicrobial rinse or add to water flosser unit 1:10 **dilution or dental professional recommendation**

Table 8.2 (continued)

Implant Type	Oral Home Care Protocol Summary

Implant-supported full-arch *removable* prosthesis (overdenture)	■ Remove the overdenture and do a visual check of attachments
	  ○ If O-rings, caps or clips are worn or missing alert dental professional
	■ Brush implants and underside of overdenture ***twice daily***
	  ○ Use soft manual, electric, or interdental toothbrush. Do not use **denture brush on overdenture**
	  ○ Soak overdenture, specific time and solution ***once a week***, remove **and rinse**
	■ Use water flosser ***twice daily*** around implants and bar of bar-supported **implants**
	■ Use a stimulator ***once daily*** to massage (stimulate) soft tissue, around implants and under the bar of bar-supported implants
	■ Rinse ***twice daily***, antimicrobial rinse prior to reinserting the overdenture
	■ Reinsert overdenture into place, leave out overnight if possible.

Peri-implant mucositis/ early peri-implantitis	■ Brush ***twice daily*** with soft manual, electric, or interdental toothbrush ■ Use water flosser ***twice daily*** ■ Use a stimulator ***once daily*** to massage (stimulate) soft tissue that **surrounds implant, if accessible** ■ Rinse ***twice daily***, antimicrobial rinse or add to water flosser unit 1:10 **dilution or dental professional recommendation** ■ Optional, apply antimicrobial gel if directed, to infected area ***twice daily* (morning/bedtime)**

Box 8.9 Motivational teaching points

1. Identify the patient's personality and receptiveness before you have the conversation.
2. Do not overwhelm the patient with too much information or overly technical dental or implantology terms.
3. Educate on one area of concern or one new home care recommendation at each visit.
4. Allow the patient to remove the prosthesis or demonstrate how they are cleaning the implant(s) at home. Ask questions and reinforce good habits.
5. Supply the patient with the brush, water flosser, mouthrinse, or other product information for implant home care.
6. Send patient home with written instructions or Apps to reinforce recommendations.

overwhelming. If you think they are confusing, think about your patients who are faced with choosing the right product for their specific implant-borne restorations or prosthesis. Evaluate home care products as they become available, stay current on new products that are safe to use on implants, and know where they are available locally. Consider stocking the products (i.e., electric toothbrush, water flosser, stimulator, mouth rinse, or other products) you and your doctor recommend for home care in the office for your patients. Providing patients with the home care tools and products necessary for home care following implant treatment reinforces your relationship. Gives the patient peace of mind and sets your office apart by going that extra mile for your patients.

Summary

Keep it simple! Individualize the at home care protocol for patients depending on the implant design, restoration/prosthesis, and access to *cleanability*. The patient's dexterity, oral systemic health, risk factors, periodontal history, and the time the patient is willing to devote to maintaining his or her implant(s) all play a role in developing a simple home care protocol. Patients rely and trust the hygienist's expertise for home care recommendations. Research and evaluate the products that would best suit your patients for their implant needs. It is critical to continue to learn and attend continuing education courses to *be the educator*. Keep up-to-date with your clinical skills and read journals to stay current on the latest home care tool options, as well as new dental products to recommend for your implant patients' oral health and overall health. Communicate to patients on the importance of good oral hygiene and the risks of peri-implant disease. The key for long-term prevention of implant complications is assessment, maintenance, home care, and patient awareness!

References

1. Kracher CM, Smith WS Oral health maintenance dental implants. Dent Assist. 2010; 79(2): 27–35.
2. Subramani K, Jung RE, Motenberg A, Hammerle CH Biofilm on dental implants: a review of the literature. Int J Oral Maxillofac Implants. 2009; 24: 616–626.
3. Berglundh T, Lindhe J, Ericsson I, et al. The soft tissue barrier at implants and teeth. Clin Oral Implants Res. 1991; 2(2): 81–90.
4. Quirynen M, De Soete M, Steenberghe D Infectious risks for oral implants: a review of the literature. Clin Oral Implants Res. 2002; 13: 1–19.
5. Greenstein G, Cavallaro J The clinical significance of keratinized gingiva around dental implants. Compend Contin Educ Dent. 2011; 32: 24–31.
6. Bidra A, Daubert D, Garcia L, et al. 2016 ACP clinical practice guidelines for recall and maintenance of patients with tooth-borne and implant-borne dental restorations. J Prosthodont. 2016; 25: S32–S40.
7. Wirthlin R, Brand J, Enriquez B, Hussain MZ Effects of stabilized chlorine dioxide and chlorhexidine mouth rinses in in vitro cells involved in periodontal healing. Periodontal abstracts. J West Soc Periodontal Abstr. 2006; 54(3): 67–71.
8. Safioti L, Kotsakis GA, Pozhitkov AE, Chung WO, Daubert DM Increased levels of dissolved titanium are associated with peri-implantitis–a case control study. J Periodontol. 2017; 88: 436–442.
9. Kotsakis GA, Caixia Lan C, Barbosa J, et al. Antimicrobial agents used in the treatment of peri-implantitis alter the physiochemistry and cytocompatibility of titanium surfaces. J Periodontol. 2016; 87(7): 809–819.
10. Fujioka-Kobayashi M, Schaller B, Pikos MA, Sculean A, Miron RJ Cytotoxicity and gene expression changes of the novel homeopathic antiseptic oral rinse in comparison to chlorhexidine in gingival fibroblasts. Materials (Basel). 2020; 13(14): 3190.
11. Lee CY, Suzuki JB The efficacy of preemptive analgesia using a non-opioid alternative therapy regimen on postoperative analgesia following block bone graft surgery of the mandible: a prospective pilot study in pain management in response to the opioid epidemic. Clin J Pharmacol Pharmacother. 2019; 1: 26–31.
12. Drake D, Villhauer AL, Dows Institute for Dental Research, College of Dentistry, University of Iowa An in-vitro comparative study determining bactericidal activity of stabilized chlorine dioxide and other oral rinses. J Clin Dent. 2011; 22: 1–5.
13. Yukna R Optimizing clinical success with implants: maintenance and care. Compend Contin Educ Dent. 1993; 15: S554–S561.
14. Suszcynsky-Meister E, Shauchuk A, Hare T, Hunger L, Valent D, Massad J, Wingrove S, St. John S. Chemical effects of stannous and sodium fluoride dental treatments on titanium alloy surfaces. AADR, 2018.
15. Nakagawa M, Matsuya S, Shiraishi T, Ohata M Effect of fluoride concentration and pH on corrosion behavior of titanium for dental use. J Dent Res. 1999; 78(9): 1568–1572.
16. Huang HH Effects of fluoride concentration and elastic tensile strain on the corrosion resistance of commercially pure titanium. Biomaterials. 2002; 23(1): 59–63.
17. Matono Y, Nakagawa M, Matsuya S, Isikawa K, Terada Y Corrosion behavior of pure titanium and titanium alloys in various concentrations of acidulated phosphate fluoride (APF) solutions. Dent Mater J. 2006; 25(1): 104–112.
18. Garcia-Godoy F, Hicks J Maintaining the integrity of the enamel surface; the role of dental biofilm, saliva and preventative agents in enamel demineralization and remineralization. JADA. 2008; 139(5): 25S–34S.

19. Sharma NC, Qaqish J, He T, et al. Superior plaque reduction efficacy of a stannous fluoride dentifrice. J Clin Dent. 2013; 24: 31–36.

20. Klukowska MA, Ramji N, Combs C, et al. Subgingival uptake and retention of stannous fluoride from dentifrice: gingival crevicular fluid concentration in sulci post-brushing. Am J Dent. 2018; 31: 184–188.

21. Kumar PS, Mason MR, Brooker MR, O'Brien K Pyrosequencing reveals unique microbial signatures associated with healthy and failing dental implants. J Clin Periodontol. 2012; 39: 425–433.

22. Grender J, Adam R, Zou Y The effects of oscillating-rotating electric toothbrushes on plaque and gingival health: a meta-analysis. Am J Dent. 2020; 33: 3–11.

23. Adam R Introducing the Oral-B iO electric toothbrush: next generation oscillating-rotating technology. Int Dent J. 2020; 70(Suppl 1): S1–S6. https://doi.org/10.1111/idj.12570.

24. Qaqish JG, Goyal CR, Schuller R, Lyle DM Comparison of a novel sonic toothbrush to a traditional sonic toothbrush and manual brushing and flossing on plaque, gingival bleeding and inflammation: a randomized controlled clinical trial. Compend Contin Educ Dent. 2018; 39(suppl 2): 14–22.

25. Van Velzen FJJ, Lang NP, Schulten EAJM, Ten Bruggenkate CM Dental floss as a possible risk for the development of peri-implant disease: an observational study of 10 cases. Clin Oral Implants Res. 2016; (5): 618–621.

26. Montevecchi M, De Blasi V, Checchi L Is implant flossing a risk-free procedure? A case report with a 6-year follow-up. Int J Oral Maxillofac Implants. 2016; 31: 79–83.

27. Montevechhi M, Valeriani L, Franchi L, Sforza NM, Plana G Evaluation of floss remnants after implant flossing in three different implant conditions: a preclinical study. Int J Oral Maxillofac Implants. 2021; 36: 569–573. https://doi.org/10.11607/jomi.8350.

28. Gorur A, Lyle DM, Schaudinn C, Costerton JW Biofilm removal with a dental water jet. *Compend Contin Educ Dent.* 2009; 30(Special issue 1): 1–6.

29. Barnes CM, Russell CM, Reinhardt RA, et al. Comparison of irrigation to floss as an adjunct to toothbrushing effect on bleeding, gingivitis and supragingival plaque. J Clin Dent. 2005; 16(3): 71–77.

30. Magnuson B, Harsono M, Stark PC, Lyle D, Kugel G, Perry R Comparison of the effect of two interdental cleaning devices around implants on the reduction of bleeding: a 30-day randomized clinical trial. Compend Contin Educ Dent. 2013; 34(Special Issue 8): 2–7.

31. Husseini A, Slot DE, Van der Weijden GA The efficacy of oral irrigation in addition to a toothbrush on plaque and the clinical parameters of periodontal inflammation: a systematic review. Int J Dent Hyg. 2008; 6(4): 304–314.

32. Linkevicius T, Puisys A, Linkeviciene L, Peciulience V, Schlee M Crestal bone stability around implants with horizontal matching connection after soft tissue thickening: a prospective clinical trial. Clin Implant Dent Relat Res. 2015; 17(3): 497–508.

33. Robert Koch Institute Infection prevention in dental medicine: hygiene requirements Federal health research Health protection. 2006; 49: 375–394.

34. Felo A, Shibly O, Ciancio SG, Lauciello FR, Ho A Effects of subgingival chlorhexidine irrigation on peri-implant maintenance. Am J Dent. 1997; 10(2): 107–110.

9 Professional In-Office Implant Maintenance and Disease Treatment

Unless you try something beyond what you have already mastered, you will never grow.
—Ronald E. Osborn

Prevention of long-term peri-implant complication starts with early *detection* of any signs of inflammation. *Diagnosis* of complications to provide early intervention and perform professional in-office maintenance *treatment* on patients at least every 6 months (1, 2). The research is clear, professional in-office implant maintenance by a dental hygienist is critical for the long-term prevention of implant complications. Lack of in-office implant maintenance shows that patients with peri-mucositis that do not have regular implant maintenance are 43% more likely to develop peri-implantitis and only 18% of patients with regular in-office implant maintenance by a dental professional develop peri-implantitis (3).

Peri-implantitis and complications can be prevented with *professional in-office maintenance, patient awareness, and early detection*. Hygienists are uniquely qualified to take the lead with evidence-based assessments, implant maintenance and home-care recommendations. Previous peri-implant therapy challenges centered on not scratching the smooth implant surfaces, but research shows that the focus needs to be oral biofilm and calculus identification and removal (4, 5) (see Figure 9.1). With the emerging evidence of corrosion on titanium implant surfaces due to chemotherapeutic agents (6, 7), it is important that the professional in-office maintenance protocol includes the correct instruments and products, proven safe to use on dental implants. Meet the peri-implant maintenance challenges head on with the guidelines and protocols outlined in this chapter.

Despite the success of implant dentistry, it is important to remember that the majority of implant patients are dental failures, patients who have lost their teeth. It is critical to identify why these patients lost their natural teeth and help them understand the importance of professional in-office implant maintenance appointments and proper implant at-home oral hygiene regimen to maintain their implants for the rest of their lives. How can the hygienist provide effective maintenance or give home care instruction if he or she has no knowledge of implant placement, restorative options, and regenerative adjunctive procedures in the patient's treatment plan? Consult with the dentist prior to the patient's first implant maintenance appointment to be prepared. Hygienists and doctors need to work together to develop a comprehensive implant maintenance plan. This plan should be based on the patient's; implant restoration/prosthesis, medical history, risk factors, and home-care.

Professional in-office regimen

A customized professional in-office implant maintenance regimen is essential for patients with single implants to complex implant-borne restorations/prosthesis to provide biological and mechanical maintenance. The American College of Prosthodontists (ACP) convened a scientific panel comprised of experts from four professional dental organizations, ACP, the American Dental Association (ADA), Academy of General Dentistry (AGD), and the American Dental Hygienists' Association (ADHA). The panel consisted of seven dentists, with Diane Daubert and Susan Wingrove representing the dental hygiene profession. The other non-dentist member was the executive director of the ACP. Together the panel developed a set of clinical practice guidelines (CPG) based on two systematic reviews of all the latest research and discussion on new research (2).

Highlights for ACP clinical practice guidelines implant-borne restorations

The scientific panel considered the benefits, harms, and contraindications for the overall oral health of tooth-borne and implant-borne restoration patients. The consequences of risk for failure of tooth-borne and implant-borne restorations were

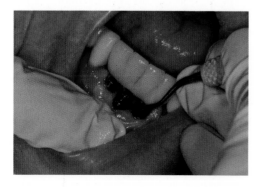

Figure 9.1 Implant maintenance with safe instruments.

a particular focus. The ACP classification and CPGs, changes how dental professionals approach maintenance and home-care recommendations with an oral biofilm focus. New protocols, technology, and products are now available to remove biofilm, prevent biofilm formation, protect teeth, implants, and restorations. Highlights of the clinical practice guidelines (CPGs) for implant-borne restoration (2), are noted in (Box 9.1).

The steps for safe, effective in-office implant maintenance are outlined in the evidence-based protocols in this chapter: review the medical history and risk factors. Assess/monitor the implant(s), provide professional oral biofilm removal, and debridement of calculus and/or residue. Polish and remove stains on implant-borne restorations/prostheses. Finely, recommend biofilm-focused implant home care that is safe for implant patients and provide a customized regimen based on type of restoration/prosthesis (2) (see Box 9.2).

Medical history

The patient's medical history and overall health should be updated and reviewed at every implant maintenance appointment. Since dental implants are medical devices, any changes in the patient's health status could impact the implants and/or treatment. Risk assessment questions are also a vital part of a comprehensive medical history. Health risk factors include uncontrolled diabetics, history of poor wound healing, or systemic diseases. Risk factors such as age, sex, obesity, smoking, functional habits, oral health (biofilm), and socioeconomic status are also important (see Chapter 2). If these factors are combined it could make any implant treatment case more complicated and potentially risky for a successful case outcome (see Chapter 4). More information on biofilm and corrosion as risk factors (see Chapter 7).

Walk the patient through the medical history and risk assessment. Record if the patient is in the care of a physician at the present time and for what medical condition. This could have an impact on the overall health of the implant, maintenance requirements, and/or the proposed treatment plan. Overall good general health is one of the keys to the success of the implant(s) and may affect the length of time between implant maintenance appointments (8).

Finally, a comprehensive, written and signed by the patient, medical history is important. Carefully read, review, and ask specific open-ended questions. Go down the list, and listen (see Chapter 2 medical history). Prevention of long-term implant complications begins with assessment, maintenance, and following home-care protocols for ceramic and titanium implants.

Assess and monitor implants and implant-borne restorations/prostheses

To assess implants, the hygienist should follow this evidence-based five-step assessment and monitoring protocol for every implant maintenance visit (see Figure 9.2). Visually inspect the soft tissue that surrounds the implant (i.e., inflammation, keratinized, or nonkeratinized). Probe and palpate for signs of infection and use floss to assess for calculus and/or residue to determine whether debridement is necessary. Continue with mobility assessment, record if patient complains of pain present, and have the doctor check occlusion at time of exam. Finally, the most critical step is to assess the bone level by taking appropriate radiograph(s) to establish the health of the implant (see Chapter 6 for more details on assessment).

Maintenance; biofilm removal, debridement, polishing, and recare

A paradigm shift has occurred in maintenance protocols. It is now equally as important to professionally remove oral biofilm as

it is to remove calculus and especially with implants. Oral biofilms will accumulate on the hard and soft surfaces in the oral cavity. Biofilm accumulation is a high risk factor for peri-implant disease and therefore, in-office professional implant biofilm elimination is critical, at least every 6 months (2).

In addition, a majority of implants placed today have a roughened surface that attracts the bone to help with osseointegration. Therefore, the implants hold more oral biofilm and microbes than a smooth surface. The microbes also differ significantly from those found in periodontal in healthy microbiome and diseased. The microbiome in peri-implantitis is a "microbially heterogeneous infection with predominantly gram-negative species and is less complex than periodontitis." (9). The microbes will migrate from natural dentition to implants and from implants (10).

Biofilm develops on all exposed titanium or ceramic implant surfaces and restorations/prostheses. Evidence supports that the restorative abutment connection, *peri-implant crevice*, is the niche for periopathogens (9) (see Figure 9.3). Therefore, the dental hygienist's role is more critical than ever in preventing and controlling bacterial infection (i.e., peri-implantitis) by directing the tip of the powder streaming device into the peri-implant crevice before debridement to professionally remove the biofilm.

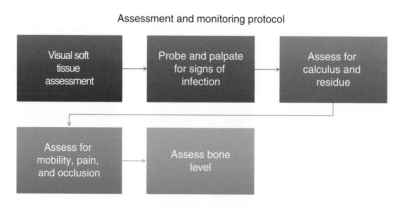

Assessment and monitoring protocol

Visual soft tissue assessment → Probe and palpate for signs of infection → Assess for calculus and residue → Assess for mobility, pain, and occlusion → Assess bone level

Figure 9.2 Assessment and monitoring protocol.

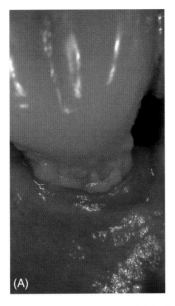
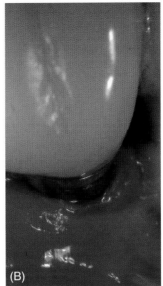

Figure 9.3 Example of biofilm (A) Before and (B) After removal with powder streaming device. Courtesy of Dr. Pam Maragliano-Muniz.

The surface chemistry and the implant–abutment configuration play a role in the bacterial accumulation. This, combined with the increased surface roughness of dental implants and the higher oral biofilm formation, solidify the importance of using a powder streaming device or polishing first to remove oral biofilm (10).

Biofilm identification and professional removal

The first step is to use a retraction device (i.e., OptraGate or cheek retractor) to protect patients lips, enhance visibility for the operator to more thoroughly access the natural teeth, tooth-borne, and implant-borne restorations (see Figure 9.4). Prior to OptraGate or cheek retractor placement, use a lip conditioner to prevent lips from drying out or any lasting effect from applying a disclosing solution or dyes.

To professionally remove biofilm, first identify the biofilm and know where to focus to be able to thoroughly remove all the biofilm present. To identify the oral biofilm present, use a disclosing solution.

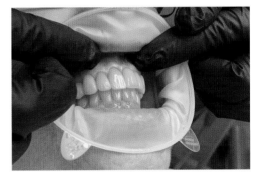

Figure 9.4 OptraGate, latex-free retraction device by Ivoclar Vivadent. Pull apart, place in the corners of mouth, position in vestibular regions for visibility. Courtesy of Wingrove Dynamics.

There are multiple disclosing solutions on the market (i.e., 2Tone by Young Dental, Tri Plaque ID gel by GC). Choose a disclosing solution that can show you the most biofilm results. These solutions can be used as an optional chair-side diagnostic tool, not just for assessing the patient's brushing performance.

The GC Tri Plaque ID gel is one example (Figure 9.5A). It is a three-way disclosing solution that shows new plaque/oral biofilm in pink and mature biofilm (48 hours) in purple which hygienists can show patients where they may need to focus more, when brushing. It also more importantly, identifies where acid producing biofilm (4.5 pH or lower) is present in a light blue color. Identifying the acid producing biofilm makes this a true diagnostic tool (see Figure 9.5C). Record the light blue areas; caries possible on natural teeth, acid producing biofilm and inflammation indicating mucositis/peri-implantitis possible for implants. Show these findings to the doctor to evaluate at the time of exam.

To use a disclosing solution as diagnostic tool, using the Tri Plaque ID gel as an example; apply the gel with a cotton applicator or microbrush (Figure 9.5B). Rinse or have patient rinse carefully and use a saliva ejector to remove any excess saliva. The oral biofilm will now be visible (Figure 9.5C). Record the light blue acid producing bio-

film areas on natural teeth/implants for the doctor to evaluate at the time of the exam. For hygienist, you are now ready to professionally remove the identified biofilm using a powder streaming device or polish with a silica xylitol prophy paste to interrupt the bacterial metabolism and disrupt the oral biofilm. This is an ideal time to talk to patient about WHY you are completing a professional biofilm removal procedure for their overall body health and how they can reinforce their good health with biofilm-focused home-care routine every 8–12 hours (see Chapter 8).

Professional oral biofilm removal; powder streaming device

According to the American College of Prosthodontists' (ACP) Clinical Practice

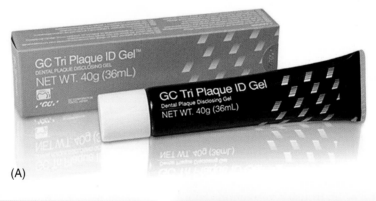

(A)

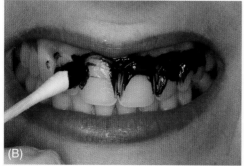

(B)

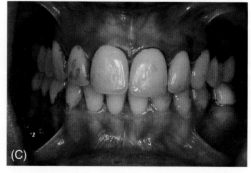

(C)

Figure 9.5 Example of chairside disclosing solution (A) Tri Plaque ID Gel by Ivoclar Vivadent (B) Application of GC Tri Plaque ID Gel. (C) Biofilm identified; pink new, purple mature, and light blue acid producing biofilm. Courtesy of Dr. Pam Maragliano-Muniz.

Guidelines professional maintenance; "Professionals should use cleaning instruments compatible with the type and material of abutments, implants, and restorations and powdered instruments such as glycine powder air-polishing system (2)."

The powder streaming device, sometimes referred to as subgingival air polishing, is a professional biofilm removal tool to remove all biofilm present (11). Traditional air polishing, also referred to as air-powder spray system, was originally developed to remove stains on natural teeth and restorations in a short amount of time. These air polishers use a powder abrasive in a stream of water and approximately 43–58 psi of air pressure and air abrasion units which use 80–160 psi of air pressure. *Both should not be confused* with a powder streaming device used subgingival and supragingival for biofilm removal.

The American Dental Hygienists' Association has published a list of guidelines for contraindications for traditional air polishers (43–58 psi) in their 2010 position paper (12). These air polishers are contraindicated for patients with respiratory, renal, or metabolic disease. They are also contraindicated for patients with restricted sodium diets, with infectious diseases, on diuretics or long-term steroid therapy, and with titanium implants (12).

Studies have also shown that air-powder spray systems with bicarbonate powder can leave deposits (i.e., residue) on the titanium implant surfaces, especially with hydroxy-apatite or titanium plasma spray (TPS) coatings (13). Therefore, traditional air-powder spray systems are *not recommended for use with titanium implants* (14, 15) and until more studies have been completed, *also not recommended for use around ceramic implants*. The deposits can also have an effect in vivo on tissue healing processes and bone regeneration. This has been confirmed on multiple studies (13, 14), however, the long-term effects of this residue are still being studied to see to what extent

this leads to implant failure. The bottom line is that traditional air polishers with bicarbonate powder are contraindicated to use subgingival and for patients with dental implants.

Currently there are multiple powder streaming devices on the market that have implant safe specialized tips, and powders to allow for the subgingival powder streaming to remove and interrupt the bacterial metabolism (see Figure 9.6).

Guided Biofilm Therapy® (GBT), an eight-step protocol developed by the Electro Medical System (EMS) company has a set regimen and two safe powder alternatives; original glycine and erythritol. Other powder streaming devices (Figure 9.6) use the original glycine powder. Both glycine and erythritol powders are specifically designed with a low micron particle size (i.e., erythritol at 14 microns and glycine at 25 microns) that have been proven in multiple studies to be safe for implants and subgingival tissue. They can also be used supragingival around natural teeth and implant-borne restorations/prostheses (11, 16).

To use a powder streaming device, patient and operator both need to be properly protected. The OptraGate is in place to protect patients lips/nose and use a high volume evacuation (HVE) to remove aerosols to protect the patient and the clinician. Powder streaming instructions for use (IFUs); select a safe subgingival powder streaming device and set-up with safe subgingival powder (i.e., erythritol or glycine powder). Insert the specialized subgingival tip, gently next to the tooth and/or implant, move the tip subgingival into the pocket/permucosal seal until resistance is felt. Pull back slightly and *activate five seconds per site* (i.e., four sites; mesial, buccal, distal, lingual), continue for all dentition present.

Remember, oral biofilm moves from tooth to tooth, tooth to implant. To achieve complete biofilm elimination, it is necessary to use the powder streaming device on the

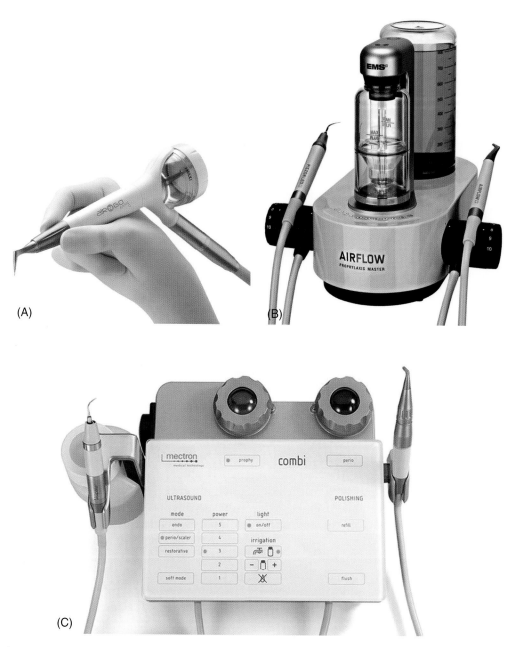

(A)

(B)

(C)

Figure 9.6 Examples of powder streaming devices. (A) ACTEON Air-N-Go Easy® (B) EMS Prophylaxis Master Airflow®Max. (C) MECTRON combi touch.

complete dentition. A supragingival tip can also be used with glycine powder on the inside of cheeks and tongue. The use of the powder streaming device for professional biofilm removal has proven to be a vital tool for implant maintenance and treatment for peri-implant mucositis (17).

Alternatively, you can use a silica xylitol prophy paste to remove the oral biofilm, interrupt the bacterial metabolism until you have a powder streaming device. Use a soft rubber cup and pumice-free xylitol (to attract the bacteria), prophy paste (see Figure 9.16) to eliminate the need to polish at the end of the implant maintenance protocol. Carefully, polish using the rubber cup to remove all biofilm present and remove any stain present on the implant-borne restorations/prosthesis. This alternative removes the oral biofilm, but is not at as effective as using a powder streaming device.

The powder streaming device is moving toward being the standard for oral biofilm removal and a critical component to implant maintenance (2). The powder streaming device does not remove calculus and/or residue. If the assessment revealed that calculus and/or residue is present on the implants, continue with proper titanium implant scalers and/or safe ultrasonic tips (see Tables 9.1 and 9.2).

Debridement instrumentation and ultrasonic research

The key to proper instrumentation for debridement of titanium and ceramic implants is the removal of calculus or residue deposits with SAFE implant hand scalers and/or ultrasonic tips that will remove calculus or residue deposits without

leaving residue on the implant(s) (see Tables 9.1 and 9.2). Debridement or any instrumentation and polishing of an implant-borne restoration is different than on natural teeth/restorations, review the literature (see Figure 9.7).

The literature and previous studies showed that titanium, graphite, and plastic implant scalers were all within safe limits for not scratching the implants surfaces however, the surface can become contaminated with trace elements that plastic, graphite, or stainless steel scalers leave behind (see Figure 9.8). Residue left behind on the implant surface can compromise the biocompatibility and long-term success of the implant (18). According to ACP Clinical Practice Guidelines, professional maintenance; "Professionals should use cleaning instruments compatible with the type and material of abutments, implants, and restorations (2)."

Implants today have a roughened surface to attract the patient's own bone to more effectively osseointegrate to the implant. When implant scalers, that are not compatible with titanium or ceramic implants, are used for debridement on a roughened implant surface, trace elements

Table 9.1 Implant safe, effective hand scalers/curettes.

Company/Instrument Name	Material	Description
American Eagle Implant	Solid titanium alloy	Multiple universal scalers
Brasseler ImplantPro™	Solid titanium alloy	Multiple universal scalers
LM Implant Misura MR™	Solid Titanium alloy	Multiple universal scalers
Nordent ImplantMate™	Solid titanium alloy	Multiple universal scalers
PDT, Inc Wingrove™	Solid titanium alloy	Designed universal scaler set

Table 9.2 Ultrasonic implant safe tips.

Company/Unit	Type of Ultrasonic	Name of Tips	Material
Acteon P5 XS BLED	Piezoelectric	Implant Protect Tips	Titanium alloy
EMS Airflow®Max	Piezoelectric	PI	PEEK
Mectron combi touch	Piezoelectric	Implant Cleaning Kit	PEEK
Parkell Integra™	Magnetostrictive	GentleClean™	Ultem PEI
W & H Ultra Proxeo	Piezoelectric	Implant-clean®	PEEK

can become lodged on the surface. This affect can cause oral biofilm to adhere, which can result in peri-implant disease. There are multiple implant scalers and ultrasonic inserts on the market today. Not all implant scalers or implant ultrasonic inserts/tips are safe and this has been confirmed on multiple studies (14, 15).

In 2009 lab observation study, Dr. James Driver PhD, UM Biological Sciences, University of Montana, imaged titanium

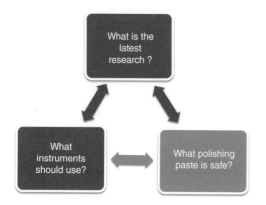

Figure 9.7 What to use, what not to use. Follow the research.

implants and current implant scalers (i.e., Hu-Friedy plastic, Paradise Dental Technologies (PDT) titanium, Graphite, and traditional stainless steel) with a Hitachi S-4700 Scanning Electron Microscope (SEM) (see Figure 9.8). His noted observations compared the titanium implant surfaces after instrumentation for surface results and residue left behind. Driver noted: "the hygiene implant instruments passage across the implant surfaces generally smoothed over rather than gouged the surface. The stainless steel instrument, however, did produce surface scratches with areas of material gouged from the titanium surface thereby forming new pockets for bacterial colonization. The plastic (unfilled resin) scaler had no effect on the implant surface but did leave plastic debris that was firmly attached to the surface as if melted or embedded to it. This plastic debris could not be removed by a jet of air commonly used to clean surfaces for SEM and could also provide additional pockets of a size suitable for bacterial colonization," (see Figure 9.8).

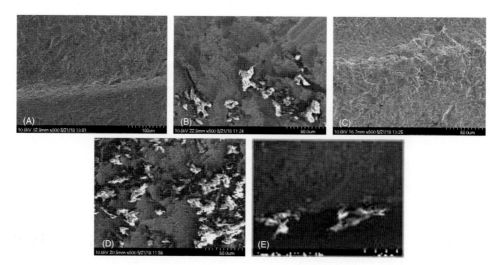

Figure 9.8 (A–E) Observational 2009 SEM study comparing debridement on implant surfaces with implant hand-scalers. Courtesy of Dr. J Driver, PhD. (A) SEM Control untouched implant surface. (B) SEM implant surface after debriding with plastic (unfilled resin) scaler. (C) SEM implant surface after debridement titanium scaler. (D) SEM implant surface after debridement with graphite scaler. (E) SEM implant surface after debridement with stainless steel scaler.

In a follow-up lab observation 2016 study, Dr. Driver using the Hitachi S-4700 SEM, evaluated titanium-alloy and ceramic (zirconia dioxide {ZrO_2}) implants surfaces after instrumentation with various composition implant scalers/curettes on the market (i.e., multiple titanium, PLASTEEL [unfilled resin], and graphite/carbon-reinforced plastic mix and titanium ultrasonic piezoelectric tips) (see Figure 9.9). The results and observations noted by Dr. Jim Driver; an overall rating equation for tools used can be demonstrated for titanium, titanium with surface coating, and ceramic implants. The titanium implant scalers (i.e., PDT Wingroves, American Eagle, both with Rockwell hardness of 28–30) and titanium piezoelectric tips (ACTEON Implant Protect tips), received the highest safety rating with least surface damage and left no debris on the titanium or ceramic implants (see Figure 9.9). Non-titanium instruments while not creating significant surface damage, left significant residue on implant surface to generate a lower overall safety rating (see Figure 9.9).

The previous 2016 study demonstrated that the titanium implant scalers and the titanium ultrasonic piezoelectric (piezo) tips were deemed as safe to debride titanium and ceramic implants. Another study, conducted in 2021 was needed to specifically evaluate ultrasonic piezo units with polyether-ether-ether-ketone (PEEK) tips on titanium and ceramic (zirconia) implants. An Ultem, polyetherimide (PEI) resin tip was also evaluated as an ultrasonic magnetostrictive (magneto) option.

There are several manufactures with ultrasonic piezo implant specific PEEK tips (i.e., EMS, Mectron, W & H). PEEK tips are semi-crystalline organic thermoplastic polymer, known for high durability, thermal resistance, and offer a non-metal debridement option. If scatter occurs, PEEK remnants are biocompatible in tissues and radiolucent on radiographs (19). The Ultem tip, made of PEI resin is an amorphous thermoplastic resin with elevated thermal resistance, high strength, stiffness, broad chemical resistance, and a magneto ultrasonic non-metal option.

The objective of the 2021 observational ultrasonic (magneto and piezo) study was to observe the implant surfaces and wear on PEEK/PEI tips after debridement on titanium and ceramic implants. A microscope, Navitar 12X zoom lens was used at 25X magnification. Control images were taken of titanium and ceramic implants and new PEEK/ PEI tips (i.e., EMS PI PEEK tip, Mectron Implant Cleaning Kit PEEK tip, W & H Implant-clean PEEK tip, and Parkell GentleCLEAN™ Ultem PEI tip). Each ultrasonic tip was used for a calibrated time and equal pressure used by the evaluator (see example of piezo and magneto results Figure 9.10).

Observational study results; minimal residue on the implant surface (footprints) were observed and PEEK tip wear varied by manufacturer. The Ultem PEI tip showed the most wear of the tips, but is recommended as one time use. All of the PEEK/PEI tips, resulted as a safe option for use with titanium implants, wear on tips varied, and no residue present on ceramic implants (see Figure 9.10). This offers ceramic (zirconia) implant patients that are concerned about metal, an excellent no-metal option for safe debridement.

Safe instrumentation on titanium implant surfaces should be performed with a titanium implant scaler or safe ultrasonic tips that are biocompatible (titanium, PEEK or PEI), to prevent instrument debris from becoming lodged on the surface (see Tables 9.1 and 9.2 for safe implant scalers/ ultrasonic options). Instrument debris left behind on the implant or in the peri-implant crevice, has been shown to harbor oral biofilm and increase the risk for peri-implantitis (5). Follow the research; more studies are needed on the long-term effects of instrumentation and residue on titanium and ceramic implants.

2016 Observational study titanium scalers / ultrasonic piezo tips –safe NO RESIDUE

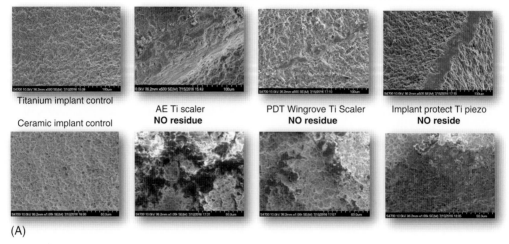

(A)

2016 Observational study plastic / graphite scalers – unsafe WITH RESIDUE

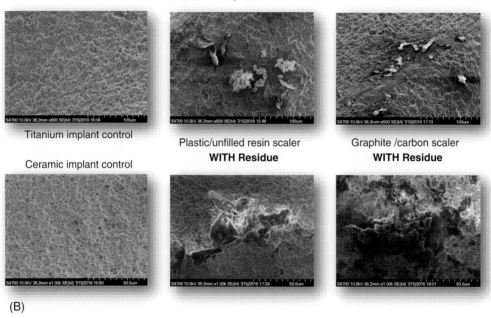

(B)

Figure 9.9 (A–B) Observational 2016 lab study results to evaluate titanium and ceramic implant surfaces using current implant scalers and ultrasonic titanium tips. Courtesy of Dr. Jim Driver. (A) Safe, NO residue results for titanium scalers and ultrasonic piezo tips. (B) Unsafe, WITH residue results for plastic (unfilled resin) and graphite scalers.

Debridement; implant type (narrow- or wide-diameter, specialty) instrumentation

Minimal or no instrumentation may be necessary for an implant with a healthy gingival attachment, no calculus or residue present. However, if the assessment revealed calculus and/or residue are present, a safe instrumentation protocol is necessary (see Chapter 6 on assessment for calculus or residue on implants). Debridement or any instrumentation of an

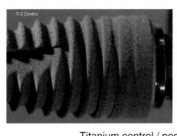

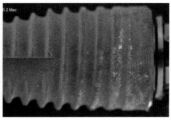

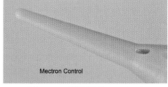

Titanium control / post-debridement

Titanium implant PEEK tip wear

MECTRON combi touch piezo
PEEK implant cleaning kit (ICP + IC1)

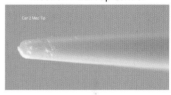

Ceramic control / post-debridement

Mectron PEEK tip control

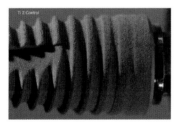

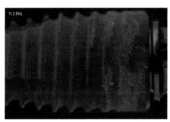

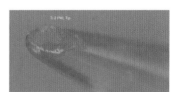

(A)

Ceramic implant PEEK tip wear

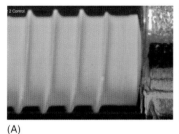

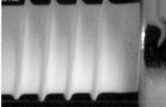

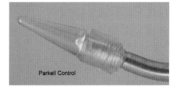

Titanium control / post-debridement

Titanium implant ultem tip wear

PARKELL integra magnetostrictive
ultem gentle clean

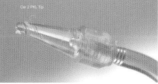

Ceramic control / post-debridement

Parkell ultem tip control

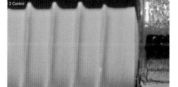

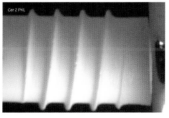

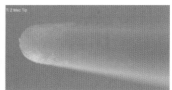

(B)

Ceramic implant ultem tip wear

Figure 9.10 Observational study results to evaluate implant surface on titanium and ceramic implant for any residue and wear on PEEK ultrasonic tips. Example of piezo and magneto results. (A) MECTRON combi touch piezo with PEEK Implant Cleaning Kit (ICP + IC1). IFUs recommend one time use of the PEEK tip, refill packages of five tips and ICP tip holder is reusable/autoclavable. (B) Parkell Integra magneto with GentleClean™ Ultem PEI tip. IFUs recommended one time use of Ultem PEI tip, refill packages of 50 tips.

implant-borne restoration is different than scaling on a natural tooth (see Chapter 3, Figure 3.1). Natural teeth are anchored in the bone by the periodontal ligament (PDL) and sulcular epithelium, while implants are osseointegrated, with direct contact between bone and the dental implant. To debride calculus on a natural tooth, place the blade of the scaler against the side of the tooth, gently move between the PDL and the tooth, and remove all calculus to the bottom of the pocket. Vertical, horizontal, or oblique stokes can all be used to remove any calculus present on a natural tooth surface, which is matrixed and thus harder to remove.

Proper *dental implant instrumentation* to debride calculus and/or residue includes removing and dislodging the microbial deposits without altering the implant surfaces or adversely affecting biocompatibility by leaving residue behind (20). Both natural teeth and implants have a sulcus, junctional epithelium, supracrestal fibers, and bone. The supracrestal fibers are different. In natural teeth, they are in a pattern of attachment and implants with an adherence. The natural teeth are held in primarily with the tissue attachment and the PDL and implants mainly by bone. Calculus deposits on implants are generally softer than those on natural teeth, and are more often found supragingival, making calculus easier to remove with short horizontal strokes (21).

Peri-implant debridement challenges include calculus and residue (i.e., cement or other residue) removal from a variety of titanium or ceramic implants and implant-borne restorations/prostheses. As well as, the challenges of how to treat peri-implant diseases (i.e., mucositis, implantitis). To tackle these challenges and choose the correct scaler/curette or ultrasonic tip to debride the implants, you need an understanding of the type of implant (i.e., titanium or ceramic), narrow-diameter or wide-diameter implant, whether exposed threads

are present, whether access will be difficult, and type of implant-borne restoration/prosthesis.

Implants; narrow-diameter, wide-diameter, or specialty

For debridement, choosing a scaler or ultrasonic tip is NOT referenced by anterior or posterior. Implants can be divided into narrow-diameter, wide-diameter, or specialty design. As well as, ball, Locator and bar-supported implants for removable overdenture patients and exposed threads and residue implants. The key to proper debridement is *light, effective horizontal strokes* with the proper titanium implant scaler and/or ultrasonic tip to remove all oral biofilm and calculus with the ultimate goal of no debris in the sulcus or residue left affixed to the implant(s). Calculus removal on implants, should fleck off easily. If the calculus seems difficult to remove, it may be residue. To choose which safe titanium implant hand scaler or ultrasonic tip to use, refer to the type of implants; narrow-diameter, wide-diameter, or specialty.

Narrow-diameter implants

Narrow-diameter implants (Figure 9.11) are implants with a narrow platform placed in both the anterior and posterior of the oral cavity; lower incisors, congenially missing laterals, and areas with limited horizontal bone. In the posterior mandible, a narrow-diameter implant can be used to replace two teeth for a patient with a narrow ridge, limited horizontal bone, and the final restoration crown is often shaped like a champagne glass (bulbous). Narrow-diameter implants are also used to support a full arch fixed final prosthesis. To debride narrow-diameter implants, select a longer, multi-bent blade titanium (Ti) implant scaler (i.e., Wingrove Ti L3–4 by PDT, Inc.).

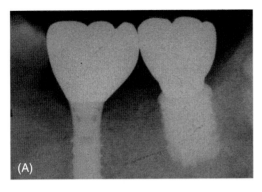
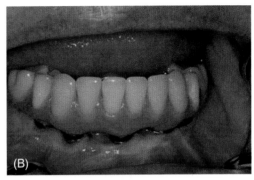

Figure 9.11 Narrow- and wide-diameter implants (A) Notice narrow-diameter implant on the left (bulbous crown to fit contacts) and wide-diameter implant on the right. These require different instruments to reach the peri-implant crevice for debridement. Courtesy of MegaGen. (B) Narrow-diameter implants supporting fixed full-arch hybrid. Courtesy of Dr. Robert Schneider.

Use short horizontal strokes to dislodge the calculus present on; narrow-diameter single implants, restorations, and implant-supported fixed final full arch prosthesis cases.

Wide-diameter implants

For wide-diameter implants, primarily placed in the mandibular posterior oral cavity (i.e., molar implants) (see Figure 9.11), select a universal titanium implant scaler (i.e., Wingrove Ti B5-6, Figure 9.12). Use the universal implant scaler in an unconventional manner, leading with the toe of the instrument. Use short horizontal strokes to dislodge the calculus, taking care not to harm the permucosal seal.

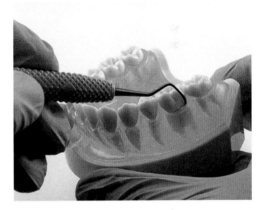

Figure 9.12 Scaling wide-diameter implant with Wingrove Titanium B5-6, PDT, Inc. Courtesy of Wingrove Dynamics.

Specialty: Exposed implant threads, bar-supported, and residue implants

To remove the calculus present on exposed implant threads (Figure 9.13) found in anterior or posterior, use a shorter radius blade tip of a titanium implant scaler (i.e., Wingrove titanium L5 mini by PDT, Inc.). For calculus removal, use tip of the instrument in a horizontal, side-to-side motion, in and out, one thread at a time. For bar-supported implants, debride around the implants with a shorter radius blade tip of a titanium implant scaler (i.e., Wingrove titanium L5 mini by PDT, Inc.). For the bar of bar-supported implants, sweep under and on the bar, using short sweeping strokes with tip of the implant scaler (i.e., Wingrove titanium N128). For residue implants, debride with short horizontal strokes (i.e., Wingrove titanium N128). To complete full debridement on residue (i.e., cement or instrument) the doctor or surgeon may need to flap the implant to see all the residue and complete a regenerative procedure (regenerate bone and tissue).

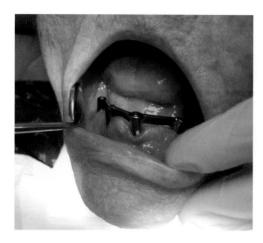

Figure 9.13 Exposed threads. To debride use tip of the instrument in a horizontal, side-to-side motion, in and out, one thread at a time. Courtesy of Wingrove Dynamics.

Every office should have a minimum of two go-to proper implant set-ups per hygienist in the office. This implant maintenance set-up, kept separately, needs to include all the necessary instruments to meet all the peri-implant maintenance challenges; titanium implant scalers and a 1 mm marking probe that can be plastic, stainless steel, or titanium (see Figure 9.14).

Lavage and debridement with safe ultrasonic tips

Continue with *lavage and debridement with safe ultrasonic tips* (see Table 9.2). Ultrasonics, magnetostrictive (magneto), and piezoelectric (piezo) are the two current options on the market today. They both have two com-

ponents; frequency and amplitude. *Frequency is described as the number of times the ultrasonic insert/tip moves and amplitude is the distance it moves.* The major difference of the two ultrasonic options is the movement. Magneto is in the form of a stack drive insert and produces *elliptical motion*. The piezo produces a *linear motion* from the piezoelectric crystals in the handpiece. Water flow is critical with any ultrasonic instrumentation and a clinician should never use an ultrasonic tip on a natural tooth or implant without water. Water cools the magneto stacks or the piezo crystals and cools the interface to the natural tooth or implant. Fictional higher heat from a magneto insert or piezo tip against the natural tooth or implant can cause damage.

The clinician should pre-set the unit water flow prior to each patient, (see Figure 9.15). *The rapid drip flow water adjustment technique is applicable for magneto and piezo ultrasonic tips.* Direct the point toward the ceiling and adjust water to a rapid drip flow on low power. Adjust water until droplets reach the point of the tip being used with a rapid drip flow. Water flow also generates aerosols and clinicians should strive to generate minimal aerosols due to microbial loads that can cause disease transmission. *For debridement of calculus from implants, the setting on ultrasonics should remain on low.* "Be methodical and precise," Noel Paschke outlines in the Paschke low and slow technique. Adjust the water flow to drop-to-drop, stay in contact with the tooth or

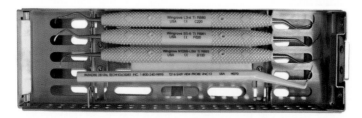

Figure 9.14 Example of the "Wingrove go-to-set"; universal set of titanium scalers specifically designed for implant maintenance, 1 mm probe and sharpening stone in a cassette. Courtesy of PDT, Inc.

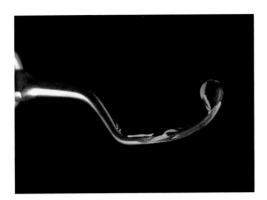

Figure 9.15 Rapid Drip Flow water adjustment technique. Direct the point of the tip toward the ceiling. Adjust water to a rapid drip flow on low power, then adjust water until droplets reach the point of the tip being used (ACTEON H3) with a rapid drip flow. Courtesy of ACTEON.

implant surface, and use a methodical, overlapping, channeling strokes (22).

Ultrasonic, piezoelectric safe tips specifically designed for implant maintenance debridement are being evaluated and becoming an integral part of implant maintenance, current examples of safe ultrasonic tips (see Table 9.2). Note, most magnetostrive inserts can be interchanged with magneto units. However, piezo tips are either S-type threads or E-type threads, referring to the thread pitch which screws into the handpiece. They are not interchangeable.

To lavage around an implant, provide intrasulcular irrigation around the implant, first set the power setting to the lowest level available or specific lavage setting on the ultrasonic unit. The power settings on ultrasonic units control the amplitude or distance an ultrasonic insert tip moves. Some units can be adjusted to turn off the amplitude (power) entirely leaving on only the lavage feature. Other units' power settings should be adjusted to the lowest power, check manufacturer IFUs document.

For lavage, set unit to lavage or lowest setting, at a drop-by-drop flow rate (see Figure 9.15). Next, adapt the tip of the ultrasonic insert tip in an apical position.

Be careful not to harm the perimucosal seal or touch the implant, implant-borne restoration or prosthesis. Lavage using a safe ultrasonic insert tip if possible, encircle the implant with the water flow to remove any debris and repeat after debridement.

A magneto or other piezo tip may be used for lavage, but CAUTION must be used to not touch the implant surface or the abutment/crown interface unless it is deemed a *implant safe tip* (see Table 9.2). Using an unsafe ultrasonic tip can cause the surface of the implant to flake causing metallosis, attachment of debris on the implant surface, or remove the oxide layer which can lead to implant complications (6, 23, 24) (see Chapter 7).

It is also important to NOT to use liquids such as Chlorhexidine (CHX) (0.12%) with a low acidic pH in the ultrasonic reservoir, as this could alter the implant surfaces as well. Therefore, if you want to irrigate with a solution during lavage procedure; water or saline is preferred (7). To *debride implants with safe ultrasonic tip*, choose a safe ultrasonic tip (see Table 9.2), set the drop-by-drop flow rate (Figure 9.15), and use short horizontal strokes.

Polishing the implant-borne restoration/ prosthesis

The goal for polishing implant-borne restorations/prostheses is to effectively disrupt the oral biofilm around implants and remove any stains present on the restorations/prosthesis. For implant maintenance, traditional air polishing is contraindicated. Hygienists not only need to understand how to clinically perform a polishing procedure on implant-borne restorations, but must know which tools to use and make the correct choice for a polishing agent (see Table 9.3 and Figure 9.16).

One polishing paste is not appropriate for all teeth, tooth-borne or implant-borne restorations and some polishing pastes can

Table 9.3 Examples of safe pumice-free prophy pastes.

Prophy Paste Name	Composition	Manufacturer
Next® Fine	Diatomaceous earth	Preventech
ProphyCare® PRO/Fine	Silica	Directa
Proxyt® Fine	Silica	Ivoclar Vivadent
MI Paste®	Recaldent™	GC America
MI Paste® Plus	Recaldent™	GC America
SoftShine®	Crushed sapphire	Waterpik

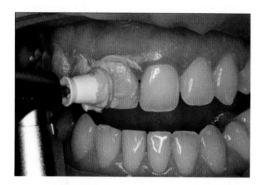

Figure 9.16 Polish restorations with soft prophy cup and pumice-free prophy paste (i.e., Proxyt® Fine). Courtesy of Ivoclar Vivadent.

be contraindicated. This is definitely not the time to pull out whatever is readily available or use coarse pumice paste to save time. When choosing a polishing agent for implant maintenance, the hygienist needs to evaluate the ingredients of the polishing agents available in paste or powder form. Most polishing agents are made up of diamond particles, aluminum oxide, silicates, pumice, and calcium carbonate. Aluminum oxide, tin oxide, and acidulated phosphate fluoride (APF)-free. Pumice-free prophylaxis paste or powder is considered the most acceptable polishing abrasives for implants (24) (see Table 9.3). The polishing tools to use on implant-borne restorations/prostheses are soft prophy cups, points or disks, not brushes.

The basic steps for proper coronal polishing around implant-borne restorations/prostheses consist of using a soft rubber cup, not brush, with appropriate pumice-free prophy paste to polish the natural

teeth, tooth-borne, and/or implant-borne restorations/prostheses (see Figure 9.16). There is no need to polish exposed implants or abutments, only implant-borne restorations/prostheses. Remove any stain present and rinse thoroughly. A soft polishing point or disc may also be used to smooth and polish an implant-supported fixed final prosthesis where access for a rubber cup may not be possible. Note that it is not necessary to repeat the polishing procedure if you chose to polish first as an alternative to using a powder streaming device at the beginning of the protocol for oral biofilm removal. After debridement and polishing are completed, apply an antimicrobial varnish or gel treatment to complete the implant maintenance protocol.

Antimicrobial varnish

Optional step, apply an antimicrobial varnish or gel to prevent colonization of oral biofilm around implants and implant-borne restorations. Multiple antimicrobial varnishes or gel are being developed. One excellent example is Cervitec® Plus varnish by Ivoclar Vivadent, a slow time release varnish of 1% chlorhexidine diacetate (CHXD) not chlorhexidine gluconate and 1% thymol (essential oil) with proven studies on biocompatibility with titanium implants (see Figure 9.17). In an in-vivo study of 30 patients, Cervitec Plus varnish reduced the presence of Porphyromonas gingivalis at the end of 1 and 3 months.

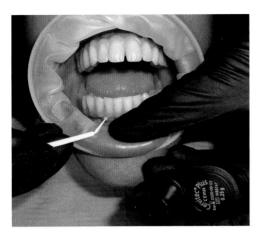

Figure 9.17 Example of antimicrobial varnish, Cervitec® Plus varnish by Ivoclar Vivadent. Courtesy of Wingrove Dynamics.

This varnish also reduces Streptococci mutans and inflammation thus benefits the overall health of the patient (25). For implants with biofilm as a major risk factor, a targeted clear, non-staining (teeth, tongue, mucosa, or restorations), antimicrobial treatment using the Cervitec Plus varnish, shows controlling *Streptococci mutans* up to 3 months with no taste alteration, is an excellent treatment that the hygienist can provide at every 3 month recare (25).

Steps to apply an antimicrobial varnish; clean the surface, rinse, and dry. Apply varnish into the permucosal seal, cervical margin. Leave to dry for 30 seconds and ask the patient to not eat or drink for 1 hour (25). Remove the OptraGate if placed or cheek retractor. Finally, *schedule an in-office implant recare appointment at least every 6 months* (2).

Professional in-office implant maintenance recare

Recare implant maintenance intervals start with loading of the implant restoration and patient is in occlusion. Start patients out with implant maintenance recare appointments every 3 months for the first year (26).

After 1 year, post loading and the crestal bone remodeling (the bone surrounding the implant maintains a mature level) of the bone and osseointegration is confirmed. After 1 year, many factors need to be evaluated to determine the patient's implant maintenance interval and evaluated on an individual basis for each patient. The recare interval is based on restoration/prosthesis type, medical history/risk factors, age, at-home oral hygiene, and biological or mechanical complications (27).

The literature supports that if the patient has a previous history of periodontal disease (has had peri-implant disease), he or she is at a 28.6% higher risk for developing peri-implantitis, compared with patients with no previous periodontal disease history at 5.8% (28, 29) (see Chapter 2 on risk assessments). These patients should remain on a *3 month implant maintenance interval* to assure the long-term success of the implant(s).

According to the ACP Clinical Practice Guidelines; "patients with implants/implant-borne restorations/prostheses are advised to present for implant assessment and maintenance at least every 6 months" (2). There is significant evidence that patients with implant-borne fixed or removable prostheses require lifelong custom patient implant maintenance regimen with a dental professional. Read the ACP clinical practice guidelines for guidelines on recare based on implant-borne restoration/prosthesis (2).

As implants are becoming prevalent, dental offices are conforming to a new system of coding for the hygienists to designate traditional prophylaxis, periodontal prophylaxis, or implant maintenance appointments. A patient's chart should be marked or a computer coding system used to identify patients with implants. The desired outcome of successful implant therapy is the maintenance of a stable, functional, aesthetically acceptable tooth replacement for the patient (30). Understanding various implant designs and having the proper instruments and products for safe implant maintenance will allow you to provide your patients with the ideal implant care to ensure the long-term success of their implants.

Single implant maintenance

The majority of implant patients that hygienists will see daily, will be single implants which include; single, mini, ball or Locator, and/or bar-supported. Follow the single implant maintenance protocol, (Box 9.3), to professionally remove the biofilm, and debride if needed with safe titanium implant scalers and/or ultrasonic tips (see Tables 9.1 and 9.2). Apply antimicrobial varnish or gel to prevent biofilm formation, around implants into the permucosal seal, cervical margin. Leave to dry 30 seconds and ask the patient to not eat or drink for 1 hour (25). Remove the OptraGate or cheek retractor and instruct patient on home care recommendations. Follow with doctor exam that includes checking the

---

Box 9.3 Single implant maintenance protocol for titanium and ceramic implants

- Assess implants and take radiographs at least once a year
- Place OptraGate or retractor for visibility and identify biofilm
- Use powder streaming device or polish to professionally remove biofilm
- Lavage; safe ultrasonic tip on low setting before/after debridement to remove debris
- Debride if calculus is present; use tip of titanium scaler and/or safe ultrasonic tip, short horizontal strokes, based on implant (narrow or wide diameter), restoration/prosthesis, or exposed threads.
- Polish restorations to remove stain present with pumice-free prophy paste
- Apply antimicrobial varnish or gel around implants to prevent biofilm formation
- Remove OptraGate or retractor and instruct on home care recommendations
- Doctor exam; check occlusion, adjust if necessary and appoint recare.

---

occlusion adjust if necessary and appoint recare at least every 6 months (2).

Mastering the Arch©

Implant-supported full-arch removable/fixed final prosthesis maintenance

Patients today want to replace lost dentition in an edentulous arch with natural looking restorations, that look and feel like natural teeth. The implant-supported full-arch removable or fixed final prosthesis offers patients an aesthetic option, retention for chewing, and the confidence to laugh or talk without worry of the denture staying in-place (see Figure 9.18).

There are two options for the implant-supported full-arch patients. The removable overdenture prosthesis with retention attachments or fixed final prosthesis only removable by a dental professional.

Full arch removable final prosthesis (Overdenture)

The patient with the removable overdenture has two to four single implants or a bar can be used to splint the implants together for more retention, to support the overdenture. The hygienist can help initiate a discussion on whether the patient is a good candidate for a removable overdenture with single implants or with a bar-supported based on; retention, oral hygiene, and if the patient is taking a medications that has a side effect of tissue growth. A patient on these types of medication is not a good candidate for the bar splinting the implants or an alternative medication can be considered with a consultation with patient's physician.

An implant-supported removable overdenture with or without a bar is a good option for a patient with previous poor dental hygiene. Having a removal full arch

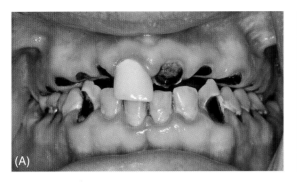
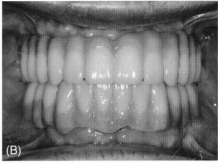

(A) (B)

Figure 9.18 Example of full-arch fixed final prosthesis case, (A) before and (B) after. Courtesy of Dr. Mark Jesin and Dr. Tom Lambert.

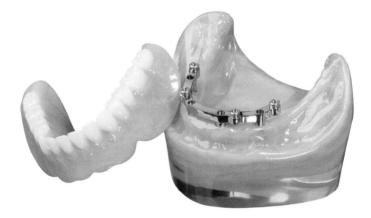

Figure 9.19 Implant bar-supported full-arch removable overdenture example. Courtesy of Glidewell.

overdenture allows the patient and the clinician to remove and keep the implants well maintained. Ultimately, the patient after consulting with the dental professionals will decide on which option they prefer, but at least they will understand the differences.

Implant maintenance for a patient with an implant-supported full-arch removable overdenture (Figure 9.19 and Box 9.4), starts with asking the patient to remove the overdenture. As the patient removes the prosthesis, observe if it difficult for him or her or if it removes too easily. Retention can be adjusted chairside by changing the attachments. After changing the attachments, always practice with the patient until the patient can place and remove the overdenture comfortably. Optimally, it should be the maximum tension for reten-

tion and that still allows the patient to remove it for at-home oral hygiene care.

Place the overdenture to clean in ultrasonic cleaner with a safe cleaner for overdentures following manufacturer and lab instructions. Assess implants following the assessment and monitoring protocol (see Figure 9.2) and take radiographs at least once a year. Place an OptraGate or cheek retractor for visibility. Biofilm can collect and result in calculus build-up on implants, bar for bar-supported implants and the overdenture. Use a powder streaming device or polish to professionally remove biofilm. If calculus is present, debride implants (mini, ball or Locator, bar-supported), use tip of titanium scaler and/ or safe ultrasonic tip with short horizontal strokes and inside the screw indentation

> **Box 9.4** Full-arch supporting implants and removable overdenture maintenance protocol
>
> - Ask patient to remove overdenture, observe if difficult or too easy to remove.
> - Flip overdenture over, assess attachments (O-rings, caps, or clips).
> - Clean overdenture in ultrasonic bath with safe solution, debride if necessary, and polish.
> - Assess implants and take radiographs at least once a year
> - Place OptraGate or cheek retractor for visibility
> - Use powder streaming device or polish to professionally remove biofilm
> - Debride if calculus is present around implants (mini, ball, Locator, and bar-supported), use tip of titanium scaler and/or safe ultrasonic tip, short horizontal strokes, inside top of the Locator screw and sweeping strokes under the bar.
> - Apply antimicrobial varnish or gel around implants to prevent biofilm formation and remove OptraGate/retractor.
> - Retrieve overdenture from ultrasonic bath, debride if needed and/or use soft brush to clean, polish overdenture to remove stains, and rinse thoroughly.
> - Replace any worn or missing attachments.
>   - Replace O-rings or Locator caps once a year, bar-clips only if missing
>   - Have patient reinsert overdenture, try in and out, check tension.
> - Doctor exam, home care recommendations, and appoint recare.

on top of the Locator attachment (Figure 9.20A). For the bar that splints the bar-supported implants, adapt a thinner curved-radius blade tip implant scaler under the bar and use a side-to-side horizontal sweeping stroke to dislodge the calculus (see Figure 9.20B).

Apply antimicrobial varnish or gel to prevent biofilm formation, around implants into the permucosal seal, cervical margin. Leave to dry 30 seconds and ask the patient to not eat or drink for 1 hour (25). Remove the OptraGate or cheek retractor and retrieve the overdenture from the ultrasonic bath. Debride the overdenture if needed with a soft titanium scaler (Rockwell hardness 28–30) and/or use soft brush to clean. Do not use a denture brush that could damage the retention attachments (i.e., O-rings, Locator caps, or bar-and-clip system). Polish the overdenture with pumice-free prophy paste or lab rag wheel, to remove any stains present and rinse thoroughly.

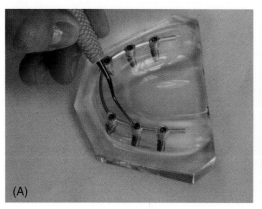 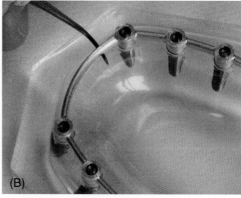

Figure 9.20 (A) Debide around and inside screw indentation on top of Locator abutment (i.e., Wingrove Titanium L5 mini) (B) Use sweeping strokes under bar of bar-supported implants (i.e., Wingrove Titanium N128). Courtesy of PDT, Inc.

After overdenture is thoroughly cleaned and polished, do a visual assessment of attachments and replace any worn or missing attachments (see Figure 9.21). Replace O-rings or Locator caps once a year and the bar-clips, only if missing. Have the patient practice taking the overdenture in and out. This allows the hygienist to see if patient has any difficulty removing the overdenture and if the retention is correct. Assist the patient on the correct technique to remove and reseat the overdenture, as this will prevent wear on the attachments (i.e., O-rings, caps, and clips).

If you notice that the patient's overdenture is difficult for him or her to remove or removes too easily, you can suggest an attachment with a different tension, which can be changed chairside. Remind the patient that a visual check of attachments (i.e., O-rings, Locator caps, or bar-and-clip system), is an integral part of his or her at-home care. If he or she notices anythingis different, he or she should notify your office and set up an appointment for a replacement according to recommendations. Time for the doctor exam, instruct the patient on any home care recommendations and appoint recare at least every 6 months (2).

Hygienists, familiarize yourself with your patient's attachments and order attachments from dental supply company or lab. Attachments are for retention of the overdenture to the implants to allow the patient to laugh, chew with confidence, the overdenture will stay in place. Assess the attachments in the overdenture (Figure 9.21) for worn or missing O-rings (Figure 9.22), Locator caps (Figure 9.23), and/or clips (Figure 9.24). Factors that will influence how often the attachments (O-rings, caps, or clips) will need to be replaced include; the convergence/divergence of the implants, the degree of angulation, and finally the patient's oral hygiene (i.e., biofilm accumulation).

Hygiene Tip:

When you first see the removal overdenture prosthesis patient, record the tension level and color of the attachments (i.e., O-ring, Locator cap, and/or bar-clip attached to the overdenture). If the patient presents for an appointment with one of these attachments worn or missing, refer to the patient's past notes for attachment record (i.e. retention level and color) for replacement.

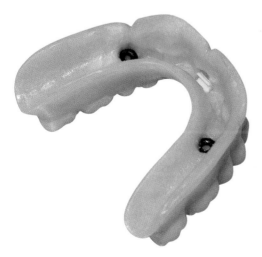

Figure 9.21 Note patient's overdenture attachments (black O-rings, yellow bar clip) in patient's record. Courtesy of Salvin Dental Specialties.

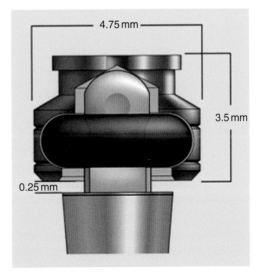

Figure 9.22 Example of O-ring system on implant. Courtesy of Glidewell.

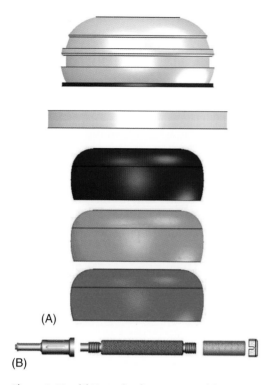

(A)

(B)

Figure 9.23 (A) Example of Locator caps (B) Locator placement and removal tool. Courtesy of Glidewell.

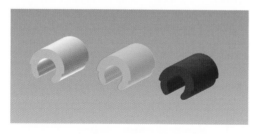

Figure 9.24 Example of clips for bar-and-clip system. Courtesy of Glidewell.

In the case of O-rings, attachments that fit on to ball implants or Locator caps for Locator implants, it is recommended to replace these once a year (31). Refer to O-rings replacement protocol (Box 9.5) and Locator cap replacement protocol (see Box 9.6 and Figure 9.25) for specifics on steps to remove and replace these attachments. For bar-clip replacement, the doctor will evaluate the clips in the bar-and-clip system on an individual basis and recommend replacement as necessary (31) (see Box 9.7).

Box 9.5   O-ring replacement protocol

- ■ Remove the worn or old O-ring carefully with a designated tool or a small-radius blade tip of an instrument.
- ■ Lubricate the new O-ring and press into place.
- ■ Have the patient practice placing and removing the overdenture before he or she leaves the operatory.
- ■ O-rings come in different colors to signify low to greatest retention; pink is the lowest retention, reserved for patients who have dexterity issues or for whom the overdenture is hard to remove. Red is moderate and black has the greatest resistance.
- ■ Replace the O-ring with the highest resistance as long as the patient's dexterity allows.
- ■ Replace if worn, missing, change in retention, or at least once a year.

Box 9.6   Locator cap replacement protocol

- ■ Remove Locator cap using designated tool or a small-radius blade tip of an instrument out of the female housing on the overdenture.
- ■ Lubricate the male Locator cap, place into the female housing on the overdenture using the placement end of the designated tool, and press into place.
- ■ Have the patient practice placing and removing the overdenture before he or she leaves the operatory.
- ■ Locator caps come in 1.5, 3.0, and 5.0 lbs. of retention force.
- ■ Extender male caps can be 0.0, 1.0, 2.0, or 4.0 lbs. for more angulation and retention options.
- ■ Retention can be determined chairside; record the doctor's recommendation for retention in patient's record.
- ■ Replace Locator cap if worn, missing, change in retention, at least once a year.

Full arch fixed final prosthesis in-place, not removed

Patients can also choose an implant-supported full-arch fixed final prosthesis, also referred to as Fixed Full Arch Hybrid.

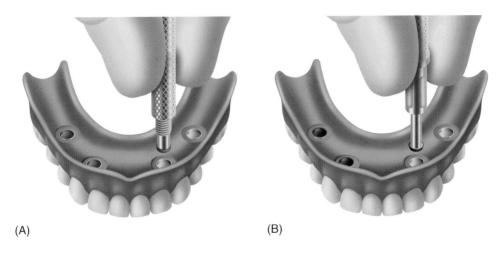

(A) (B)

Figure 9.25 Locator cap replacement (A) Remove worn Locator cap. (B) Replace with new cap into the Locator attachment in overdenture. Courtesy of Zest Anchors, LLC.

Box 9.7 Bar-clip system replacement protocol

■ Remove bar-clip using designated tool or a small-radius blade tip of an instrument.
■ Lubricate the new clip and press into place.
■ Have the patient practice placing and removing the overdenture before he or she leaves the operatory.
■ Clips come in different colors that range from low to increased retention, with yellow universally moderate and normally used. Low retention reserved for patients who have dexterity issues and for whom the overdenture is hard to remove.
■ Replace the bar retention clips when chipped, missing, or to change retention.

Box 9.8 Full-arch final prosthesis in-place, *not removed*, maintenance protocol

■ Assess for any inflammation or infection, access is limited. Take radiographs at least once a year, ideally when prosthesis is removed.
■ Place OptraGate or assistant for visibility.
■ Use powder streaming device or polish to professionally remove biofilm.
■ Lavage; safe ultrasonic tip on low setting before/after debridement to remove debris.
■ Debride with soft titanium scaler and/or safe ultrasonic tip, short horizontal strokes around implants and under the prosthesis on facial and lingual as access permits.
■ Polish prosthesis to remove stain present with pumice-free prophy paste.
■ Apply antimicrobial varnish or gel around implants to prevent biofilm formation.
■ Remove OptraGate or retractor and instruct on home care recommendations.
■ Doctor exam; check occlusion, adjust if necessary and appoint recare.

The implant-supported fixed final prosthesis is only removable by a dental professional and needs to be evaluated on WHEN to remove the prosthesis for assessment and monitoring and professional in-office maintenance. Performing an assessment and maintenance on a fixed full arch final prosthesis patient is possible with *prosthesis in place*. For assessment; note any signs of inflammation or infection, but access is limited. Panoramic or cone beam computed tomography (CBCT) at least once a year and *maintenance every 2–6 months*. Most often, the hygienist will complete the assessment and implant maintenance with the implant-supported fixed final prosthesis in place (Box 9.8), every 2–3 months and at least every 6 months (2). Removal of the fixed final prosthesis is now suggested every 6–18 months and new screws considered each time removed (2).

The maintenance protocol for implant-supported fixed final prosthesis when the final prosthesis is left in-place and not removed, (see Box 9.8). The steps for maintenance begins by placing an OptraGate, latex free retraction device for visibility (see Figure 9.26). It is extremely hard to get access to the implants supported the final prosthesis without a retraction device or an assistant.

To begin the maintenance for the full arch final prosthesis patient when the prosthesis is not removed, assess for any signs of inflammation or infection, access is limited. Take radiographs at least once a year, ideally when prosthesis is removed. Place an OptraGate or have an assistant help for access and visibility to the implants, difficult to complete the maintenance without. Use a powder streaming device to remove biofilm, not possible to polish as an alternative. Lavage before/after debridement with safe ultrasonic tip on lavage setting to remove any debris, caution should be used

not to touch implants or implant-borne prosthesis if the ultrasonic tip is not safe for implant debridement. Assess if calculus is present, debride with soft titanium (Rockwell hardness of 28–30) implant scaler or safe ultrasonic tip (see Figure 9.26) around the implants and the underside of the prosthesis on facial and lingual as access permits. Polish prosthesis to remove any stain present with pumice-free paste and apply an antimicrobial varnish or gel around the implants to prevent biofilm formation (see Figure 9.17). Remove the OptraGate if placed and instruct patient on home care recommendations. Doctor exam, check occlusion, adjust if necessary and schedule recare every 2–3 months or at least every 6 months.

Full-arch fixed final prosthesis removed and reseated

Professional in-office assessment and maintenance for fixed full-arch hybrid at *least* every 6 months (2), most clinicians have recommended that the fixed full arch hybrid patients present for implant maintenance every 2–3 months based on patient's risk factors and home care. The evaluation or assessment of patients tissues, abutments, and implants is a critical component in the in-office professional implant maintenance visit. To truly evaluate the final prosthesis, implants, and implant abutments on an implant-supported fixed final prosthesis patient, the prosthesis needs to be removed. It is now suggested to remove the final prosthesis on a case by case basis for patients *every 6 to 18 months* to evaluate; the prosthesis, patients tissues under the prosthesis, implants and their abutments that hold the prosthesis in place.

There are multiple opinions on when to remove the implant-supported fixed final prosthesis *every 6 months, once a year or 18 months*. Factors include origin of the

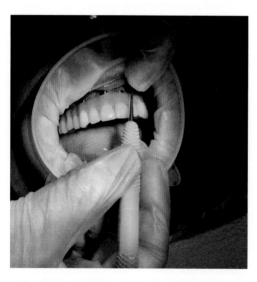

Figure 9.26 Implant maintenance fixed final prosthesis in-place, not removed. Using a titanium scaler, WinTiL3-4 by PDT, Inc. to debride implants and prosthesis. Courtesy of Dr. Marco Padilla and Heather Rogers, RDH.

implants, the prosthesis, and the patient's medical or dental risk factors. Occlusion is also important, if the patient presents with grinding or clenching or hard contact noted on the blue indication paper assessment, removal on a routine basis to monitor the abutments is needed. They may loosen or fracture abutments and the only way to evaluate the abutments or implants is by removal of the fixed final prosthesis. The removal can be done by the dentist or trained hygienist where their state/country license allows. Specific tools and materials are needed for removal and reseating the implant-supported final prosthesis (see Figure 9.27 and Box 9.9).

Acquire the correct implant screwdriver per implant manufacturer and prosthesis design. Consult with doctor on whether to order new screws ahead of visit based on patient prosthesis design and implant company. Note; the ACP' Clinical Practice Guidelines (CPG) recommends to use new screws each time removed (2).

Attain a designated instrument (i.e., spoon excavator, explorer, or drill) to remove the access plug (i.e., composite or Fermit temporary material) and cotton pliers or explorer to remove tape or cord that covers protects the screws (see Figure 9.28).

Box 9.9 Tools and materials for removal/reseating of fixed final prosthesis

1. Acquire correct implant screwdriver per implant manufacturer and prosthesis type.
2. Order new screws ahead of the visit based on patient, prosthesis design, implant company, and ACP Guidelines that recommend to use new screws each time removed.
3. Attain an instrument (i.e., spoon excavator, explorer, or drill) to remove access plug and cotton pliers or explorer to remove tape/cord that protects the screws.
4. Secure Teflon tape or packing cord to replace the removed tape/cord to access the screws and instrument (i.e., plugger or condenser) to place tape/cord.
5. Procure access plug replacement material, instrument to place, and curing light if plug material requires.

Secure new Teflon tape or packing cord to replace the removed tape/cord to access the screws and instrument (i.e., plugger or condenser) to place tape/cord. Procure access plug replacement material (i.e., Fermit or composite) (see Figure 9.27B), instrument to place, and a curing light to cure replacement plug material if required (see Box 9.9).

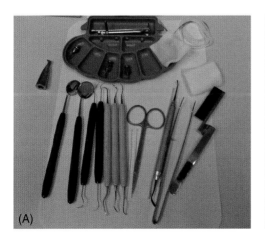 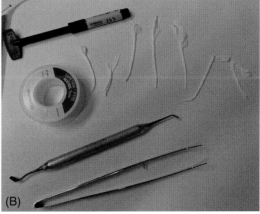

Figure 9.27 Example of specific tools and materials for removal (A) and (B) reseating the implant-supported final prosthesis. Courtesy of Wingrove Dynamics.

Fixed final prosthesis removal

To begin appointment, ask the doctor to greet and complete a preliminary exam with the prosthesis in place; check occlusion, recommend removal, specify any specific maintenance or any other directives (see Box 9.10). Hygienists, remove the access plug or have the doctor use the drill if necessary to remove the composite. Use the cotton pliers or explorer to remove the Teflon tape or cord that has been protecting the screws (Figure 9.28).

Now that the screws are exposed, remove the screws one by one with the correct implant screwdriver and place on wet gauze. The gauze soaked in an antimicrobial rinse, NOT CHX Gluconate, helps to start the disinfection process and prevents the screws from rolling off the tray. Let the screws soak in antimicrobial gauze, wipe clean and disinfect before replacing or replace with new screws based on ACP'

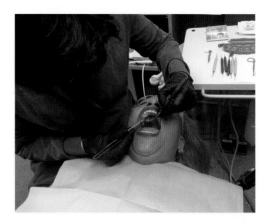

Figure 9.28 Removal of final fixed prosthesis, remove tape in the access hole with cotton pliers to expose the screw. Courtesy of Wingrove Dynamics.

Clinical Practice Guidelines (CPG) (2), doctor's directive, and implant manufacturer recommendations.

Assessment after the fixed final prosthesis is removed

The assessment process begins with removing the prosthesis to gain access and properly assess the abutments and implants, not possible with the final prosthesis in place (see Box 9.11). Assess the final prosthesis for cracks, fractures, and/or debris. Place prosthesis carefully in a bag or container with *safe prosthesis cleaner designated by prosthesis composition* in the ultrasonic bath and activate for 10–15 minutes.

Perform a visual soft tissue and abutment assessment with magnification loupes, light, and/or intraoral camera. Assess tissue surrounding the implants for inflammation, red halos, keratinized or non-keratinized soft tissue and note in the patient's record.

Before you examine the abutments, you need to know about the abutments you are examining. There are many types of abutments and custom abutments available on the market. To clarify what to look for, *angled abutments will have two screws.*

Box 9.10 Fixed final prosthesis removal protocol

1. Doctor greets and completes exam with prosthesis in place; checks occlusion, recommends removal, specifies any specific maintenance or any other directives.
2. Remove access plug material (i.e., temporary or composite) covering the screw with instrument or have doctor use the drill to remove composite.
3. Remove Teflon tape strip or cord to expose each screw with cotton pliers or an explorer.
4. Remove all the screws with correct implant screwdriver and place on wet gauze.
   - ■ Gauze soaked in antimicrobial rinse, NOT CHX Gluconate. This starts disinfection process and prevents screws from rolling off the tray.
5. Let the screws soak in antimicrobial gauze. Wipe clean and disinfect before replacing OR replace with new screws based on CPG, doctor's directive, and implant manufacturer recommendations.

Box 9.11 Assessment after fixed final prosthesis is removed protocol

1. **Assess the prosthesis** for cracks, fractures, and/or debris.
   - ■ Place prosthesis carefully in bag or container with safe prosthesis cleaner in ultrasonic bath and activate for 10–15 minutes.
2. **Visual soft tissue and abutment assessment** with magnification loupes, light and/or intraoral camera.
   - ■ Assess tissue surrounding the implants for inflammation, red halos, keratinized or non-keratinized and note in patient's record.
   - ■ Examine the abutment for any fractures. If fractures are present doctor may need to replace abutment or schedule for replacement.
3. **Percussion;** gently tap each abutment with a blunt-end instrument.
   - ■ **Listen for normal solid sound or hollow sound** that could be a sign abutment is loose, loss of implant osseointegration, or a zygomatic implant which may sound different. Note any hollow sound in record for doctor to evaluate.
   - ■ **Check the** N° **torque level of each screw in an angle abutment or straight abutment**

   itself. **If loose, tighten** per correct N° torque guidelines from the manufacturer, retest, and note in patient's record for doctor to evaluate.
4. **Mobility;** place two blunt-end instruments on each abutment, move back/forth and note any mobility in patient's record. If mobility, take a radiograph to assess bone level. Doctor evaluates for occlusal trauma, loose screw or bone loss.
5. **Probe/Palpate** implants for signs of infection.
   - ■ **Probe;** wait at least 1-year after the implants have been loaded. Make base-line custom probe depth 1-year after loading to monitor the probe depths at every removal recare.
   - ■ **Palpate;** place a finger on tissue of each side of abutment, draw upward on lower arch and downward on upper arch. Note in patient's record any signs of infection (i.e. bleeding or exudate).
6. **Radiographs** at least once a year for signs of bone loss and/or residue present.
   - ■ Take a Panorex, CBCT, or individual PA's as prescribed by doctor.

One screw to attach the abutment to the implant and one prosthetic screw that attaches the prosthetic to the abutment when reseating the final prosthesis (see Figure 9.29A). *Straight abutments, there is only one prosthetic screw* to use upon reseating the final prosthesis when maintenance is complete (see Figure 9.27B). Hygienists, check the torque of the abutment itself to the implant or have the dentist check at the time of exam. Fractures are uncommon for a straight abutments. *The biggest indicator that there may be a problem is if the patient's prosthetic screws will not torque upon reseating the final prosthesis.* Alert the doctor if the implant will not torque into place at the time of exam. The doctor will assess at the time of exam and may replace the abutment that did not torque in place or schedule for replacement. *Examine the abutments for any fractures.* If fractures are present or the

abutment will not torque in place, the doctor may need to replace abutment or schedule for replacement.

Complete a *percussion test* to assess for possible complications with implant integration and to assess if abutments or angled abutment screws are loose. Begin by gently tapping on each abutment with a blunt-ended instrument and listen to the sound. *Listen for a normal solid sound* (i.e., tapping on a window) or *hollow sound* that could be a sign abutment is loose, loss of implant osseointegration, or a zygomatic implant which may sound different. Record in patient's notes any sound differences for the doctor to evaluate at the time of the exam.

Next, *check the N° torque level of each abutment screw* for angled abutments or the abutment itself for straight abutment (no separate screw). If either is loose, tighten or have the doctor tighten per

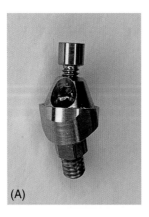
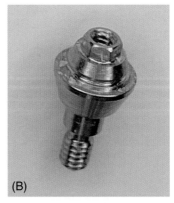

(A)   (B)

Figure 9.29 (A) Angled abutment with two screws. (B) Straight abutment with one screw. Courtesy of Jeff Carlson CDT.

correct N° torque guidelines from the manufacturer and re-test. Note any loose abutment or angled abutment screw or any hollow sound from any abutment in the patient's record that needs to be evaluated further by the doctor at time of the exam.

Check mobility with two blunt-ended instruments (i.e., mirror handle or other blunt-end instrument), move back/forth gently, and note any mobility in patient's record. Ask the patient if they are experiencing anything that does not feel normal to them. The patient may comment to you that they noticed that the prosthesis is loose or the occlusion check with the prosthesis in place may have appeared to be out of balance or hitting harder than normal for that patient. If mobility is present, take a radiograph to assess bone level. Doctor will evaluate at the time of exam for signs of occlusal trauma, loose screw, or lack of osseointegration (i.e., bone loss).

Probe and palpate each implant for signs of infection. It is important to note that it is recommended to wait until 1-year after the implants have been loaded to probe. *Make a base-line custom probe depth at 1-year after loading to monitor the probe depths at each removal appointment thereafter.* Palpate, only possible if prosthesis is removed. *Place a finger on the tissue of each side of the abutment, draw upward on lower arch and downward on the upper arch.* Note in the patient's record

any signs of infection (i.e., bleeding or exudate) to show doctor at the time of exam.

The final step is to *take a radiograph at least once a year* for signs of bone loss and/or residue present or more often as prescribed by doctor. Take a Panorex, CBCT, or individual periapical (PA) radiographs as prescribed by the doctor. Assessment is now complete, note findings for the doctor to evaluate at time of exam and continue with implant maintenance (see Box 9.11).

Implant maintenance and reseat fixed final prosthesis

For maintenance on the implants that support the fixed final prosthesis after the fixed final prosthesis is removed, follow the maintenance and reseating protocol, (see Box 9.12). Begin by *placing an OptraGate* (latex-free by Ivoclar Vivadent) if possible for retraction and *use a powder streaming device* with erythritol or glycine powder to remove oral biofilm around each implant/abutment. *Lavage after debridement* with safe ultrasonic tip on lavage or lowest setting to remove any debris present without touching the implants or abutments.

Assess if calculus is present and *debride implants* with titanium scalers or safe ultrasonic tips ONLY, with short horizontal

---

Box 9.12 Full-arch fixed final prosthesis removed and reseated maintenance protocol

- Place OptraGate for retraction and visibility if possible
- Use powder streaming device to professionally remove biofilm
- Lavage; safe ultrasonic on low setting before/after debridement to remove any debris.
- Debride implants with titanium scaler and/or safe ultrasonic tip, short horizontal strokes.
- Apply antimicrobial varnish or gel around implants to prevent biofilm formation.
- Retrieve prosthesis from the ultrasonic bath unit and rinse thoroughly.
  - Debride, if calculus is present on prosthesis, with soft titanium scaler.
  - Remove any stain present, pumice-free prophy paste chair-side or in-office lab steamer or rag wheel, if available.
- Rinse the prosthesis with antimicrobial rinse and carefully remove any debris in the screw openings.

- Doctor exam; evaluate prosthesis, patient tissue, abutments, implants, and hygienist's record notes.
- Reseat prosthesis in place in the patient's mouth with the proper screws and hand tighten carefully to avoid any tissue distention or impingement.
- Torque each screw with proper torque wrench to complete placement in the correct N° torque per doctor directive and implant manufacturer.
- Take a radiograph to confirm full arch final prosthesis is seated correctly.
- Fill in screw access holes with Teflon tape strip or cord. Place plug material (i.e., Fermit or composite) with a condenser to seal the access hole and if needed light cure, per manufacturer directions.
- Doctor final exam; check occlusion, adjust if necessary, appoint recare.

---

strokes (see Tables 9.1 and 9.2). *Rinse, dry, and place antimicrobial varnish or gel* (i.e., Cervitec Plus by Ivoclar Vivadent) to prevent oral biofilm formation around each abutment for up to three months (25). Let the patient know not to eat or drink for 1 hour.

Remove the OptraGate if used and retrieve the prosthesis from the ultrasonic bath, rinse thoroughly. Debride prosthesis if necessary with soft (Rockwell hardness 28–30) titanium scaler (i.e., Wingrove Ti Implant Scaler by PDT or Brasseler ImplantPro Scaler), being careful not to scratch the prosthesis. *Remove any stains present on the prosthesis* with a pumice-free prophy paste chairside or in-office lab steamer or use a rag wheel if available. *Rinse the prosthesis with an antimicrobial mouth rinse and carefully remove any debris in the screw openings* and return to the patient. Ready for *doctor exam* to evaluate prosthesis, patient tissue, abutments, implants, and review patient record notes from hygienist's assessment.

Hygiene Tip:

To reseat the prosthesis hand tighten screws first (Figure 9.30A). Note the correct torque for the specific implant manufacture recommendation ahead of appointment and if possible use a breakaway wrench or pre-set at the correct torque setting ahead to move from screw to screw, in a timely manner.

Once the doctor exam is complete, follow protocol to reseat the prosthesis (see Box 9.12). Begin the protocol to reseat the prosthesis in the patient's mouth with proper screws and hand tighten first carefully to avoid any tissue distention or impingement (see Figure 9.30A). Torque each screw with proper torque wrench to complete placement in the correct N° torque per doctor directive and implant manufacturer. Note the correct torque for specific implant manufacture recommendation ahead of appointment and if possible use a breakaway wrench or pre-set at

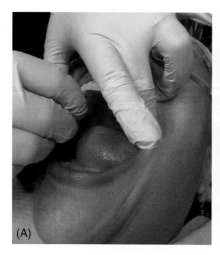
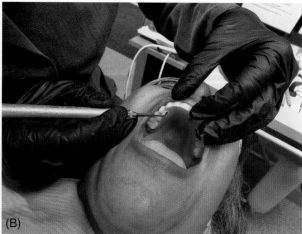

Figure 9.30 (A) Hand tighten screws, then torque in place with correct N° torque per doctor directive and implant manufacturer. (B) Reseat final prosthesis, place access hole plug material with condenser to seal access hole. Courtesy of Wingrove Dynamics.

the correct torque setting ahead to move from screw to screw in a timely manner.

Important, *take a radiograph to confirm the full arch final prosthesis is seated correctly. Fill in the screw access holes* with Teflon tape strip or cord with cotton pliers and/or packing instrument (i.e., plugger or condenser). Place plug material (i.e., Fermit temporary material or composite) with a plugger or condenser to seal the access holes and light cure if required to set material per manufacture directions (see Figure 9.30B). Reseat is now completed, ready for the doctor's final exam to check occlusion, adjust if necessary and appoint recare at least every 6 months (2).

Peri-implant disease assessment and treatments

Protocols for peri-implant disease treatment will be ever changing and evolving, but hygienists will play the *starring role* in assessing and providing treatment for mucositis and peri-implantitis. The American Academy of Periodontology (AAP) and the European Federation of Periodontology (EFP) developed a Classifications of Periodontal and Peri-Implant Disease and Conditions and published in 2018. This classifications follow a medical model that allows clinicians to explain treatment to patients based on stage, extent, and progression. This World Workshop on the Classification of Disease and Conditions provided 19 review papers and 4 consensus reports that outline classifications and conditions affecting the periodontium and biofilm induced and non-biofilm induced inflammation (32, 33).

As hygienists we need to understand these classifications and conditions. Peri-implant disease calcification has four major categories; Peri-implant health, Peri-implant mucositis, Peri-implantitis, and Peri-implant soft-, and hard-tissue deficiencies (32, 33). The case definitions, diagnostic considerations, and notes for clinical application to write in patient record for each category are outlined in Table 9.4.

Conditions of *peri-implant soft- and hard-tissue deficiencies* include a review of patient medical history, dental history, and risk factors, that took place after tooth loss and resulted in tissue and bone loss (i.e., from periodontal disease). Regeneration has shown that for true regeneration, both tissue and bone health of the implant is

Table 9.4 Clinical applications peri-implant therapy/note for patient's record/recare.

Implant Health Category	Inflammation/soft tissue, Probe Depth (PD), Bleeding on Probing (BOP), Suppuration (exudate)	Bone Loss (BL)	Notes/Clinical Application: All Implant Categories: Baseline probe depth and radiograph at 1-year post-load, Recare at least every 6 months
Peri-implant healthy	Absence of inflammation, BOP, swelling, and exudate.	No bone loss <2.0 mm	Absence of BL beyond the crestal bone level changes from remodeling at 1-year. Monitor, Recare at least every 6 months
Peri-implant mucositis	Inflammation, BOP, plaque pathological factor, and/or exudate	No bone loss from previous exam, base-line, <2.0 mm	Record Gingival Index 1–3: mild, moderate, severe. Treat, reevaluate, recare 3 months
Peri-implantitis	Inflammation, BOP, plaque pathological factor, and/or exudate Note any increased PD from previous exam	Subsequent progressive BL from previous exam >2.0 mm	**Early:** PD >4 mm, BL <25% of implant length Treat, Recare 3 months **Moderate:** PD >6 mm, BL 25–50% of implant length Surgical TX **Advanced:** PD >8 mm, BL >50% of implant length. Surgical TX
Peri-implantitis in absence of previous examination	Inflammation, BOP, and/or any suppuration PD ≥6 mm and/or recession	Radiographic BL ≥3.0 mm	Make baseline PD and radiograph Diagnosis of Peri-Implantitis; Treat, recare 3 months or Surgical treatment

©Susan Wingrove/Based on New Classification for Peri-Implant Diseases and Conditions/19 review papers and four consensus reports (32–37).

vital to the success and prevention of peri-implant complications (see Chapter 7).

Soft-tissue deficiency conditions that can cause recession of the peri-implant mucosa are; malposition of implants, thin tissue biotype, lack of keratinized tissue or buccal bone, status of periodontal attachment on adjacent teeth, and surgical tissue trauma (36). *Hard-tissue deficiency* conditions include; injury, longitudinal root fracture, medications, previous smoker, pneumatization of the maxillary sinus, and systemic disease reducing the amount of naturally formed bone including periodontal disease (36). In addition, *previous dental history factors* are also a consideration. The agenesis of teeth, loss of periodontal support, endodontic infections, thin buccal bone plate, buccal/lingual tooth position in relation to the arch, pressure from soft-tissue supported removable prosthesis, extraction with trauma to the tissues, or a combination of factors, to monitor accordingly (36, 38).

For all implant-borne restoration patients records should contain for each implant; *a radiograph at time of implant placement, loading and 1-year post-load as a baseline. Probe depth reading in as many of the six-sites as possible at 1-year post-load should also be included.* Monitor your patient's 1-year post-load radiograph and probe depth for the life of the implant. Encourage patients to achieve keratinized tissue with stimulation using a rubber tip stimulator once daily for comfort, aesthetics, and ease of oral biofilm control. Combine this with good at-home oral hygiene regimen for long-term implant prevention of peri-implant complications, (1, 33, 37).

Peri-implant health is defined as an absence of visual signs of inflammation and bleeding or exudate on probing or palpating. Implants can still be considered healthy, with normal or reduced bone support from crestal bone remodeling at baseline. For patients to remain in the healthy category; no increased probe depth from previous exams or bone loss from radiographic base-line following crestal bone remodeling at 1 year post-load.

No specific probe depth is universal for a determination of health for implants. A custom probe reading for each patient is unique to them. Ideally this base-line probe depth would be recorded at 1 year post-load after crestal bone remodeling has been established. This base-line probe and a 1 year post-load radiograph follow the patient for life of the implant. At every recare implant maintenance visit, compare the patient's base-line probe depth and radiograph to the new probe depth and radiograph (33, 35). Studies show the prevalence of peri-implant mucositis is statistically, 50–80% and if not treated can develop into peri-implantitis in more than 40% of patients (38–40).

Peri-mucositis is defined as inflammation, bleeding on probing and/or palpation that can be biofilm induced and non-biofilm (i.e., cement or instrument residue) induced inflammation that can subsequently or not progress to bone loss in both titanium and ceramic implants. Peri-mucositis also defined as the absence of bone loss beyond the base-line crestal

bone level changes on the 1 year radiograph post-load. Record the Gingival Index #1–3 (i.e., mild, moderate, or severe) of the implant(s) inflammation level in the patient's record and if possible take an intraoral camera image to compare at next reevaluation.

Oral biofilm is the primary etiology for mucositis that can lead to peri-implantitis (33), but residue left behind can also cause a non-biofilm induced inflammation response that leads to bone loss if untreated (5). If residue (i.e., cement or instrument residue) is suspected, a peri-implantitis evaluation is recommended with a CBCT. Complications that affect implants vary from; biofilm as a major risk factor and if the implant-supported restoration/prosthesis is cleanable. Also, patient's tobacco use, lack of keratinized and attached peri-implant mucosa (41), and if any non-calculus residue is present (5). For more details on oral biofilm as a risk factor and corrosion complications (see Chapter 7).

Oral biofilm associated pathological condition in tissue can be reversed with a peri-mucositis treatment such as powder streaming with glycine powder, according to the 2012 Consensus Conference of the European Association for Osseointegration; "peri-implant mucositis can be successfully treated non-surgically, the treatment modalities should disrupt the sub-mucosal biofilm" (17). Followed by good oral hygiene by the patient every 8–12 hours. For peri-mucositis and early peri-implantitis treatment protocol (see Box 9.13). The reevaluation is critical for peri-mucositis/early peri-implantitis patients. On the reevaluation appointment, palpate and floss the implants to determine if inflammation is still present. If present, the inflammation may be due to a residue (i.e., cement or instrument) and the implant may need to be surgically flapped or a periodontal endoscope used to evaluate for peri-implantitis (see Chapter 7 for more on complications).

Box 9.13 Peri-mucositis/early peri-implantitis treatment protocol

■ Place OptraGate or retractor for visibility.
■ Use erythritol or glycine in powder streaming device as a treatment (17).
■ Lavage; safe ultrasonic on low setting before/after debridement to remove debris.
■ Debride implants, if calculus present with titanium scalers and/or safe ultrasonic tips.
■ Polish restorations/prosthesis to remove stain present with pumice-free paste.
■ Place antimicrobial varnish or gel around implants to prevent biofilm formation.
■ Remove OptraGate or retractor and instruct on home care recommendations
  ○ Brush, water flosser, and antimicrobial rinse twice daily.
■ Re-evaluate in 3–6 weeks, refer for peri-implantitis evaluation if inflammation and/or residue is still present.

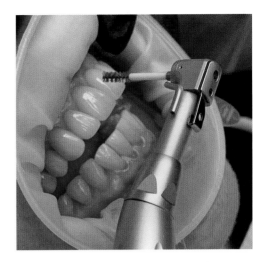

Figure 9.31 Labrida BioClean chitin brush. Courtesy of Wingrove Dynamics.

Peri-implantitis is also oral biofilm induced or non-biofilm induced that occurs in the tissue that surrounds dental implants and *has progressive radiographic bone loss* (42). Also defined as a patient with increased probe depth, inflammation, and progressive bone loss beyond the crestal bone level changes at 1-year baseline. In the absence of previous records, radiographs on a new implant patient, refer to peri-implantitis in the absence of previous examination (Table 9.4). Any implant with probe depths equal of greater than 6 mm, bone loss greater than 3 mm on radiograph and inflammation present, a doctor needs to assess this patient as a peri-implantitis treatment patient.

A promising new non-surgical treatment for peri-implant disease is the Labrida BioClean™ brush. This should not be considered as a replacement for surgical treatment for peri-implantitis when necessary. The BioClean chitin brush is designed to use for effective cleaning of the implant surface and soft tissues during an implant maintenance appointment to treat peri-implant mucositis with pocket depths 3 mm

or greater and pre-surgical early peri-implantitis. It has been shown in studies to effectively treat *peri-mucositis with greater than 3 mm pockets* (43) and *mild peri-implantitis with 1–2 mm bone loss and pocket depth 4 mm or deeper* (44). Studies are ongoing for *peri-implantitis with 2–4 mm bone loss and pockets 4 mm or deeper*.

The LABRIDA BioClean brush is made of chitosan, a marine biopolymer that is biocompatible with implants and resorbs quickly (see Figure 9.31). It is non-allergenic (45) with bacteriostatic and anti-inflammatory properties (46). Chitin, a structural scaffold polymer of protective shrimp shells can be extracted and converted into the high-performing biopolymer chitosan. The extraction and conversion process includes demineralization, deproteinization, and deacetylation of the shells. The chitin is so chemically modified that chitosan is not considered to be of animal origin, therefore not considered as an allergen risk for patients with a shellfish allergy.

For the Labrida BioClean treatment, first assess that the patient is a *peri-mucositis patient with pocket depth >3 mm* or a *mild peri-implantitis patient with 1–2 mm bone loss and pocket depth >4 mm*. Select one brush, single use ONLY for one patient. The brush can be used on two to four implants. *Soak chitosan brush in sterile saline for at least 2 minutes before use.* Insert the chitosan brush into the oscillating dental bur handpiece (600–1000 rpm) without touching the chitosan fibers. Carefully seat into the peri-implant crevice and with light pressure debride for 2 minutes, using up-and-down probing movements. The chitosan brush can be rinsed in sterile saline during treatment to remove debris. Once treatment is completed, irrigate with sterile saline. Take radiographs to monitor bone loss and seek peri-implantitis surgical treatment as necessary. Repeat at 3- to 6-month implant maintenance recare intervals depending on clinical response (see Box 9.14).

Labrida BioClean brush in vitro studies show that the chitosan brush fibers, if released during treatment, are gentle to the peri-implant soft tissues, harmless to the implant surface (46), and will resorb or dissolve. The chitosan brushes should be stored in the sealed provided aluminum bag, chitosan fibers are sensitive to low air humidity (may dry out). The chitosan brush is attached to a stainless steel stem with a soft polypropylene sleeve to protect the implant surface, and need to be used in standard angled oscillating dental bur handpiece (600–1000 rpm). The Labrida BioClean brushes are single use ONLY for one patient, can be used on two to four implants (see Box 9.14 for treatment protocol and Figure 9.32 treatment case).

Cement residue assessment and treatment

The three main reasons that implants are at risk from excess cement complications are; biology, tissue depth, and cement types, with the added dimension of a direct link to peri-implant disease (47) (see Figure 9.33). Cement extrusion subgingivally on an implant may result in soft tissue swelling, soreness, bleeding and/or exudate on probing or palpating, and can lead to implant failure (5, 48). Therefore, hygienists will have an active role in nonsurgical cement residue identification, with the first step being to do a visual assessment and clinically check radiograph (see Figure 9.34).

To assess for cement, residue, and/or calculus on implants, carefully floss the implant with dental tape. Insert the floss in contact on the mesial and distal without removing the floss, crisscross in front, move in shoe-shining motion. Important to remove the floss from the mesial then the distal, NOT pulling the floss through which can leave floss remnants behind. Check the floss; if frayed, roughened, or if blood is present on the floss. This can indicate that cement or other residue, causing inflammation is present. Note on patient's record and alert doctor to evaluate at time of exam.

Box 9.14 Labrida BioClean peri-mucositis/early peri-implantitis treatment protocol

- Assess patient; *peri-mucositis with pocket depth >3 mm, mild peri-implantitis with 1–2 mm bone loss and pocket depth >4 mm.*
- Select one chitosan brush, single use ONLY for one patient, on 2–4 implants.
- *Soak chitosan brush in sterile saline for at least 2 minutes before use.*
- Insert the chitosan brush into the oscillating dental bur handpiece (600–1000 rpm), Do not touch the chitosan fibers.
- Carefully seat into the peri-implant crevice, use light pressure and debride for 2 minutes, using up-and-down probing movements.
- Rinse the chitosan brush in sterile saline during treatment to remove debris.
- Once treatment is completed, irrigate with sterile saline.
- Take radiographs to monitor bone loss and seek peri-implantitis surgical treatment as necessary.
- Repeat at 3- to 6-month implant maintenance recare intervals depending on clinical response.

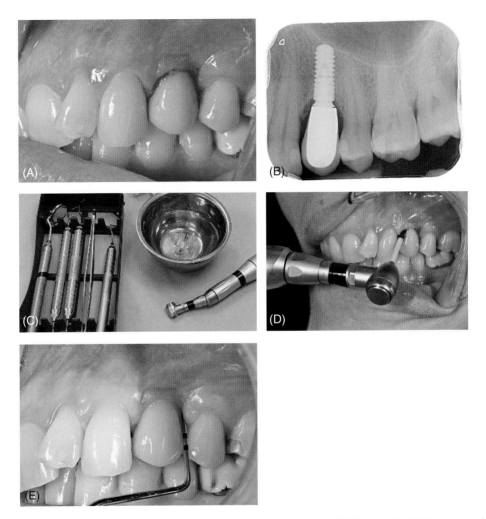

Figure 9.32 Labrida BioClean treatment case. Courtesy of Dr. Caspar Wohlfahrt. (A) Initial exam, patient presents with diagnosis peri-mucositis, Tooth 24 FDA, Stage 1 Grade A, BOP severe (Gingival Index 3), Probe depths 5–7 mm, (B) Initial Radiograph, (C) Set up: LBC, Oscillating Handpiece, sterile saline (D) Debride implant (E) TX results; improvement of probe depths of 2–5 mm and BOP minimal (Gingival index 0–1). Recare set 3 months.

There are many instances where the cement is not detectable, even with blood present on the floss. The cement forms a thin layer around the abutment, and the cement often reaches the threads of the implant, making removal very difficult because it is usually embedded on the rough surface. Detection may also be possible radiographically (see Figure 9.34). However, due to the lack of radiopacity in many of the implant-specific cements, this may not be possible (49, 50). In many cases, bone loss is evident on the radiograph and a flap is raised to evaluate the implant, and this is when the cement is discovered (see Figure 9.33).

The dentist or specialist, completes a flap surgical procedure to achieve full access to the affected implant with the residue present. The goal is removal of cement and/or residue and now recommended to do this with care using titanium implant scaler,

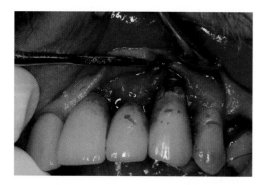

Figure 9.33 Note the cement residue present. Courtesy of Dr. John Remien.

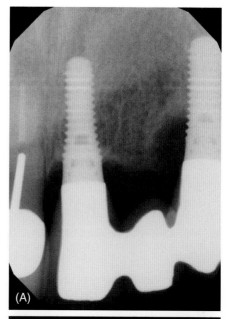

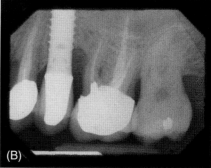

not stainless steel ultrasonics that could lead to removal of the oxide layer on titanium implant making it prone to corrosion. After the residue is removed, a regenerative technique is needed to regenerate the tissue and bone lost, a guided tissue or bone regeneration procedure (GTR, GBR). A healing time of generally 3 months is needed to save the implant (see cement treatment case Figure 9.35).

Summary

Early detection and treatment of implant complication is the key to long-term implant success. Peri-implant mucositis can occur in 43–47% of implants, and peri-implantitis in 20–22%, in the 5–10 years after implant placement (51). Follow the research-based, biofilm-focused ACP' Clinical Practice Guidelines for maintenance and recare (2) and use the tools and technology now available for safe, effective peri-implant therapy. Review the prevention protocols outlined in this text-

Figure 9.34 Radiographs. Courtesy of Dr. John Remien. (A) Notice the saucer-like radiolucent area, equal on both sides of the implant, indicative of cement. (B) Notice bone loss that is not symmetrical, only on one side of the implant, indicative of calculus.

book for; implant assessment, professional in-implant maintenance, and home-care recommendations to prevent peri-implant complications for predictable long-term implant success.

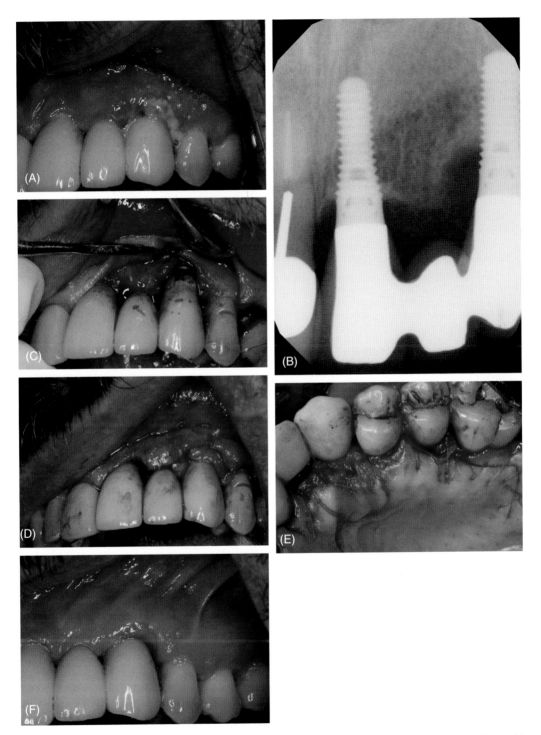

Figure 9.35 Cement treatment case. Courtesy of Dr. John Remien. (A) Pre-op (B) Pre-op X-ray, radiographic bone loss from cement. (C) Flapped to reveal cement and debride. (D) GBR, regenerative products, and connective tissue pedicle graft. (E) Sutured. (F) Post-op at 3 months.

References

1. Wingrove S. Long-term prevention of peri-implant complications: assessment, maintenance, and home-care protocols. Straumann. com/490.600-en_low.pdf
2. Bidra A, Daubert D, Garcia L, et al. 2016 ACP clinical practice guidelines for recall and maintenance of patients with tooth- borne and implant-borne dental restorations. J Prosthodont. 2016; 25: S32–S40.
3. Jepsen S, Berglundh T, Genco R, et al. Primary prevention of peri-implantitis: managing peri-implant mucositis. J Clin Periodontol. 2015; 42(Suppl 16): S152–S157.
4. Salvi GE, Ramsier CA Efficacy of patient-administered mechanical and/or chemical plaque control protocols in the management of peri-implant mucositis. A systematic review. J Clin Periodontol. 2015; 42(Suppl 16): S187–S201.
5. Wilson TG Jr The positive relationship between excess cement and peri-implant disease: a prospective clinical endoscopic study. J Periodontol. 2009; 80: 1388–1392.
6. Safioti L, Kotsakis GA, Pozhitkov AE, Chung WO, Daubert DM Increased levels of dissolved titanium are associated with peri-implantitis – a case control study. J Periodontol. 2017; 88: 436–442.
7. Kotsakis GA, Lan C, Barbosa J, et al. Antimicrobial agents used in the treatment of peri-implantitis alter the physiochemistry and cytocompatibility of titanium surfaces. J Periodontol. 2016; 87(7): 809–819.
8. Palmer RM, Pleasance C Maintenance of osseointegrated implant prosthesis. Dent Update. 2006; 33: 84–86.
9. Kumar PS, Mason MR, Brooker MR, O'Brien K Pyrosequencing reveals unique microbial signatures associated with healthy and failing dental implants. J Clin Periodontol. 2012; 39(5): 425–433.
10. Subramani K, Jung RE, Molenberg A, Hammerle CH Biofilm on dental implants: a review of the literature. Int J Oral Maxillofac Implants. 2009; 24: 616–626.
11. Daubert D Subgingival air polishing- Use of glycine powder with new technique may offer benefits to periodontal and implant maintenance therapy. Dimens Dent Hyg. 2013; 11: 69–73.
12. ADHA Org. American Dental Hygienists' Association Position Paper on Polishing. Accessed 2010, https://www.adha.org/resources-docs/7115_Prophylaxis_Postion_Paper.pdf
13. Bergendahl T, Forsgren L, Kvint S, Lowstedt E The effects of air abrasive instrument on soft and hard tissues around osseointegrated implants. Swed Dent J. 1990; 14: 219–223.
14. Dmytryk JJ, Fox SC, Moriarty JD The effects of scaling titanium implant surfaces with metal and plastic instruments on cell attachment. J Periodontol. 1990; 61: 491–496.
15. Ramaglia L, di Lauro AE, Morgese F, Squillace A Profilometric and standard error of the mean analy- sis of rough implant surfaces treated with different instrumentations. Implant Dent. 2006; 15: 77–82.
16. Hagi TT, Hofmanner P, Salvi GE, Ramseier C, Sculean A Clinical outcomes following subgingival application of a novel erythritol powder by means of air polishing in supportive periodontal therapy: a randomized, controlled clinical study. Quintessence Int. 2013; 44: 753–761.
17. Klinge B, Meyle J Working group 2. Peri- implant tissue destruction. The third EAO Consensus Conference 2012. Clin Oral Implants Res. 2012; 23(Suppl 6): 108–110.
18. Fox SC, Moriarty JD, Kusy RP The effects of scaling titanium implant surface with metal and plastic instruments: an in vitro study. J Periodontol. 1990; 61: 485–490.
19. Kurtz SM, Devine JN PEEK biomaterials in trauma, orthopedic, and spinal implants. Biomaterials. 2007; 28(32): 4845–4869.
20. Meschenmoser A, d'Hoedt B, Meyle J, et al. Effects of various hygiene procedures on the surface characteristics of titanium abutments. J Periodontol. 1996; 67: 229–235.
21. Darby ML, Walsh MM. Dental Hygiene Theory and Practice, 1st ed. Philadelphia: WB Sauders, 1995.
22. Paschke N A path to fewer aerosols with ultrasonics. RDH Mag. 2021; 1: 28–30.
23. Hallmon W, Waldrop T, Meffert R, Wade BW A comparative study of the effects of metallic, nonmetallic, and sonic instrumentation on titanium abutment surfaces. Int J Oral Maxillofac Implants. 1997; 5: 296.
24. Matarasso S, Quaremba G, Coraggio F, et al. Maintenance of Implants: an in vitro study of titanium implant surfaces subsequent to the application of different prophylaxis procedures. Clin Oral Implant Res. 1996; 7(1): 64–72.
25. George AM, Kalangi SK, Vasudevan M, Krishnaswamy NR Chlorhexidine varnishes effectively inhibit Porphyromonas gingivalis and Streptococcus mutans – an in vivo study. J Indian Soc Periodontol. 2010; 14(3): 178–180.

26. Misch CE Prosthetic options in implant dentistry. Int J Oral Implantol. 1991; 7: 17–21.

27. Meffert R Periodontitis versus peri-implantitis: the same disease? The same treatment? Oral Biol Med. 1996; 7: 278–291.

28. Renvert S, Persson GR Periodontitis as a potential risk factor for peri-implantitis. J Clin Periodontol. 2009; 36(10 Suppl): 9–14.

29. Kotosovili S, Karousis I, Trianti M, Fourmousis I Therapy of peri-implantitis: a systemic review. J Clin Periodontol. 2008; 35: 621–629.

30. Parameter on placement and management of the dental implant. J Periodontol. 2000; 71: 870–872.

31. Staubli P, Bagley D. Attachments and Implants Reference Manual, 8th ed. San Meteo, CA: Strong Design, 2007.

32. Caton G, Armitage G, Berglundh T, et al. A new classification scheme for periodontal and peri-implant diseases and conditions – introduction and key changes from the 1999 classification. J Clin Periodontol. 2018; 45(Suppl. 20): S1–S8.

33. Berglundh T, Armitage G, Araujo MG, et al. Peri-implant diseases and conditions: consensus report of workgroup 4 of the 2017 World Workshop on the Classification of Periodontal and Peri-Implant Diseases and Conditions. J Periodontol. 2018; 89(Suppl 1): S313–S318.

34. Froum SJ, Rosen PS A proposed classification for peri-implantitis. Int J Periodontics Restorative Dent. 2012; 32: 533–540.

35. Renvert S, Rutger PG, Pirih F, Camargo P Peri-implant health, peri-implant mucositis, and peri-implantitis: case definitions and diagnostic considerations. J Clin Periodontol. 2018; 45(Suppl 20): S278–S285.

36. Hämmerle CHF, Tarnow D The etiology of hard- and soft-tissue deficiencies at dental implants: a narrative review. J Periodontol. 2018; 89(Suppl 1): S291–S303.

37. Wingrove S. Clinical applications for the 2018 classification of peri-implant diseases and conditions. Perio-Implant Advisory Website: Published November 6, 2018.

38. Koldsland OC, Scheie AA, Aass AM, et al. Prevalence of peri-implantitis related to severity of the disease with different degrees of bone loss. J Periodontol. 2010; 81(2): 231–238.

39. Costa FO, Takenaka-Martinez S, Cota LOM, et al. Peri-implant disease in subjects with and without preventive maintenance: a 5-year follow-up. J Clin Periodontol. 2012; 39(2): 173–181.

40. Monje A, Wang H-L, Nart J Association of preventive maintenance therapy compliance and peri-implant diseases: a cross-sectional study. J Periodontol. 2017; 88(10): 1030–1041.

41. Roccuzzo M, Grasso G, Dalmasso P Keratinized mucosa around implants in partially edentulous posterior mandible: 10-year results of a prospective comparative study. Clin Oral Implants Res. 2016; 27(4): 491–496.

42. Schwarz F, Derks J, Monje A, Wang H-L Peri-implantitis. J Periodontol. 2018; 89(Suppl 1): S267–S290.

43. Wohlfahrt JC, Aass AM, Koldsland OC Treatment of peri-implant mucositis with a chitosan brush—A pilot randomized clinical trial. Int J Dent Hyg. 2019; 17: 170–176.

44. Wohlfahrt JC, Evensen BJ, Zeza B, et al. A novel non-surgical method for mild peri-implantitis – a multicenter consecutive case series. Int J Implant Dent. 2017; 3: 38.

45. Muzzarelli RA Chitin and chitosans as immuno-adjuvants and non-allergenic drug carriers. Mar Drugs. 2010; 8(2): 292–312.

46. Arancibia R, Maturana C, Silva D, et al. Effects of chitosan particles in periodontal pathogens and gingival fibroblasts. J Dent Res. 2013; 92(8): 740–745.

47. Larsen OI, Enersen M, Kristoffersen AK, et al. Antimicrobial effects of three different treatment modalities on dental implant surfaces. J Oral Implantol. 2017; 43: 429–436.

48. Maximo MB, de Mendonca AC, Santos RV, Figueiredo LC, Feres M, Duarte PM Short-term clinical and microbiological evaluations of peri-implant diseases before and after mechanical anti-infective therapies. Clin Oral Implants Res. 2009; 20: 99–108.

49. Pauletto N, Lahiffe BJ, Walton JN Complications associated with excess cement around crowns on osseointegrated implants: a clinical report. Int J Oral Maxillofac Implants. 1999; 14: 865–868.

50. Gapski R, Neugeboren N, Pemeraz AZ, Reissner MW Endosseous implant failure influenced by crown cementation: a clinical case report. Int J Oral Maxillofac Implants. 2008; 23: 943–946.

51. Lee CT, Huang YW, Zhu L, Weltman R Prevelences of peri-implantitis and peri-implant mucositis: systematic review and meta-analysis. J Dent. 2017; 62: 1–12.

Appendix: Terminology and Resources

Implant dentistry terminology

Abutment The component part that screws directly into the implant to retain the crown, bridge, and/or overdenture prosthesis in place. Different types of abutments are stock, standard, fixed, angled, tapered, and nonsegmented.

Acquired factors Factors that are not inherited and are acquired after birth.

Allograft Bone harvested from the same species, human bone/cadaveric bone and human tissue usually obtained from a tissue bank used in regeneration and preservation procedures.

Alloplast Synthetic bone, hydroxyapatite, and biocompatible substances, with similar properties to bone used in regeneration and preservation procedures.

Amniotic stem cells Able to differentiate into various tissue types such as skin and bone to aid with regeneration.

Amplitude is the distance, movement the ultrasonic tip/insert moves.

Atraumatic extraction Extraction of a tooth without breaking the buccal plate and/or nontraumatic extraction to preserve the bone, tissue and place implants.

Attachment Used for retention of prosthesis. Can also have bar attached (i.e., Hader bar), which is referred to as attachment-retained prosthesis.

Augmentation Used to correct concavities with the goal of bone formation to correct concavities in the buccal plate and add vertical and/or horizontal bone where significant bone loss has occurred.

Autograft Patient's own bone harvested from a donor site to be used in regeneration and preservation procedures.

Barrier membrane Device to prevent tissue (fast) growth in an area where (slow) bone growth is desired.

Biocompatibility The ability of a material to perform with an appropriate host in response to a specific application.

Biologic growth factor Any highly specific biologic that stimulates the division and differentiation of a particular type of cells for regeneration.

Peri-Implant Therapy for the Dental Hygienist, Second Edition. Susan S. Wingrove.
© 2022 John Wiley & Sons, Inc. Published 2022 by John Wiley & Sons, Inc.
Companion website: www.wiley.com/go/wingrove/implant

Biological complications Complications in the function of the implant from an infection, fistula, soft-tissue hyperplasia, or loss of the implant including the peri-implant hard and soft tissues that surround the implant.

Biological width In regard to implants, it is the vertical dimension of the interface between the implant and the peri-implant mucosa.

Biological width impingement A chronic inflammation with possible vertical bone loss that can occur if the distance between the bone margin and the margin of the restoration is compromised or impinged upon.

Bone morphogenic protein (BMP) Endogenous family of proteins that have great potential for bone grafting procedures.

Blade-form implants Wide, flat metal plate or blade in cross section available in different heights and lengths, some with tapered sides to replace one to multiple teeth with a single blade for narrow bones in maxillary or mandible.

Bruxism A severe, dehibilitating disease that does not have a known etiology, affecting occlusion.

CAD/CAM Computer manufacturing tool for generating laboratory products.

Cancellous bone Interior spongy bone, highly vascular, contains red bone marrow where the production of blood cells occurs.

Cantilever An extension to a restoration to aesthetically replace a missing tooth with no support underneath.

CAT scan Computerized axial tomography scan; computer generated with X-ray for 3-D image.

CBCT Cone-beam computed tomography; software-based treatment planning.

Ceramic implants Zirconia-based, machined (ZrO_2m), or sandblasted (rough ZrO_2r). No oxide layer, nontoxic metal-free implant option.

Chlorhexidine gluconate (CHX) Antimicrobial mouth rinse often recommended for inflammation and antimicrobial properties. Available in alcohol or nonalcohol versions.

Chlorine dioxide Nonalcohol antimicrobial mouth rinse often recommended for inflammation and antimicrobial properties.

Connecting bar An attached system between two or more implants to be utilized for stability for implant prosthesis.

Coping Component for dental implant and/or abutment.

Commensals A relationship in which one organism derives benefits from another organism without hurting or helping it.

Corrosion The degradation of the implant surface. The breakdown or dissolution of the biocompatible interface represented by titanium dioxide layer of the surface.

Cortical bone Forms the outer hard shell of bones; made up of mainly calcium.

Cover screw A screw that is used at first-stage surgery to seal the platform of an implant, preventing bone and/or, soft tissue from infiltrating the internal aspect of the implant during osseointegration.

Crestal The coronal aspect of the ridge of the jaw.

Crestal bone remodeling The bone surrounding the implant once it maintains a mature level.

Crown lengthening Procedure to sculpt the gingival margin to balance the smile line and expose more of the crown of the tooth prior to restoration(s) being placed on the teeth. Can be cosmetic to remove the excess soft tissue only, or functional, which involves removal of soft tissue and some bone to prevent biological width impingement.

Defect The loss of bone or tissue.

Dehiscence Bone loss around an implant or tooth.

Demineralized bone matrix (DBM) Inorganic mineral is removed, leaving behind collagen matrix. More biologically active, mechanical properties are diminished.

Denture A removable prosthesis fabricated to replace totally edentulous arch of missing teeth.

Diagnostic wax-up Models that are waxed-up to illustrate and treatment plan complex cases.

Dysbiosis A loss of microbial diversity with an imbalance that means a decrease in beneficial bacteria, an increase in pathogenic species and the onset of disease.

Dysbiotic state The innate host response becomes dysfunctional and the once ordered inflammatory mediator expression that was protective in health becomes destructive in disease.

Edentulous Missing all teeth in an arch or entire mouth.

Embryonic stem cells Derived from the early stage of an embryo.

Endosteal implant (root form) Generally made of titanium alloy, and are designed to replace the root of one or more teeth.

Exudate Infection in form of cellular debris, fluid, and blood that oozes from the tissues surrounding the teeth and/or implants.

Fenestration Incomplete closure of soft tissue.

Fixed prosthesis A fixed, nonremovable restoration by patient but is removable by a dental professional.

Fixed removable prosthesis A restoration that attaches to implants and is removable by patient and dental professional.

Frequency The number of times, movement the ultrasonic insert/tip moves.

Gingival graft A procedure using the patient's own keratinized tissue around an implant or edentulous ridge.

Growth factor Stimulates, like a signal, the division and differentiation of particular types of cells to regenerate bone and/or tissue that was lost.

Guided bone regeneration (GBR) Bone regeneration procedure that is used in an edentulous area with a barrier membrane to seal off the area to allow bone to regenerate while keeping the connective tissue out, so osteogenesis is achieved. Refers to mainly ridge augmentation and bone regenerative procedures.

Guided tissue regeneration (GTR) Repair and regeneration of connective soft tissue, periodontal ligament, and damaged bone.

Hard-tissue deficiency Conditions reducing the amount of naturally formed bone including periodontal disease, injury, longitudinal root facture, medications, previous smoker, pneumatization of the maxillary sinus, and systemic disease.

Healing abutment A component that connects to the implant and extends through the gingival tissue to assist and retain the tissue contour/emergence profile to receive the final abutment and restoration.

Healing cap Also referred to as cover screw; is used at first-stage surgery to seal the platform of an implant preventing bone and/or soft tissue from infiltrating the internal aspect of the implant during osseointegration.

Hydroxyapatite Synthetic bone component that is inorganic, mainly calcium; used as an alloplast and can be used as a dental implant coating.

Implant A biocompatible device placed in the bone to replace the root lost, preserve the bone level, and support the prosthesis.

Implant body Component part of the implant system that is within the bone.

Implant thread(s) The screw-like component part of the body of the endosteal, root-form implant.

Impression posts The component used during the impression procedure for the final restoration/prosthesis to transfer the precise position of the implant to the model.

Insulin growth factor (IGF-I and II) Promotes protein, extracellular matrix synthesis to increase membrane glucose transport for regeneration.

Keratinized Stippled, healthy; in relation to tissue.

Laboratory analogs Component made to represent exactly the top of the implant fixture in the laboratory model.

Lavage Use of an ultrasonic tip /insert to provide intrasulcular irrigation around an implant not to harm the perimucosal seal or touch the implant, implant-borne restoration, or prosthesis.

Magnetostrictive (magneto) An ultrasonic device, tips that are stacks drive inserts and produces elliptical motion.

Mechanical complications Complications for implants affected by stress or occlusal forces resulting in failure and generally becoming mobile.

Microbiome The genetic material of all the flora that are shared by all or most humans.

Mineralized bone matrix (MBM) Bone with all the organic materials removed, leaving behind an osteoconductive matrix.

Mini implant Root form implant of small diameter used in orthodontics and reten-

tion of overdentures that can also be used as a temporary implant to support a provisional while other implants are healing.

Occlusal loading Attaching the restoration to the implant, which allows the maxillary and mandibular aches to come in contact.

Oral biofilm A layer of bacteria that can accumulate inside oral cavity. Sticky white dental plaque that contains a wide variety of microorganisms including bacteria but also fungi, viruses, and/or other species.

Osseointegration The firm, direct, and lasting biological attachment of an implant to vital bone with no intervening connective tissue

Ossification Formation of or conversion into bone or a bony substance.

Osteoblasts Bone cells.

Osteoconductive Guiding the reparative growth of the natural bone.

Osteogenesis Living bone cells in the graft material contribute to bone remodeling that only occurs with autografts.

Osteoinduction Encouraging undifferentiated cells to become active osteoblasts.

Osteonecrosis of the jaw (ONJ) Necrosis of the jaw caused by taking bisphosphonates. Bisphosphonate-related osteonecrosis of the jaw (BRONJ) is also referred to as BON.

Osteotomy A site prepared in the bone for the placement of a dental implant or graft.

Overdenture A denture (prosthesis) used in implant dentistry with attachment mechanisms built in, to attach to implants for retention.

Palpate Place a finger on soft, to identify any signs of infection (i.e., bleeding or exudate).

Panoramic radiograph Maxillary and mandibular jaw radiograph that also shows the anatomy necessary for diagnostic treatment planning of implants.

Pedical graft An adjacent tissue flap reflected with base attached to donor site, laterally or coronally positioned to cover the surgical site or for aesthetic soft-tissue contouring.

Peri-implant crevice The restorative abutment connection to the implant, a niche where perio-pathogens, biofilm collects.

Peri-implant disease Collective term for inflammatory lesions that may affect the peri-implant area, mucositis, and peri-implantitis.

Peri-implantitis A pathological condition in the tissues around dental implants, characterized by inflammation of the peri-implant mucosa and loss of supporting peri-implant bone.

Perimucosal seal The tissue seal that separates the connective tissues from the outside environment around a dental implant.

Peri-mucositis An inflammatory lesion of the mucosa surrounding an implant without the loss of supporting peri-implant bone.

Periosteum Fibrous vascular membrane that fits tightly on the outer surface of the bone.

Piezoelectric (piezo) An ultrasonic device, tips produce linear motions with the piezoelectric crystals in the handpiece.

Platelet-derived growth factor (PDGF) Growth factors derived from whole human blood through the process of a gradient density centrifugation that stimulates regeneration.

Platelet-rich fibrin (PRF) Enriched fibrin glue that induce an improved peri-implant bone reaction, often coated on implants.

Platelet-rich plasma (PRP) Whole human blood that is used to signal and assist regeneration; often sprayed on implants to stimulate bone formation.

Platform switching Using a small diameter abutment on a larger diameter implant may preserve crestal bone and prevent bone loss by locating the connection away from the bone.

Preservation Ridge or socket procedure to retain the bone and avoid resorption.

Progressive loading Refers to the gradual increase in the application of load on a prosthesis and thus to a dental implant.

Prosthesis A restoration that is removable or nonremovable to the implant to replace the teeth.

Prosthesis-retaining screws Screws used to secure the prosthesis to the implant(s) metal framework.

Provisional Temporary prosthesis to use while healing.

Regeneration To replace bone and tissue that was lost with factors that stimulate the division and differentiation of particular cells.

Restoration Dental filling, crown, bridge, or prosthesis.

Ridge augmentation A procedure to bring back the lost bone and rebuild the ridge height and width because a socket prevention procedure was not completed originally.

Risk factor An environmental or social habit that can affect overall health.

Rockwell hardness The hardness scale based on indentation hardness of a material. The hardness of a metal, increased number means an increase in hardness.

Scaffold Framework to maintain the shape or maintain an original shape for regeneration to occur.

Sinus augmentation (sinus lift) Augmentation of the antral floor with autogenous bone and/or bone substitutes to accommodate dental implant insertion. Improves bone height in posterior maxilla for more favorable implant placement.

Socket preservation Procedure to place graft particulates or scaffold in a tooth socket done at time of extraction to preserve the alveolar ridge.

Soft-tissue deficiency Conditions that can cause recession of the peri-implant mucosa. Examples; malposition of implants, thin tissue biotype, lack of keratinized tissue or buccal bone, status of periodontal attachment on adjacent teeth, and surgical tissue trauma.

Soft-tissue grafts Used to improve gingival margin symmetry by covering the roots that are exposed to improve aesthetics and/or correct soft-tissue ridge deficiencies.

Surgical guide (template) A guide used to assist in the preparation for implant surgery. It indicates drilling position and angulation for implant placement.

Subperiosteal implants A custom-casted framework of surgical grade metal or alloy that lies on top of the jawbone.

Temporary anchoring devices (TADs) TADs are titanium mini-screws, used primarily by orthodontists. They are screwed directly into the bone through the gingiva to facilitate tooth movement and to anchor an orthodontic appliance. Once treatment is complete, the clinician can remove the TAD without trauma or need for bone grafting.

Titanium plasma spray (TPS) Titanium powder sprayed on a titanium implant to create a dense and porous covering to attract bone at a faster rate to help with osseointegration.

Torque Used to tighten or loosen components under resistance; expressed in Newton centimeters.

Transforming growth factor beta (TGF--β1) Stimulates wound matrix and B3; inhibits scar formation.

Transosteal/staple implant An orthopedic device that is inserted through the inferior border of the mandible and designed to function for an edentulous atrophic mandible.

Uncover procedure A small surgical procedure performed in order to expose the head of the implant and connect a healing abutment or cover screw.

Wax sleeves Attach to the abutment by the relating screw for the laboratory model.

Xenograft Bone or tissue transplant from another species (animal), used in regeneration and preservation procedures.

Zygomatic implant Root formed implant used in maxillary molar area at an angle for use with All-on-4™ or full fixed implant prostheses.

Resources

Companies

Aidian (QuikRead®), www.aidian.eu
American Eagle, www.am-eagle.com
BioHorizons, www.biohorizons.com
Brassler, www.brasslerusa.com
Colgate, www.colgate.com
CloSYS (Rowpar), www.closys.com
Crest + Oral-B/P& G, www.dentalcare.com
Dentsply, www.dentsply.com
Directa, www.directadental.com
Electro Medical Systems (EMS), www.ems-company.com
GC America, www.gcamerica.com
Glidewell Dental, www.glidewelldental.com

Hu-Friedy, www.hu-friedy.com

Ivoclar Vivadent, www.ivoclarvivadent.com

Keystone Dental, www.keystonedental.com

Kilgore International, www.kilgore-international.com

Mectron, www.dental.mectron.com

Medical billing, www.tipsmedicalbilling.com

MegaGen, www.megagenus.com

Nobel Biocare, www.nobelbiocare.com

Noess, www.neoss.com

Nordent, www.nordent.com

OralDNA testing, www.oraldna.com

Orsing, www.orsing.se

Paradise Dental Technologies (PDT), www.pdtdental.com

Parkell, www.parkell.com

Phillips, N. America (Sonicare®), www.soni-care.phillips.com

Practicon, www.practicon.com

Premier, www.preusa.com

Preventech, www.preventech.com

Proxysoft (Thorton), www.proxysoft.com

Salvin Dental Specialties, www.salvin.com

Straumann, www.straumann.us

Sunstar Americas, www.sunstar.com

Surgical Esthetics, www.surgicalesthetics.com

Swiss Dental Solutions (SDS), www.swissdentalsolutions.us

TePe Oral Health Care, www.tepe.com

Troll Dental, www.trolldentalusa.com

Waterpik, www.waterpik.com

W & H, www.wh.com

Young dental, www.youngdental.com

Zeramex, www.zeramexusa.com

Zirc, www.zirc.com

Organizations associated with implant dentistry

Academy of Osseointegration (AO), www.osseo.org

American Academy of Implant Dentistry (AAID), www.aaid-implant.org

American Academy of Periodontology (AAP), www.perio.org

American Dental Education Association (ADEA), www.adea.org

American Association of Oral and Maxillofacial Surgeons (AAOMS), www.aaoms.org

American College of Prosthodontists (ACP), www.prosthodontics.org

American Dental Association (ADA), www. ada.org

American Dental Hygienists' Association (ADHA), www.adha.org

American and International Dental Implant Association (ADIA), www.americandentalimplantassociation.com

International Academy of Ceramic Implantology, www.iaoci.com

International College of Prosthodontists (ICP), www.icp-org.com

International Federation of Dental Hygienists (IFDH), www.ifdh.org

Western Society of Periodontology (WSP) www.wsperio.org

Index

Peri-Implant Therapy for the Dental Hygienist, Second Edition. Susan S. Wingrove.
© 2022 John Wiley & Sons, Inc. Published 2022 by John Wiley & Sons, Inc.
Companion website: www.wiley.com/go/wingrove/implant